William M. Powell

Saunders' Pocket Medical Formulary

William M. Powell

Saunders' Pocket Medical Formulary

ISBN/EAN: 9783742829986

Manufactured in Europe, USA, Canada, Australia, Japa

Cover: Foto ©Lupo / pixelio.de

Manufactured and distributed by brebook publishing software
(www.brebook.com)

William M. Powell

Saunders' Pocket Medical Formulary

SAUNDERS'

POCKET

MEDICAL FORMULARY.

WITH AN APPENDIX

CONTAINING POSOLOGICAL TABLE: FORMULÆ AND DOSES
FOR HYPODERMIC MEDICATION; POISONS AND THEIR
ANTIDOTES; DIAMETERS OF THE FEMALE PELVIS
AND FŒTAL HEAD; OBSTETRICAL TABLE; DIET
LIST FOR VARIOUS DISEASES; MATERIALS
AND DRUGS USED IN ANTISEPTIC
SURGERY;
TREATMENT OF ASPHYXIA FROM DROWNING; SURGICAL
REMEMBRANCER; TABLES OF INCOMPATIBLES;
ERUPTIVE FEVERS; WEIGHTS AND
MEASURES, ETC.

BY

WILLIAM M. POWELL, M.D.,

AUTHOR OF "ESSENTIALS OF DISEASES OF CHILDREN;" ONE OF THE
ASSOCIATE EDITORS OF THE "ANNUAL OF THE UNIVERSAL MEDI-
CAL SCIENCES;" ATTENDING PHYSICIAN TO THE CHILDREN'S
SEASHORE HOUSE FOR INVALID CHILDREN, AND THE MER-
CER HOUSE FOR INVALID WOMEN AT ATLANTIC CITY,
N. J.; MEMBER OF THE PHILADELPHIA
PATHOLOGICAL SOCIETY.

FIFTH EDITION.
THOROUGHLY REVISED

PHILADELPHIA:
W. B. SAUNDERS,
925 WALNUT STREET.
1899.

This Little Work

PREFACE TO THE FIFTH EDITION.

In the issuance of a new edition of the Formulary the opportunity has been taken to make extensive revision and addition, in order to bring the book in line with the advances that have been made in therapeutics. Accordingly, a large number of new formulæ have been incorporated, while many of older date and lesser usefulness have been replaced by others of recent origin and established worth. The Table of Doses has been amplified and modified, in conformity with the changes wrought by time; and the sections on Antagonists and Incompatibles and Poisons and Antidotes have been considerably expanded. The section on Drugs and Materials used in Antiseptic Surgery has also been thoroughly revised. No part of the book has escaped scrutiny, and it is hoped that it will retain the popularity it has so long enjoyed.

v

PREFACE.

In offering this Formulary to the Profession, the compiler wishes to state that he has endeavored to introduce, so far as possible in the many prescriptions contained therein, a considerable number, of the more important recently discovered drugs.

Especial thanks are due to Dr. Richard C. Norris, of Philadelphia, for his aid in furnishing the diameters of the female pelvis and fœtal head, and to the many professional friends, who have provided the author with valuable prescriptions from their private practice, hitherto unpublished.

Indebtedness is acknowledged to the following text-books: Starr on Diseases of the Digestive Organs in Infancy and Childhood; J. Lewis Smith, Meigs and Pepper, Ashby and Wright, Ellis, Eustace Smith, Goodhart and Starr, and to Keating's Encyclopædia of Diseases of Children; The Annual of the Universal Medical Sciences; Wood's, Bartholow's, Hare's, Ringer's, Potter's, and Napheys' Therapeutics; Duhring, Shoemaker, Stelwagon, and Van Harlingen on Skin Diseases; Goodell's Gynæcology; Hirst's System of Obstetrics; Ashhurst's, Agnew's, and Martin's Surgeries; Sajous on Nose and Throat; Seiler on the Throat; and Pepper's System of Practice of Medicine, etc.

In conclusion, the author would gladly acknowledge any corrections or additions.

W. M. POWELL.

26 South Indiana Avenue,
Atlantic City, N. J.
Sept. 1891.

AUTHORITIES.

Abadie.
Abercrombie.
Agnew.
Ainslie.
Aitken.
Aldridge.
Alison.
Alrich.
Andeer.
Anders.
Anderson.
Anglada.
Annals of Gynæcology and Pædiatry.
Annual of the Universal Med. Sciences.
Armaignac.
Aschenbach.
Ashhurst.
Atkinson.
Atlee.
Aubert.
Audhoui.
Aulde.
Austie.

Baer.
Baker.
Balfour.
Balzer.
Barbacci.
Bareges.
Barker.
Barnes.
Barrett.
Barthez.
Bartholow.
Barwell.
Basham.
Bazin.
Beall.

Bean.
Beauperthuy.
Bellevue Hospital.
Benedict.
Bennett, W. H.
Bernardy.
Bertarelli.
Bezold.
Bibron.
Billroth.
Bird, Golding and George.
Bixby.
Blachez.
Blackwood.
Blasius.
Bonjean.
Boteler.
Bouchard.
Bouchut.
Brande.
Breima.
Brensinger.
Brinton.
Brockes.
Brodie.
Brondel.
Brooke, H. G.
Browne, Crichton.
Brown-Séquard.
Bruns.
Brunton.
Bucknell.
Bulkley.
Bumstead and Taylor.
Bundy.
Burgess.
Burnett.

Campi.
Canada Lancet.

FORMULÆ.

ABORTION.

1—℞ Tr. opii, ... ♏xx–xxx.
   Sig.: Mix with one or two ounces of starch-water
and inject into the rectum.   PARVIN.

ABSCESSES.

2—℞ Acid. carbolici, . . . gr. viij.
    Aq. destillat., . . . f ℨj.—M.
   Sig.: Inject ♏x into swelling, and repeat every
three days.   MARTIN.

3—℞ Sodii hypophosphitis, . . ℈iv.
    Calcii hypophosphitis, . . ℈viij.
    Syr. simp., ... f ℥iss.
    Aq. fœniculi, . . q. s. ad f ℥iv.—M.
   Sig.: Two teaspoonfuls four times a day.
      CHURCHILL.

4—℞ Iodoformi, ... ℨj.
    Glycerinæ, ... f ℨj.—M.
   Sig.: Inject into the abscess cavity after evacua-
ting the pus.   BILLROTH.

5—℞ Calcii sulphureti, . . gr. vj.
    Pulv. glycyrrhizæ, . . q. s.—M.
   Et ft. pil. No. xii.
   Sig.: One pill every three hours.   WAUGH.

ACIDITY (See also Pyrosis).

6—℞ Sodii bicarb., ... ℨj.
    Pulv. rhei, ... ℥ss.
    Spt. menthæ pip., . . . f ℨij.
    Aquæ, . . . q. s. ad f ℥iv.—M.
   Sig.: Tablespoonful after meals.
      BELLEVUE HOSPITAL.

7—℞ Hydrarg. cum cretæ, . . gr. viij.
       Bismuth. subnit., . . . gr. xij.
       Pulv. nucis myristicæ, . . gr. iij.—M.
   Et ft. chart. No. vi.

Sig.: One powder night and morning. (*For children.*)   GERHARD.

8—℞ Liq. calcis,
       Aq. cinnam., . . . āā f℥ij.—M.

Sig.: One or two teaspoonfuls in ice-water as
required.   STARR.

9—℞ Sodii bicarb., ... ℨiij.
   Div. in chart. No. xii.

Sig.: One powder in wineglassful of cold water
after meals.   CLARK.

ACNE (See also Skin Diseases).

10—℞ Huile de cade, . . . ℨss.
       Adipis preparat., . . . ℨj.—M.
   Et ft. unguentum.

Sig.: Apply night and morning.   TILBURY FOX.

11—℞ Magnesii sulph., . . . ℥j.
       Ferri sulph., ... gr. viij.
       Acidi sulphurici arom., . . f℥j.
       Aquæ menth. pip., . . f℥iv.

Sig.: Tablespoonful in cup of water, p. r. n.
                        DÜHRING.

12—℞ Hydrarg. chlorid. corrosiv., . gr. j-ij.
       Resorcini, ... ℨss-ℨj.
       Aquæ lauro-cerasi, . . f℥ij.
       Lanolin., . . . q. s. ℥iij.—M.

Sig.: Apply night and morning.

13—℞ Bismuthi subnitrat.,
       Hydrarg. ammoniat.,
       Ichthyolis, ... āā gr. xlviij.
       Vaselin., ... ℥j.—M.

Sig.: Apply night and morning.

ACNE (Continued).

Apply externally:

14—℞ Acidi borici, ... Ɵj.
  Lanolini, ... ℥ij.
  Ol. eucalyptol, . . . gtt. v.
  Ung. zinci oxidi, . . . ℥j.
  Bismuthi subnit., . . . ℥j.—M.
 Sig.: Ft. unguentum.   Shoemaker.

15—℞ Hydrarg. oxidi rubri,
  Hydrarg. ammon., . . āā gr. v.
  Adipis, ... ℥j.—M.
 Sig.: Apply night and morning. (*In obstinate cases.*)
             Fox.

16—℞ Liq. potassæ, ... f℥j.
  Aq. rosæ, ... f℥iv.—M.
 Sig.: Apply with sponge twice daily.
           Bartholow.

17—℞ Sulphuris iodid., . . . ℥ss.
  Adipis, ... ℥j.—M.
 Sig.: Apply freely night and morning.   Ringer.

AGALACTIA.

18—℞ Ex. pilocarpi fl., . . . f℥ij.
 Sig.: Teaspoonful two or three times a day.
           Bartholow.

ALBUMINOID KIDNEY.

19—℞ Ammon. chlor., . . . ℥iij.
  Aq. menthæ pip., . . . f℥iij.—M.
 Sig.: Teaspoonful in water three times a day.

ALBUMINOID LIVER.

20—℞ Syr. ferri iodid., . . . f℥ij.—M.
 Sig.: Ten drops in water three times a day.
           Hughes.

ALBUMINURIA (Bright's Disease).

21—℞ Auri et sodii chlor., . . . gr. iij.
  Hydrarg. chlor. corr., . . gr. v.
  Ex. gentian, . . . q. s.—M.
 Ft. pil. No. lx.
 Sig.: One pill morning and evening. Bartholow.

22—℞ Ol. erigeronitis, . . . f℥ss.
 Sig.: Five drops on a lump of sugar every three or
four hours. (*In chronic forms.*)   Bartholow.

3

23—℞ Pulv. scillæ,
  Pulv. digitalis,
  Caffein. citrat., . iāi gr. xxx.
  Hydrarg. chlorid. mit.,   . gr. v.—M.
Ft. pil. No. xxx.
Sig.: One pill thrice daily, after meals.

24—℞ Potass. acetat., . . . gr. x–xx.
  Infus. digitalis, . . . f$\mathfrak{Z}$ij.
  Infus. juniperi, . . . f$\mathfrak{Z}$ij.—M.
Sig.: Every two or three hours.

25—℞ Mist ferri et ammon. acetat.
  (U. S. P.), ... f$\mathfrak{Z}$vj.
Sig.: One to two teaspoonfuls well diluted three
times a day.   BASHAM.

26—℞ Ferri sulph., ... gr. xv.
  Magnes. sulph., . . . f$\mathfrak{Z}$ij.
  Potass. bicarb., . . . $\mathfrak{Z}$iij.
  Infus. buchu, ... f$\mathfrak{Z}$viij.—M.
Sig.: Tablespoonful once or twice daily in water.
(*When constipation exists.*)   FOTHERGILL.

27—℞ Pulv. jalapæ comp., . . $\mathfrak{Z}$ss–$\mathfrak{Z}$j.
Sig.: Take before breakfast.

28—℞ Acid. gallici, ... $\mathfrak{Z}$j–$\mathfrak{Z}$ij.
  Acid. sulphuric. dil., . . f$\mathfrak{Z}$ss.
  Tr. lupuli, . . . f$\mathfrak{Z}$j.
  Infus. lupuli, . . . ad f$\mathfrak{Z}$vj.—M.
Sig.: Tablespoonful three times a day. (*If urine
is smoky.*)   AITKEN.

ALCOHOLISM.

29—℞ Tr. nucis vomicæ, . . ♏lxxx.
  Tr. gentian co.,
  Tr. calumbæ co., . . āā f$\mathfrak{Z}$ij.—M.
Sig.: Dessertspoonful before each meal, in water.
             LOOMIS.

30—℞ Spt. ammon. aromat., . . f$\mathfrak{Z}$ij.
  Tr. camphoræ, . . . f$\mathfrak{Z}$iss.
  Tr. hyoscyami, . . . $\mathfrak{Z}$iiss.
  Spts. lavandulæ co., q. s. ad f$\mathfrak{Z}$ij.—M.
Sig.: Teaspoonful every hour or two until relieved.
             AITKEN.

ALCOHOLISM (Continued).

31—℞ Zinci oxidi,   .   .   gr. xxiv.—M.
Div. in pil. No. xii.
Sig.: One pill three times a day.   MORRIS.

32—℞ Zinci oxidi,   .   .   ℥j.
Piperinæ,   .   .   Əj.—M.
Et ft. pil. No. xx.
Sig.: One pill three or four times a day. (*In chronic form.*)   CHAPMAN.

33—℞ Tr. capsici,
Tr. zingiber.,   .   .   .   āā f℥j.
Tr. valerianæ ammon.,
Tr. gentian. comp.,   .   āā f℥ij.—M.
Sig.: Take dessertspoonful in a teacupful of hot tea three or four times a day.   GERHARD.

34—℞ Sodii brom., ...   ℥ss.
Chloral. hydrat.,   .   .   .   ℥iiss.
Syr. aurant. cort.,   .   .   f℥ss.
Aquæ, ...   ad f℥iv.—M.
Sig.: Tablespoonful at night. Repeat if necessary.   AITKEN.

ALOPECIA (See also Skin Diseases).

35—℞ Ext. jaborandi fluid.,
Tinct. cantharidis,   .   .   āā f℥ss.
Glycerinæ,
Olei vaselini,   .   .   .   āā .℥j.—M.
Sig.: Apply locally with a sponge at night.
    BARTHOLOW.

36—℞ Tr. macis, ...   f℥iss.
Ol. olivæ,   .   .   .   ad f℥ij.—M.
Sig.: Apply two or three times a day to affected spots.   HEBRA.

37—℞ Ext. pilocarpi, fld.,   .   .   f℥j.
Tinct. cantharidis,   .   .   f℥ss.
Linimentum saponis,   . q. s.   f℥iv.—M.
Sig.: Rub in the scalp daily.   BARTHOLOW.

38—Tr. cantharidis, ...   f℥iss.
Tr. capsici, ...   ♏xx.
Glycerinæ, ...   f℥ss.
Spt. odoratæ,   .   .   .   ad f℥vj.—M.
Sig.: Apply two or three times daily.   GROSS.

ALOPECIA (Continued).

39—℞ Quiniæ sulphat., . . . ℈ss.
   Tr. cautharidis, . . . f℥j.
   Spt. ammon. aromat., . . f℥j.
   Ol. ricini, ... f℥iss.
   Spt. myrciæ, ... f℥vss.
   Ol. rosmarini, . . . gtt. v.—M.
  Sig.: Shake well. Apply with stiff brush two or
three times a day.   GERHARD.

40—℞ Tr. cantharidis, . . . f℥ss.
   Ol. ricini, ... f℥iv.—M.
  Sig.: Rub well into roots of hair night and morning.
                            WARING.

AMENORRHŒA.

41—℞ Ex. Aloes aqueosi, . . . ℈j.
   Ferri sulphat. exsiccat.,. . ℈ij.
   Asafœtidæ, ... ℈iv.—M.
  Ft. pil. No. c.
  Sig.: One to three pills three times a day. GOODELL.

42—℞ Hydrarg. bichlorid., . gr. j.
   Sodii arsenit., . . gr. iiss.
   Strychn. sulph., . . gr. ¼.
   Potass. carb. pur., . . gr. ix.
   Ferri sulph. exsic., . gr. ix.—M.
  Et ft. pil. No. x.
  Sig.: One thrice daily after meals.
                            WINTON.

43—℞ Terebinthinæ alb.,
   Pulv. aloes,
   Ferri sulph. exsic., . . āā ℈j.—M.
  Et ft. pil No. xx.
  Sig.: One pill three times a day.   PARVIN.

44—℞ Syr. ferri hypophosphit.,
   Syr. sodii hypophosphit.,
   Syr. mangani hypophosphit.,
   Glycerin., ... āā f℥j.
   Aq. lauro-cerasi, . . . ℔xl.—M.
  Sig.: A teaspoonful after each meal.

45—℞ Tr. ferri chlor., . . . f℥iij.
   Tr. cantharidis, . . . f℥j.
   Tr. guaiac ammon., . . f℥iss.
   Tr. aloes, ... f℥ss.
   Syrupi, . . . q. s. ad f℥vj.—M.
  Sig.: Tablespoonful three times a day.   DEWEES.

46—℞ Liq. potass. arsenitis, . . f℥j.
Vini ferri amar., . . . f℥vj.—M.
Sig.: Tablespoonful three times a day, after meals.
F. P. HENRY.

47—℞ Tr. ferri chlor., . . . f℥iv.
Acid. phosphor. dil., . . f℥vj.
Spts. limonis, ... f℥ij.
Syr. simp., . . q. s. ad f℥vj.—M.
Sig.: Dessertspoonful, well diluted, after meals.
GOODELL.

48—℞ Quiniæ sulph., . . . gr. xx.
Ferri sulph. exsiccat., . . gr. xl.
Strychninæ sulph., . . gr. ss.—M.
Et div. in pil. No. xx.
Sig.: One pill three times a day. BARTHOLOW.

49—℞ Ferratin., ... ℨiij.
Ext. aloes, . . . gr. xiv.
Ext. rhei comp., . . gr. ix.—M.
Div. in tabellæ No. xxx.
Sig.: One or two to be taken twice a day.

50—℞ Ferri sulphat.,
Sodii chlorid., . . . āā gr. xij.
Magnesii sulphat., . . . ℥iss.
Acid. sulphuric. dil., . . . f℥iss.
Infus. quassiæ, . . . q. s. f℥vj.—M.
Sig.: A tablespoonful before meals.

51—℞ Sodii arseniat., . . . gr. j.
Aquæ, ... ℥x.—M.
Sig.: Teaspoonful daily during meal times.

52—℞ Acid. phosphorici dil.,
Acid. nitro-muriatic dil.,
Acid. sulphuric. aromat.,
Tr. ferri chloridi, . . āā f℥ss.—M.
Sig.: From twenty to thirty-five drops in half a glassful of cold, sweetened water.
Given as a tonic in the anæmia of children, especially when this is associated with loss of appetite and general debility. MAYS.

53—℞ Ferri sulph. exsiccat.,
Potassi carb., . . . āā gr. j.—M.
Ft. pil. j. t. d. DA COSTA.

54—℞ Ext. cinchonæ,
    Ext. gentianæ,
    Ext. rhei,
    Ferri et potassæ tart.,   .   5ā   gr. lxxv.
    Ext. nucis vomicæ,   .   .   gr. vijss.
    Ol. anisi, ...   gtt. v.
    Glycerinæ, ...   q. s.—M.
Et div. in pil. No. c.
Sig.: Two pills before each meal.   HUCHARD.

55—℞ Acidi arseniosi,   .   .   .   gr. j.
    Ferri sulphat. exsiccat., .   .   gr. ss.
    Pulv. pip. nigr.,   .   .   .   ℨj.
    Pil. aloes et myrrhæ,   .   .   ℨj.—M.
Et div. in pil. No. xl.
Sig.: One twice a day after meals.   FOTHERGILL.

56—℞ Hydrarg. chloridi corrosivi,   .   gr. ij.
    Liquoris arsenici chloridi,   fℨj.
    Tincturæ ferri chloridi,
    Acidi hydrochlorici diluti,   āā   fℨiv.
    Syrupi simplicis,   .   .   .   fℨiij.
    Aquæ,   .   .   .   q. s. ad   f℥vj.—M.
Sig.: Dessertspoonful in a wineglassful of water
after each meal.

57—℞ Liq. potass. arsen.,   .   .   fℨj.
    Tr. ferri chlor.,
    Acid. phos. dil.,   .   .   āā   f℥ss.
    Aquæ,   .   .   .   q. s. ad   f℥ij.—M.
Sig.: Teaspoonful in water taken through a glass
tube t. i. d. after meals.   NICHOLS.

ANÆSTHESIA, LOCAL.

In such cases as opening a bone felon, scraping a
small fistula in the gums, removal of epithelioma in
the face, or, in fact, any small operation requiring
a local anæsthetic lasting from two to six minutes,
Dobish recommends the use of the following solution
in a Richardson spray :—

58—℞ Chloroformi,   .   .   fℨiss.
    Æther. sulphuric., .   .   fℨiv.
    Menthol,   .   .   .   gr. xv.—M.
Sig.: As a spray.

ANEURISM.

59—℞ Potass. iodid., . . . ℨss.
Syr. simp., ... f℥j.
Aq. menthæ pip., . . ad f℥iij.—M.
Sig.: A teaspoonful three times daily, gradually
increased to double the quantity. BALFOUR.

60—℞ Tr. digitalis, ... f℥ss.
Ex. ergotæ fl., . . . f℥iiiss.—M.
Sig.: Teaspoonful in water three times a day.
DA COSTA.

ANGINA PECTORIS.

61—℞ Sol. nitro-glycerin (1 per cent.), f℥ss.—M.
Sig.: One to two drops internally. (*When pallor
of face exists.*) PEPPER.

℞ Methylal, ... f℥ix.
Amyl nitrite, ... f℥j.—M.
Sig.: Drop thirty or forty drops on handkerchief
and inhale. RICHARDSON.

62—℞ Tr. digitalis, ... f℥iiss.
Spt. chloroform., . . . f℥vj.
Ex. buchu fl., . . . f℥j.
Spt. juniperi comp., q. s. ad f℥iv.—M.
Sig.: Dessertspoonful three times a day.
FOTHERGILL.

63—℞ Amyl nitrite, ... ℳv.
Sig.: For inhalation. MURCHISON.

ANTHRAX.

64—℞ Acid. carbol., ... ℳx–xxx.
Aquæ, ... f℥j.—M.
Sig.: Inject with hypodermic needle five drops into
and around the pustule. MARTIN.

65—℞ Hydrarg. bicyanid., . . . gr. v.
Aq. destillat., ... f℥j.
Cocain. salicylat., . . . q. s.—M.
Sig.: Inject subcutaneously from 10 to 20 minims
and cover the affected area with sublimate compresses.

APHTHÆ.

66—℞ Sodii salicylat., . . . ℨiss.
Aquæ rosæ, ... f℥j.—M.
Sig.: Apply several times daily. HIRTZ.

9

APHTHÆ (Continued).

67—℞ Potass. chlorat., . . . ꝰij.
    Tr. ferri chlor., . . . ʒj.
    Syr. simp., ... f ʒvj.
    Aq. cinnam., . . q. s. ad f ʒij.—M.
Sig.: Teaspoonful every two hours for a child of
two years.   STUBBS.

68—℞ Potass. chlorat., . . . gr. xx.
    Vini opii, ... ♏v.
    Glycerinæ, ... f ʒj.
    Aq. rosæ, . . q. s. ad f ʒj.—M.
Sig.: Use as mouth-wash.   STARR.

69—℞ Mel boracis, ... ʒj.
Sig.: Apply several times daily to patches.
          RINGER.

70—℞ Potass. iodid., . . gr. i.–v.
    Aquæ, ... f ʒj.—M.
Sig.: Use locally.   BARTHOLOW.

71—℞ Zinci chlor., ... gr. iij.
    Alcoholis dil., . . . f ʒviij.—M.
Sig.: Use as mouth-wash.   SIMON.

APOPLEXY.

72—℞ Tr. veratri viridis, . . . f ʒss.—M.
Sig.: Three to five drops every three or four hours.
          HUGHES.

73—℞ Ol. tigli, ... gtt. j.
    Glycerinæ, ... ♏xij.—M.
Sig.: Place on tongue.

ASTHMA.

74—℞ Potassii iodid., . . . ʒijss.
    Tinct. lobeliæ, . . . f ʒiv, ♏x.
    Syr. sarsaparillæ comp., q. s. ad f ʒij.—M.
Sig.: Teaspoonful every two hours till relieved.
          ANDERS.

75—℞ Tr. sanguinariæ,
    Tr. lobeliæ,
    Ammon. iodid., . . āā ʒj.
    Syr. tolu., ... f ʒvj.—M.
Sig.: Teaspoonful every two to four hours.
          BARTHOLOW

76—℞ Ammon. brom., . . . ϶viij.
    Ammon. chlor., . . . ℥iss.
    Tr. lobeliæ, ... f℥iij.
    Spt. æther. comp., . . . f℥j.
    Syr. acaciæ, . . . ad f℥iv.—M.
Sig.: Dessertspoonful in water every hour or two
during paroxysms.   PEPPER.

77—℞ Potass. brom., . . ℥ss.
    Ex. grindeliæ rob. fl.,
    Syr. ipecac., . . . āā f℥j.
    Aquæ, ... f℥ij.—M.
Sig.: Teaspoonful every four hours. ROCHESTER.

78—℞ Ammon. iodid., . . ℥ij.
    Ex. grindeliæ rob. fl., . f℥ss.
    Ex. glycyrrhizæ fl., . f℥iv.
    Tr. lobeliæ,
    Tr. belladonnæ, . . āā f℥ij.
    Syr. tolu., . . q. s. ad f℥iv.—M.
Sig.: Teaspoonful three times a day; extra doses
during paroxysms.   COVERT.

79 -℞ Tr. lobeliæ æthereal, . . . ℳxv.
    Spt. ætheris, ... ℳxx.
    Tr. chloroform. comp., . . ℳv.
    Aq. camphoræ, . . . ad f℥j.—M.
Sig.: To be taken when breathing is difficult.

80—℞ Amyl nitritis, . . . f℥j.
Sig.: Inhale three to five drops from a handkerchief.   FRASER.

81—℞ Ex. euphorbiæ piluliferæ fl., . f℥j.
Sig.: Thirty to sixty drops, as required. PAYNE.

82—℞ Pulv. stramonii fol.,
    Pulv. belladonnæ fol., . āā ℥j.
    Pulv. potass. nit., . . . ℥iss.
    Pulv. opii, ... gr. xv.—M.
Sig.: Burn a little and inhale the fumes.

83—℞ Hyoscin. hydrobromat., . . gr. $\frac{1}{200}$.
    Strychnin. sulphat., . . gr. $\frac{1}{60}-\frac{1}{40}$.
    Morphin. sulphat., . . gr. $\frac{1}{3}-\frac{1}{4}$.—M.
Sig.: For hypodermic injection.

                  COHEN.

BED SORES.

84—℞ Hydrarg. perchlor., . gr. ij.
    Spt. rect., . . . f℥j.—M.
Sig.: Use locally.   ERICHSEN.

85—℞ Alumin.,
    Sodii chloridi, . āā ℥ss.
    Aquæ,
    Alcoholis, . . . āā Oj.—M.
Sig.: For local use, twice daily. (*To prevent bed-sores.*)   FORBES.

BILIOUSNESS..

86—℞ Sodii sulphat.,
    Potass. et sodii tart., . āā ℥j.
    Infus. cascarillæ, . . . f℥viij.—M.
Sig.: Two tablespoonfuls three times a day.
          FOTHERGILL.

87—℞ Fellis bovini purif., . . ℨj.
    Manganesii sulph. exsiccat., . ℈ij.
    Resinæ podophylli, . . gr. v.—M.
Et ft. pil. No. xx.
Sig.: One pill three times a day.   DA COSTA.

88—℞ Ex. colocynth. comp., . . gr. iiss.
    Podophyllin, ... gr. ¼.—M.
Et ft. pil. No. i.
Sig.:

89—℞ Ammonii iodid., . . . ℨj.
    Liq. potass. arsenit., . . . f℥ss.
    Tr. calumbæ, ... f℥ss.
    Aq. destillat., ... f℥iss.—M.
Sig.: One teaspoonful three times daily, before meals.

BITES (Insects).

91—℞ Pulv. ipecac., . ℥ss.
    Spt. vini rect.,
    Ether sulphur., . āā f℥ss.—M.
Sig.: Apply to bite.   NEAL.

BITES (Snakes).

92—℞ Tr. iodinii, ... f℥j.
Sig.: Apply freely to wound. S. WEIR MITCHELL.

BITES (Continued).

93—℞ Aq. ammoniæ, . . ♏xxx.
    Aquæ, ... f℥iss.—M.
    Sig.: Inject in vein.   HALFORD.

BLADDER. AFFECTIONS OF (See Catarrh).

BOILS (See Abscesses.)

BREATH, FETID.

94—℞ Sodii bicarbonat.,
    Saccharin.,
    Acid. salicylic, . . āā ℨj.
    Alcoholis, ... ℥vj.—M.
    Sig.: A teaspoonful in a glass of water to rinse the mouth. .

95—℞ Sodii biborat., . . . gr. xv
    Thymol, ... gr. viiss.
    Aquæ, ... f℥viij.—M.
    Sig.: Mouth wash.

BRIGHT'S DISEASE (See Albuminuria.)

BROMIDROSIS.

96—℞ Ex. geranii mac. fl., . f℥ij.
    Sig.: Use externally.   PEPPER.

BRONCHITIS.

97—℞ Vini ipecacuanhæ, . . . f℥ij.
    Liq. potass. citrat., . . f℥iv.
    Tr. opii camphorat.,
    Syr. acaciæ, . . . āā f℥j.—M.
    Sig.: Tablespoonful three times a day in the first
stage.   DA COSTA.

98—℞ Tr. veratri viridis, . . . ♏xij.
    Syr. scillæ comp., ... f℥ij.
    Syr. tolu., ... f℥xiv.—M.
    Sig.: Teaspoonful every two or three hours for a
child five years old, in the first stages.
    J. LEWIS SMITH.

99—℞ Apomorph. mur., . . . gr. ss.
    Pot. bromidi., . . . ℨij.
    Syr. senegæ, . . q. s. ad f℥ij.—M.
    Sig.: Teaspoonful every two hours. (*First or dry
stage.*)

100—℞ Am. mur.,
  Am. brom., . . . āā ℨj.
  Spts. ætheris nit., . . . f℥ss.
  Syr. pruni virg.. . q. s. ad f℥ij.—M.
 Sig.: Teaspoonful t. i. d. (*Second stage.*)

101—℞ Terebene, . . ℨijss.
  Mucl. acacia,
  Aquæ, ... āā f℥ss.
  Syr. zingiberi, . q. s. ad f℥ij.—M.
 Sig.: Teaspoonful t. i. d. (*In bronchitis with profuse mucopurulent expectoration.*)   NICHOLLS.

102—℞ Ammoniæ muriat., . . ℨj.
  Ext. euphorbiæ pil. fld., . f℥ij.
  Tinct. digitalis, . . . f℥iss.
  Syr. tolu., ... f℥j.
  Syr. simplici, . . . q. s. f℥ij.—M.
 Sig.: A teaspoonful every two or three hours. (*In subacute bronchitis.*)   MAYS.

103—℞ Potass. citrat., . . . ℥ss.
  Apomorphiæ hydrochlor., . gr. j.
  Syr. ipecac., . . . f℥ss.
  Succi limonis, . . . f℥ij.
  Syr. simp., . . q. s. ad f℥iv.—M.
 Sig.: Dessertspoonful, in water, every three hours. (*In first stage.*)   WOOD.

104—℞ Ammon. chlor., . . . ℨij.
  Mist. glycyrrhizæ comp., . f℥iij.—M.
 Sig.: Dessertspoonful three times a day. (*In chronic form.*)   DA COSTA.

105—℞ Ammon. carb., . . . Ɖij.
  Spt. chloroform, . . . f℥ss.
  Infus. senegæ, . . . f℥viij.—M.
 Sig.: Two tablespoonfuls every four to six hours.
      FOTHERGILL.

106—℞ Tr. aconiti, ... gtt. xij.
  Syr. ipecac., ... f℥ss–j.
  Liq. potassii citratis, q. s. ad f℥iij.—M.
 Sig.: One teaspoonful every three hours.

107—℞ Terebene, ... f℥ss.
 Sig.: Two to five drops on sugar every four hours according to child's age.   CARMICHAEL.

108—℞ Codein. hydrochlorat, . . gr. ⅛.
       Apomorphin.hydrochlor., . . gr. 1/30-1/20.
       Acid. hydrocyanic. dil., . . ℳj.
       Syr. pruni Virginiani, . . f℥ss.
       Aquæ, . . . q. s. ad f℥j.—M.
   Sig.: A teaspoonful every three or four hours.

109—℞ Ammonii chloridi, . . . ℥iss.
       Tinct. hyoscyami, . . . f℥iv.
       Vini ipecac., ... f℥iss.
       Syr. hypophos. comp., . . f℥j.
       Aq. destillat., . . . ad ℥iv.—M.
   Sig.: Two teaspoonfuls every four hours. (*In chronic
   form.*)   AMERICAN MEDICO-SURGICAL BULLETIN.

111—℞ Morphin. bimeconatis, . . gr. j.
       Ammon. muriatis, . . . ℥j.
       Aquæ camphoræ, . . . f℥iss.
       Aquæ, . . . q. s. ad f℥iij.—M.
   Sig.: One teaspoonful as required.
                        JOUR. OF RESP. ORGANS.

112—℞ Liq. ammon. acetat., . . f℥ss.
       Syr. ipecac., ... f℥j.
       Liq. morphiæ sulph. (U. S. P.), ℳxl.
       Syr. acaciæ, ... f℥j.
       Aquæ, ... f℥iss.—M.
   Sig.: Teaspoonful every two hours for a child of
   two years.   MEIGS and PEPPER.

113—℞ Ammon. muriat., . . . ℥j.
       Syrup. senegæ, . . . f℥ss.
       Tr. opii camphorat., . . f℥j.
       Syrup. tolutan., . . . f℥ss.
       Aq. gaultheriæ, . q. s. ad f℥ij.—M.
   Sig.: Teaspoonful every two hours.   REX.

114—℞ Syrup. tolu.,
       Syrup. pruni virg.,
       Tinct. hyoscyami,
       Spirit. ætheris comp.,
       Aquæ, ... āā f℥j.—M.
   Sig.: Dose, a teaspoonful.   JANEWAY.

15

BRONCHITIS *(Continued)*.

116—℞ Ammon. carb., . . . gr. xxiv.
  Syr. tolu., ... f℥vj.
  Spt. vini gal., . . . f℥iij.
  Syr. senegæ, ... f℥iiss.
  Syr. acaciæ, . . q. s. ad f℥iij.—M.

Sig.: Teaspoonful every two hours. (*In capillary*
form.)   GOODHART and STARR.

117—℞ Acid. hydrocyan. dil., . . ℳxvj.
  Syr. prun. virg.,
  Aq. camphoræ, . . āā f℥j.—M.

Sig.: Teaspoonful every two or three hours.
          HARTSHORNE.

118—℞ Tr. sanguinariæ,
  Tr. lobeliæ, . . . āā f℥j.
  Vini ipecac., ... f℥ij.
  Syr. tolu., ... f℥ss.—M.

Sig.: Teaspoonful every three hours. BARTHOLOW.

119—℞ Vini ipecac., ... f℥ij.
  Vini antimonialis, . . . f℥j.
  Vini xerici, ... f℥iij.—M.

Sig.: Three drops every hour to a child six months
old.   DESSAU.

120—℞ Ammon. carb., . . . ℈ij.
  Spt. chloroform., . . . f℥ss.
  Infus. senegæ, . . . f℥viij.—M.

Sig.: Tablespoonful every four to six hours.
          FOTHERGILL.

BRUISES.

121—℞ Potass. chlorat., . ℥ss.
  Tr. iodi.,
  Aquæ, . . . āā f℥ss.—M.

Sig.: Apply locally.   BRENSINGER.

122—℞ Tr. capsici,
  Tr. myrrh.,
  Tr. opium, . . āā f℥ij.
  Tr. guaiac., . . . f℥j.
  Spts. camphor., . . f℥ij.—M.

Sig.: Use locally.

123—℞ Tr. aconiti rad.,
  Tr. opii,
  Chloroform., . . . āā f℥ij.—M.

Sig.: Shake well before using. (*Poison*.)
          WHELPLEY.

ADDITIONAL FORMULÆ.

BUBO.

124—℞ Tr. iodi., ... f℥j.

Sig.: Paint well every other day until skin becomes tender.   VAN BUREN.

125—℞ Cadmii iodid., . . . gr. xxx.
      Adipis, ... ℥j.—M.

Sig.: Apply twice daily.   MARTIN.

126—℞ Hydrogen peroxide (March-
      and's solution), . . . f℥vj.

Sig.: Apply with an atomizer after suppuration has begun.   RINGER.

BUNIONS.

127—℞ Argenti nitratis, . . . ℥j.
      Aquæ, ... f℥j.—M.

Sig.: Paint twice daily.   MARTIN.

128—℞ Acid. tannic.,
      Ungt. petroleii, . . āā ℥ss.—M.

Sig.: Apply to joint after the skin has been removed by blistering.   GROSS.

129—℞ Tr. iodinii,
      Tr. belladonnæ, . . āā f℥j.—M.

Sig.: Apply twice daily.

BURNS.

130—Wash with 1-4000 bichloride lotion ; dust lightly with iodoform ; apply protective and dress antiseptically. Or, instead of the antiseptic dressing, use—

131—℞ Acid. boric.,
      Ungt. petrolei, . . āā ℥j.—M.

Sig.: Apply on lint.   MARTIN.

132—℞ Acid. borici, ... ℥j.
      Aquæ, ... f℥iv.—M.

Sig.: A piece of oiled silk a trifle larger than the lesion is dipped in the solution and applied ; then a larger piece of lint dipped in the same solution placed over the silk and held loosely by a bandage.   LISTER.

133—℞ Sodii bicarb., . . . ℥ij.
      Aquæ, ... Oij.—M.

Sig.: Apply freely on lint.   MARTIN.

BURNS *(Continued).*

134—℞ Ol. lini,
    Liq. calcis, . . . āā f℥ij.
    Acid. carbol., ... gtt. xv.—M.
    Sig. : Wring out dressings of sterile gauze in this
mixture and apply.   CHARITY HOSPITAL, N. Y.

135—℞ Acid. carbol., . . . gr. viij.
    Vaseline, ... ℥ij.—M.
    Sig.: Spread on lint and apply where the skin is
broken.   BELLEVUE HOSPITAL, N. Y.

136—℞ Europhen., . . gr. v.
    Vaselin.,
    Lanolin., ... āā ℥j.—M.
    Sig.: Apply three or four times daily.

137—℞ Cerat. resinæ, . . ℥j.
    Ol. terebinth., . . f℥j.—M.
    Sig.: Apply freely on lint.   AGNEW.

138—℞ Acid. salicyl., . . . ℥j.
    Ol. olivæ, ... f℥iij.—M.
    Sig.: Apply to burn covering with lint.
    BARTHOLOW.

139—℞ Cocaini, ... gr. x–xx.
    Boroglyceridi, . . f℥ij.—M.
    Sig.: Apply locally on absorbent cotton.   ELLER.

CALCULI, BILIARY.

140—℞ Morphiæ sulphat., . . . gr. vj.
    Atropiæ sulphat., . . . gr. ⅕.
    Aq. destillat., . . . f℥ss.—M.
    Sig.: Ten minims hypodermically during par-
oxysm.   BARTHOLOW.

141—℞ Ol. olivæ, ... Oj.
    Sig.: Take in divided doses before breakfast.
    D. D. STEWART.

142—℞ Chloroformi, ... f℥iij.
    Sig.: Inhale in small quantities until paroxysm
ceases.   RINGER.

143—℞ Sodii phosphatis, . . ℥ss.
    Ft. in chart. No. xii.
    Sig.: One powder before each meal.   BARTHOLOW.

CALCULI, RENAL AND VESICAL, WITH ACID URINE.

144—℞ Lithii citratis, . . . ʒss.
Syr. aurant. cort., . . . fʒj.
Aquæ, ... ad fʒij.—M.
Sig.: Teaspoonful in water three times a day.

GUY.

145—℞ Sodii benzoat.,
Lithii carbonat.,
Ex. stigmat. maydis, āā ʒj.
Ol. anisi, . . . gtt. iv.—M.
Et ft. pil. No. lxxx.
Sig.: One pill four times a day. HUCHARD.

146—℞ Liq. potassæ, ... fʒij.
Infus. buchu, ... fʒviij.—M.
Sig.: Three tablespoonfuls an hour after meals.

REECE.

CALCULI, RENAL AND VESICAL, WITH ALKALINE URINE.

147—℞ Ammon. benzoat., . . . ʒij.
Syr. simp., ... fʒiss.
Aquæ, ... ad fʒvj.—M.
Sig.: Tablespoonful three times a day. SEYMOUF

148—℞ Acid. nitric. dil.,
Acid. hydrochlor. dil., . āā fʒiij.
Syr. aurant. cort.,
Aq. aurant. flor., . . āā fʒj.
Aquæ, ... fʒxiiiss.—M
Sig.: Wineglassful three times a day. DRUITT

149—℞ Strychniniæ sulphat., . . gr. j.
Acid. nitric. dil., . . . fʒj.
Aquæ, ... fʒxij.—M.
Sig.: Two tablespoonfuls three times a day.

BIRD

CANCER.

150—℞ Syr. ferri et manganesii iodid., fʒss.
Syr. simp., ... fʒiss.
Aq. destillat., . . . fʒij.—M.
Sig.: Dessertspoonful three times a day. STILLÉ

151—℞ Bismuth. salicylat.,
Magnesiæ (English),
Sodii bicarb., . . āā ʒiiss.—M.
Et ft. chart. No. xxv.
Sig.: One before each meal. DUJARDIN-BEAUMETZ.

19

152—℞ Bismuth. subnit., . . . ℥ij.
     Acid. hydrocyanic. dil., . . f℥ss.
     Syr. acaciæ,
     Aq. menthæ pip., . . āā f℥ij.—M.

Sig.: Tablespoonful three times a day in milk. (*In cancer of stomach.*)   BARTHOLOW

153—℞ Iodoformi, ... gr. xv.
     Ex. opii, ... gr. viij.
     Ess. menthæ., . . . gtt. x.
     Ol. theobromæ, . . . ℥ijss.—M.
    Ft. supp. No. xii.

Sig.: A suppository to be introduced into the vagina in cases of cancer of the cervix uteri. In case this remedy be insufficient, one may prescribe hypodermic injections of morphine in the following formulæ :—

154—℞ Morphinæ sulphat., . . gr. xvj.
     Sulph. (neut.) atropinæ, . gr. vj.
     Aq. destill., . . . ℥ij.—M.

Sig.: Inject six drops of this solution into the vicinity of the great trochanter to calm the pains of uterine cancer.   L'UNION MÉDICALE.

155—℞ Morphiæ sulphat., . . . gr. j.
     Bismuth. subnit., . . . ℥ij.—M.
    Et ft. chart. No. vi.

Sig.: One powder three times a day. (*In gastric cancer.*)   BARTHOLOW.

156—℞ Sodii chloratis, ... ℥v.
     Syr. aurantii corticis, . . f℥j.
     Aq. destillat., ... f℥iij.—M.

Sig.: From two to eight teaspoonfuls daily.

157—℞ Sodii chloratis, ... ℥iiss.
     Bismuthi subnitratis, . . ℥iiss.
     Iodoformi, ... ℥j.—M.

Sig.: Apply a small quantity on a tampon to the cervix. (*Cancer of the uterus.*)

158—℞ Zinci chlor., ... ℥ij.
     Pulv. rad. althææ, . . ℥vj.
     Aq. destillat., . . . q. s.—M.
    Et ft. magma.

Sig.: Apply to affected part. (*In epithelioma.*)   CANQUOIN.

CANCER (Continued).

159—℞ Liq. ferri subsulphatis, . . f℥j.
Aq. destillat., . . . f℥iij.—M.
Sig.: To inject into the uterus, in hemorrhage from cancer. BARNES.

CARBUNCLE.

160—℞ Acidi carbolici, . . . gr. viij.
Aq. destil., ... f℥j.—M.
Sig.: Make several injections into different parts of the induration. Not more than ℥j of this solution should be used at one treatment. The injection may be repeated, if necessary, in three days.

161—℞ Tr. iodi., ... f℥ss.—M.
Sig.: Paint around the carbuncle until vesication is produced. FURNEAUX-JORDAN.

162—℞ Pulv. opii,
Unguent. hydrarg.,
Saponis duræ, . . āā ℥ss.—M.
Sig.: Apply spread on thick leather.

163—℞ Europhen., . . . ℈iv.
Ol. olivæ, . . . ℥ijss.
Lanolin., . . .
Vaselin., . . āā ℥vj.—M.
Ft. ung.
Sig.: Apply topically and cover with sterilized gauze. (*To abort furuncles.*)

164—℞ Calcii sulphidi, . gr. iij.
Ft. pil. No. xxx.
Sig.: One pill every two hours. RINGER.

165—℞ Cerat. resinæ comp., . ℥j.
Ol. olivæ, . . . f℥ij.—M.
Sig.: Apply on lint. WITHERSTINE.

166—℞ Resorcin, ... ℈iss-℥iss.
Lanolini, ... ℥j.—M.
Sig.: Apply after making parallel incisions into carbuncle. (*Abortive.*) WEISS.

CARIES.

167—℞ Syr. hypophos. comp.,
Ol. morrhuæ, . . . āā f℥iv.—M.
Sig.: Dessertspoonful four times daily.

21

CARIES *(Continued).*

168—℞ Syr. calcii lactophosphat. (U.

  S. P.), ... f℥vj.—M.

 Sig.: A teaspoonful three or four times a day.

              BARTHOLOW.

169—℞ Hydrogen peroxide (Mar-

  chand), ... f℥vj.—M.

 Sig.: Apply with an atomizer or small syringe.

170—℞ Cupri sulphat.,

  Zinci sulphat., . . āā gr. xv.

  Liq. plumbi subacctat., . . f℥ss.

  Aceti alb., ... f℥iiiss.—M.

 Sig.: Inject through the sinuses. (Liqueur de Vil-
late.)   NOTTA.

CATARRH, NASAL AND FAUCIAL.

171—℞ Cocain. hydrochlor., . .

  Morphin. hydrochlor., . āā gr. j.

  Pulv. camphoræ, . . . gr. x.

  Pulv. benzoini, . . . gr. xv.

  Pulv. acid. boric., . . . gr. xxx.

  Bismuthi subnit., . . . ℥j.—M.

 Sig.: Use as snuff. (*Coryza.*)

172—℞ Sulph. zinci, . . . ⁻. grs. xv.

  Thymoli, ... gr. ⅓.

  Alcoholis,

  Glycerinæ, . . . āā f℥iss.

  Aq. menth. pip., . . f℥x.—M.

 Sig.: Use as gargle.

    MEDICAL AND SURGICAL REPORTER.

173—℞ Pulv. aluminis, . . . gr. v.-xxx.

  Aquæ, ... f℥j.—M.

 Sig.: Use with spray three or four times a day.
(*Coryza.*)   J. S. COHEN.

174—℞ Salol., ... gr. xv.

  Acid. salicyl., . . . gr. iij.

  Acid. tannici, . . . gr. j.

  Acid. borici, . . . ℥j.—M.

 Sig.: Use hourly as a snuff for half a day. (*To
abort coryza.*)

175—℞ Menthol., ... ℥ss.

  Chloroform., ... f℥v.—M.

 Sig.: Inhale four or five drops, rubbed on palms of
hands several times a day. (*Coryza.*)

CATARRH (Continued).

176—℞ Tr. aconiti rad., . . . f℈j.
   Tr. belladonnæ, . . . f℈ij.—M.
   Sig.: Three drops every hour. (*Pharyngitis and acute tonsillitis.*) RINGER.

177—℞ Cocain. muriat., . . . gr. vj.
   Bismuth. subcarb., . . ℈ss.
   Talc, ... f℥iss.—M.
   Sig.: Enough to cover a silver five-cent piece insufflated into each nostril every two hours. (*For acute coryza.*) SAJOUS.

178—℞ Acid. carbol. liq. . . . ℳxxx.
   Sodii biborat.,
   Sodii bicarb., . . . āā ℈j.
   Glycerinæ, ... f℈iiiss.
   Aquæ, . . . q. s. ad f℥iv.—M.
   Sig.: To be used as a spray. DOBELL.

179—℞ Sodii salicylat., . . . ℈ij.
   Sodii biborat., . . . ℈iij.
   Glycerinæ, ... f℈iv.
   Aquæ, . . . q. s. ad f℥vj.—M.
   Sig.: Dessertspoonful in a pint of water, used as a douche. BEAN.

CATARRH, BRONCHO-PULMONARY.

180—℞ Morphiæ sulphat., . . . gr. ss.
   Quiniæ sulphat., . . . gr. x.—M.
   Et ft. chart. No. i.
   Sig.: Take at bedtime. BARTHOLOW.

181—℞ Tr. opii, ... gtt. iij.
   Spt. frumenti, . . . f℥j.
   Aq. bullientis, . . . f℥iv.
   Sacch. alb., . . . q. s.—M.
   Sig.: Take at bedtime. (*Incipient catarrh.*) RINGER.

182—℞ Ammon. carbonat., . gr. xxxij.
   Ex. senegæ fl.,
   Ex. scillæ fl., . . . āā f℈j.
   Tr. opii camph., . . . f℈vj.
   Aquæ, ... f℈iv.
   Syr. tolu., . . q. s. ad f℥iv.—M.
   Sig.: Teaspoonful every three or four hours. STOKES.

23

CATARRH (Continued).

183—℞ Tr. eucalypti,
    Syr. simp., . . . āā f℥j.—M.
    Sig.. Teaspoonful every three hours.   GUBLER.

CATARRH, GALL-DUCTS.

184—℞ Ammon. iodid., . . . ℨj.
    Liq. potass. arsenitis, . . f℥ss.
    Tr. calumbæ, ... f℥ss.
    Aquæ destillat., . . . f℥iss.—M.
    Sig.: Take a teaspoonful three times a day before meals. (*With jaundice.*)   BARTHOLOW.

185—℞ Sodii phosphatis, . . . ℨij.
    Ft. iu chart. No. xvi.
    Sig.: One powder every four hours.   BARTHOLOW.

186—℞ Ammon. chlor., . . . ℥ss.
    Ex. taraxaci fl., . . . f℥iij.—M.
    Sig.: Teaspoonful three times daily.   BARTHOLOW.

CATARRH, GASTRO-INTESTINAL.

187—℞ Creosot. (beechwood), . . gtt. iij.
    Alcohol., . . . ♏xv.
    Gummi Arabic., . . . ℨijss.
    Syrupi, ... f℥j.
    Aquæ aurantii flor., . . f℥ijss.
    Aquæ, . . . q. s. ad f℥ij.—M.
    Sig.: A teaspoonful for children, a tablespoonful for adults, before each meal.

188—℞ Acid. nitrohydrochlor. dil., . f℥ss.
    Tr. nucis vomicæ, . . f℥ij.
    Liq. potassii arsenitis, . . gtt. lxxij.
    Ess. pepsin., . q. s. ad f℥vj.—M.
    Sig.: Dessertspoonful thrice daily, after meals.

189—℞ Tr. opii deod., . . . gtt. xvj.
    Bismuth. subnit., . . . ℨij.
    Syr. simp., ... f℥iv.
    Aq. cinnam., . . . f℥iss.—M.
    Sig.: Teaspoonful every two to four hours. (*For child one year old.*)   J. LEWIS SMITH.

CATARRH (Continued).

190—℞ Bismuthi subnit., . . . gr. x.
Potassii bromidi, . . . gr. xv–xx.
Acid hydrocyanici dil., . . ℳv.
Spt. chloroformi, . . . ℳx.
Mucilag. acaciæ, . . . f℥ij.
Aquæ, . . . q. s. ad ℥j.—M.

Sig.: To be taken every three or four hours, about ten minutes before each meal. (*Acute gastric catarrh.*)

BRUNTON.

CATARRH, GENITO-URINARY.

192—℞ Ex. buchu fl., . . . f℥j.
Potass. citrat., . . . ℥iij.
Spt. æther. nitro., . . . f℥ss.
Syr. limonis, . . q. s. ad f℥iij.—M.

Sig.: Teaspoonful every three hours. (*Subacute cystitis.*)

WOOD.

193—℞ Potass. citrat., . . . ℥ss.
Spt. chloroform., . . . f℥iiss.
Tr. digitalis, ... ℳlxxx.
Infus. buchu, . . . f℥viij.—M.

Sig.: Two tablespoonfuls three or four times a day.

FOTHERGILL.

194—℞ Atropiæ sulphat., . . . gr. j.
Acid. acetici, ... gtt. xx.
Alcoholis,
Aquæ, ... āā f℥ss.—M.

Sig.: Four drops in water before each meal. (*In acute cystitis.*)

GOODELL.

195—℞ Iodoformi, ... gr. i¾.
Ex. hyoscyami, . . . gr. j.
Ol. theobromæ, . . . gr. xiv.—M.

Sig.: Make one suppository and introduce high up into the rectum.

The bladder should be washed morning and evening with lukewarm water. If there be any urethral irritation, a pill containing one and three-fourths grains of terpin should also be taken morning and evening.

196—℞ Tr. aconit., ... f℥j.
Spt. æther. nitros., . . f℥j.
Liq. potass. citrat., q. s. ad f℥vj.—M.

Sig.: Dessertspoonful every four hours until all fever ceases and the pulse is quiet. (*Cystitis.*)

HARE.

198—℞ Potass. bicarbouat.,   .   . ℥iv.
     Ex. hyoscyami fl., .   .   . fʒij.
     Ex. ergotæ fl.,   .   . fʒiv.
     Syr. simp.,   .   .   . fℨij.
     Aquæ,   .   .   . q. s. ad fℨvj.—M.

Sig.: Dessertspoonful every two to four hours.
(*Cystitis.*)   MARTIN.

199—℞ Argenti nitrat.,   .   .   . gr. vij.
     Aq. destillat.,   .   .   . fℨiiiss.—M.

Sig.: Inject into the bladder every third or fourth
day after washing it out with warm water.   RICORD.

200—℞ Copaibæ,
     Spt. lavand. co.,   .   . āā ℥ij.
     Syr. acaciæ,   .   .   . fℨss.
     Syr. simp.,   .   .   . fℨiij.
     Aquæ, ... fℨiv.—M.

Sig.: Tablespoonful twice daily.   WOOD.

201—℞ Uvæ ursæ,   .   .   . ℥j.
     Lupulin.,   .   .   . ℥ss.
     Aq. bullient., .   .   . Oj.
     Dein. adde—
     Sodii bicarb., .   .   . ℥ij.
     Tinct. opii camph., .   . fℨij.—M.

Sig.: fℨij every four hours.   BRINTON.

CHANCRE.

202—℞ Ol. lavand., ... ♏xx.
     Iodoformi,
     Lycopodii,   .   .   . āā ℥ij.—M.

Sig.: Dust on part and cover with lint.

203—℞ Cupri subacetat.,
     Hydrarg. chlor. mit.,   . āā gr. x.—M.

Sig.: Dust over sore.   ELLIS.

204—℞ Hydrarg. chlor. mit.,   .   . gr. viij.
     Liq. calcis,   .   .   . fℨij.—M.

Sig.: Shake and use as a wash. (Black wash.)

205—℞ Hydrarg. chlor. corros., .   . gr. iv.
     Liq. calcis,   .   .   . fℨij.—M.

Sig.: Shake and use as a wash. (Yellow wash.)

206—℞ Hydrogen peroxide,   f℥j.
    Sig.: Use as a wash and apply on lint. If too strong, may be diluted.   RINGER.

207—℞ Hydrarg. chlor. mit.,   .   . ℥ss.
    Sig.: Dust on and cover with dry lint.
                         VAN BUREN and KEYES.

CHANCROID.

208—Actual cautery and dress antiseptically.

209—℞ Acidi sulphurici,
       Pulv. carbonis ligni,   .   āā   ℥ss.—M.
    Q. s. ft. magma.
    Sig.: Dry the sore and apply thoroughly by means of a wooden spatula. Allow artificial eschar thus formed to separate spontaneously, using no dressing.
                           RICORD.

210—Cauterize with nitric acid, protecting the surrounding parts by oil.

211—℞ Iodoform., ... ℥ij.
       Ol. menth. pip.,   .   .   . ♏x.—M.
    Sig.: Dust on sore and cover with moist lint.

212—℞ Bismuth. subiodid.,   .   . ℥ij.
    Sig.: Dust on sore and cover with dry lint.
                          CHASSAIGNAC.

213—℞ Pulv. acidi salicylici,   .   . ℥ij.
    Sig.: Dust on sore and cover with dry lint.
                          ANGLADA.

214—℞ Succi limonis,   .   .   . f℥iss.
       Vini opii, ... ♏xlv.
       Liq. plumbi subacetat., .   . f℥j.
       Aq. destillat., ... f℥v.—M.
    Sig.: Soak pledgets of lint in the solution and apply locally. (*In phagedenic form.*)   RODET.

CHILBLAINS.

215—℞ Calcis chloratæ,   .   .   . ℥j.
       Boracis pulv.,   .   .   . ℥j.
       Adipis, ... ℥j.—M.
    Sig.: Use locally.   TROUSSEAU.

CHILBLAINS (Continued).

216—℞ Resorcin.,
Ichthyol.,
Acid. tannic., . . . āā ℥iss.
Aquæ, ... f℥j.—M.
Sig.: To be painted on (after shaking) every night.
BOECK.

CHLOROSIS (See Anæmia).

CHOLERA.

217—℞ Strychniæ sulph., . . . gr. ¼.
Acid. sulphuric. dil., . . f℥ss.
Morphiæ sulph., . . . gr. ij.
Aq. camphoræ, . q. s. ad f℥iv.—M.
Sig.: Teaspoonful every hour or two, well diluted.
BARTHOLOW.

218—℞ Acid. hydrochlor. dil., . ‗ ℳxv.
Pepsin., ... gr. xx.
Tr. opii, ... ℳxx.
Aq. menth. piper., . . . f℥ijss.
Syr. aurantii cort., . . . f℥j.—M.
Sig.: Teaspoonful hourly at first; 4 times daily later.

219—℞ Tr. opii,
Tr. capsici,
Spt. camphoræ, . . āā f℥j.
Chloroform., ... f℥iij.
Alcoholis, . q. s. ad ft. f℥v.—M.
Sig.: Twenty to forty minims diluted. SQUIBB.

CHOLERA INFANTUM.

220—℞ Naphthalini, . . . gr. xx–lxx.
Ol. bergamii, . . . gtt. i–ij.—M.
Et ft. chart. No. xii.
Sig.: One powder every two or three hours.
HOLT.

221—℞ Tr. opii deod., . . . gtt. xvj.
Spt. ammon. aromat., . . f℥j.
Bismuth. subnit., . . . ℥ij.
Syr. simp., ... f℥iv.
Mist. cretæ, ... f℥iss.—M.
Sig.: Teaspoonful every two or three hours for a
child of one year. J. LEWIS SMITH.

222—℞ Cupri arsenit., . . gr. 1/60 –gr. 1/40.
Sacchar. lact., . q. s.—M.
Ft. chart. No. v.
Sig.: One every hour, two hours, or three hours.

28

223—℞ Acid. sulphuric. aromat.,   . ℥xxiv.
     Liq. morphiæ sulphat., .   . f℥j.
     Elix. curacoæ,   .   .   . f℥ij.
     Aquæ,   .   .   . q. s. ad f℥iij.—M.

Sig.: Teaspoonful every three hours for a child one year old.   GOODHART and STARR.

224—℞ Hydrarg. cum cretæ,   .   . gr. ij.
     Sacch. lactis, .   .   . gr. x.—M.
Et ft. chart. No. xii.

Sig. One powder every hour.   RINGER.

225—℞ Acid. sulph. aromat.,   .   . gtt. xxiv.
     Ol. caryophylli,   .   .   . ℥viij.
     Tr. opii camph.,   .   .   . f℥j.
     Spt. chloroform.,   .   .   . gtt. xlviij.
     Syr. zingiberis,   . q. s. ad f℥iij.—M.

Sig.: Teaspoonful every two hours for a child of one year.   HARE.

CHOLERA MORBUS.

226—℞ Tr. opii deod.,   .   .   . f℥ij.
     Acid. sulphuric. aromat.,   . f℥iij.—M.

Sig.: Twenty drops every hour or two in ice water.
     BARTHOLOW.

227—℞ Acid. nitrosi, ... f℥j.
     Tr. opii, ... gtt. xl.
     Aq. camphoræ,   .   .   . f℥viij.—M.

Sig.: One-fourth to be taken every three or four hours.   HOPE.

228—℞ Acid. sulph. aromat.,   .   . f℥ij.
     Ex. hæmatoxylon,   .   . f℥ij.
     Spt. chloroform.,   .   . f℥ss.
     Syr. zingiberis,   . q. s. ad f℥iij.—M.

Sig.: Teaspoonful every two hours.   HARE.

CHORDEE.

229—℞ Ex. opii,   .   .   . gr. vj.
     Ex. hyoscyami,   .   . gr. iij.
     Ol. theobrom.,   .   . q. s.—M.
Et ft. suppos. No. vi.

Sig.: Introduce one into the rectum at bedtime, and repeat if necessary.   MARTIN.

CHORDEE *(Continued).*

230—℞ Ex. opii, ... gr. j.
    Camphoræ, ... gr. x.
    Ol. theobrom., . . . q. s.—M.
  Et ft. suppos. No. i.
  Sig.: Use at bedtime.   RICORD.

231—℞ Pulv. opii, . . . gr. vj.
    Pulv. camphoræ, . . gr. xij.
    Sacch. alb., . . . q. s.—M.
  Et ft. cap. No. vi.
  Sig.: One capsule at bedtime, and repeat in two hours if necessary.   STURGIS.

CHOREA.

232—℞ Chloral. hydrat., . . . ʒij.
    Sodii bromid., ... ʒiv.
    Aq. destillat., . . q. s. ad f℥ij.—M.
  Sig.: Teaspoonful every five hours in water, for three doses.   HARE.

233—℞ Zinci bromid., . . . ʒj.
    Syr. simp., ... f℥j.—M.
  Sig.: Ten drops three times a day, increased as rapidly as the stomach can bear it.
        W. A. HAMMOND.

234—℞ Lobelinæ hydrobrom., . . gr. j.
    Aquæ, ... f℥v.—M.
  Sig.: Three to fifteen minims hypodermically.
        BARTHOLOW.

235—℞ Eserinæ sulphat., . . . gr. j.
    Aquæ destillat., . . . f℥vj.—M.
  Sig.: Six minims hypodermically twice daily with tonics.   RIESS.

236—℞ Liq. potass. arsenitis, . . f℥ss.
  Sig.: One to five drops three times a day gradually increased.   WOOD.

237—℞ Ferri citrat., ... ʒij.
    Syr. simp., ... f℥iv.
    Aq. aurant. flor., . . . f℥iss.—M.
  Sig.: Teaspoonful before or after meals. (*When anæmic.*)   HARTSHORNE.

238—℞ Ex. cimicifugæ fl., . . . f℥ij.
  Sig.: Half teaspoonful increased to a teaspoonful three times a day. (Six to ten years old.)
        JESSE YOUNG.

CHOREA (*Continued*).

239—℞ Liq. pot. arsenit., . . . ℳiij.
    Chloral. hydrat., . . . gr. v.
    Aq. menth. pip., . q. s. ad f℥j.—M.
    Sig.: Dose, one drachm.   VANDERBILT CLINIC.

240—℞ Lactophenin.,
    Quinin. hydrobromid., . āā gr. ijss.—M.
    Sig.: To be taken three times a day.

241—℞ Lactophenin.,
    Quinin. hydrobromid., . āā gr. xij.
    Olei theobromæ, . . . ℥ijss.—M.
    Sig.: A suppository to be used at bedtime.

COLIC.

242—℞ Spt. chloroform.,
    Tr. cardamom. co., . āā f℥ij.—M.
    Sig. Teaspoonful every half hour until relieved.
                             BARTHOLOW.

243—℞ Tr. opii deod., . . . gtt. xij.
    Magnesii calcinat., . . gr. xii–xxiv.
    Sacch. alb., ... ℥j.
    Aq. anisi, ... f℥iss.—M.
    Sig.: Shake well. One teaspoonful for a child of
one year.   J. L. SMITH.

244—℞ Camphoræ monobromatæ, . gr. i–ij.
    Ex. hyoscyami fl., . . . gtt. v–viij.
    Syr. lactucarii (Aubergier's), f℥ij.—M.
    Sig.: One teaspoonful p. r. n. (*In infantile colic.*)

245—℞ Tr. assafœtidæ, . . . f℥ss.
    Tr. opii, ... f℥j.
    Decocti hordei, . . . Oss.—M.
    Sig.: One injection. (*For adults with flatulence.*)
                                 HOOPER.

246—℞ Aq. camphoræ, . . . f℥ij.
    Sig. Teaspoonful when necessary.   NELIGAN.

247—℞ Chloroformi, ... f℥iss.
    Tinct. opii deod., . . . f℥j.
    Camphoræ, ... gr. xv.
    Olei cajuputi, ... f℥j.
    Aquæ, . . . q. s. ad f℥ij.—M.
    Sig.: Dessertspoonful every two or three hours.

COLICA PICTONUM.

248—℞ Magnesii sulphat., . . ℥j.
   Acid. sulphuric. dil., . . f℥j.
   Aquæ, ... f℥iv.—M.
Sig.: Give one tablespoonful three times a day,
preceded by ten grains of iodide of potash.
            BRUNTON.

249—℞ Strychniæ sulphat., . . gr. j.
   Confection. rosæ, . . . ℥ss.—M.
Et ft. pil. No. xx.
Sig.: One pill three times a day. (In lead palsy.)

250—℞ Radicis rhei, ... ℈ij.
   Fol. sennæ, ... ℥iij.—M.
Et ft. infusum ad f℥iv. Dein. adde—
Magnesii sulphat., . . f℥j.—Solv.
Sig.: Tablespoonful every two hours until bowels
are moved, then every six hours.   GERHARD.

251—℞ Aluminis, ... ℥ij.
   Magnesii sulphat., . . . ℥j.
   Syr. simp., ... f℥iij.
   Aq. rosæ, ... f℥v.—M.
Sig.: Two tablespoonfuls in two wineglassfuls of
water daily, before breakfast.   ALDRIDGE.

252—℞ Pulv. opii, . . . gr. xij.
   Ex. belladonnæ, . . gr. ij.
   Ol. tiglii, . . . gtt. xij.—M.
Et ft. pil. No. xii.
Sig.: One pill every two hours until relieved.
            LOOMIS.

CONDYLOMATA, COMMON.

253—℞ Acid. acetici glacialis, . . f℥j.
Sig.: Apply a drop once daily.   GERHARD.

254—℞ Acid. chromici, . . . gr. c.
   Aq. destillat., ... f℥j.—M.
Sig.: Apply locally with glass rod.   BARTHOLOW.

255—℞ Acid. salicylici,
   Spt. vini rec., . . . ꜹꜹ ℥ss.
   Ætheris sulph., . . . ♏lxxv.
   Collodii, ... f℥iiss.—M.
Sig.: Apply daily with camel's-hair brush.
            VIDAL.

CONDYLOMATA, VENEREAL.

256—℞ Hydrarg. chlor. mit., . . ℥ij.
  Sig.: Wash with solution of chlorinated soda, then
  dust with the powder. RICORD.

257—Wash well with soap and water, then with bichloride, 1–1000 ; then touch with the following
  solution :—
  ℞ Hydrarg. chlorid. corrosiv., . ℈j.
    Aq. destillat., ... f℥j.—M.
    GROSS.

258—℞ Pulv. sabinæ,
    Pulv. aluminis, . . āā ℨj.—M.
  Sig.: Dust on the parts every night. (*In condylomata of the vulva.*) BLACHEZ.

CONJUNCTIVITIS.

259—℞ Atropiæ sulphat., . . . gr. ss–j.
    Morphiæ sulphat., . . . gr. ii–iv.
    Zinci sulphat., . . . gr. ii–viij.
    Aq. rosæ, ... f℥j—M.
  Sig.: For the eye. BARTHOLOW.

260—℞ Zinci sulphat., . . gr. ss.
    Sodii biborat., . . gr. ij.
    Aq. camphoræ,
    Aquæ, ... āā ℨij.—M.
  Filter.
  Sig.: Two or three drops in the eyes twice or three
  times daily. DIXON.

261—℞ Argenti nitratis, . . . gr. ii–v.
    Aq. destillat., ... f℥j.—M.
  Sig.: Two drops in eyes daily. (*In granular conjunctivitis.*) NOYES.

262—℞ Hydrastin. sulphat.,
    Acid. boric.,
    Sodii biborat., . . . āā gr. v.
    Tinct. opii deod., . . . f℥ss.
    Aq. destillat., ... f℥j.—M.
  Sig.: Inject beneath the lids every hour, the eyes
  being cleansed frequently in the intervals with tepid
  water and vaselin applied to the edges of the lids.
  (*For purulent conjunctivitis in children.*) SCOTT.

263—℞ Acid. boracici, . . . gr. vj.
    Aq. camphoræ,
    Aq. destillat., . . . āā f℥j.—M.
  Sig.: Bathe the eyelids and drop two drops in the
  eye three times a day. FOX.

33

264—℞ Pulv. aloë Socot., . . . gr. vij.
      Pulv. rhei, ... gr. xxiv.
      Ex. belladonnæ, . . . gr. j.—M.
  Et ft. pil. No. xii.
  Sig.: One or two pills as required.   DA COSTA.

266—℞ Ex. belladonnæ, . . gr. ¼.
      Pil. aloes et myrrh., . gr. ix.
      Ol. cari, . . . gtt. ij.—M.
  Et ft. pil. No. vi.
  Sig.: One pill at bedtime for a child of six years.
                    GOODHART and STARR.

267—℞ Ex. cascaræ sagrad. fl., . . f℥j.
  Sig.: Three drops three times a day, to be increased, if necessary, for a child of five years.

268—℞ Pulv. acaciæ, ... ℥iv.
      Ol. ricini, ... f℥j.
      Elix. saccharini, . . . ♏xx.
      Ol. amygdalæ amaræ, . . ♏j.
      Ol. caryophylli, . . . ♏ij.
      Aq. destillat., . . q. s. ad f℥ij.—M.
  Dissolve the gum in sufficient water, add the oil
gradually, and finally the flavoring agents.
  Sig.: From a dessertspoonful to a tablespoonful, as
required.
  (*A palatable emulsion of castor-oil.*)

269—℞ Mannæ opt.,
      Magnesii carb., . . āā ℥j.
      Ex. sennæ fl., ... f℥iij.
      Syr. zingiber., . . . f℥j.
      Aquæ, . . . q. s. ad f℥iij.—M.
  Sig.: One or two teaspoonfuls three times a day
for a child of two years.   GOODHART and STARR.

270—℞ Aloes purificat., . . . gr. xx.
      Ex. belladonnæ, . . . gr. iv.
      Ex. nucis vomicæ, . . . gr. v.
      Oleo resinæ capsici, . . gr. iv.—M.
  Et ft. pil. No. xx.
  Sig.: One pill at bedtime.   WAUGH.

271—℞ Tr. aloes et myrrh.,   .   .   f℥j.

Sig.: One to three drops in sweetened water three times a day, according to age of child.

272—℞ Mannæ opt., ... ℨj.
Syr. simp., ... f℥ss.
Aq. cinnam., .   .   q. s. ad   f℥j.—M.

Sig.: Teaspoonful three times a day for an infant.
STARR.

273—℞ Ext. cascar. sag fl.,   .   . ℥ss.
Tr. nucis vom.,   .   .   . ℨv.
Tr. bellad.,   .   .   . ℨij.
Glycerini,   .   .   q. s. ad   ℥ij.—M.

Sig.: Teaspoonful t. i. d.   (*Habitual constipation*.)

274—℞ Ex. nucis vom.,
Aloes Soc.,
Ferri sulph.,
Pulv. ipecac.,
Pulv. myrrh.,   .   . āā   gr. ss.—M.
Ft. pil. No. i.

Sig.: To be taken after meals.   CLARK.

275—℞ Pil. hydrarg.,
Ext. coloc. comp., .   . āā   gr. j.
Pulv. jalapæ, ... gr. ss.
Pulv. hyoscyami, .   .   . gr. j.—M.
Et ft. pil. No. i.

Sig.: Pill at bedtime.   PANCOAST.

276—℞ Ex. belladonnæ,   .   .   . gr. j.
Glycerinæ, ... f℥j.
Vini ferri amar.,   .   q. s. ad   f℥iij.—M.

Sig.: Teaspoonful three times a day at the age of six years.   GOODHART and STARR.

277—℞ Magnesiæ sulphatis,   .   . ℥j.
Ferri sulphatis,   .   .   . gr. iv.
Sodii chloridi,   .   .   . ℨss.
Acidi sulphurici diluti, .   . f℥j.
Infus. quassiæ,   q. s. ad   f℥iv.—M.

Sig.: Tablespoonful in goblet of water half hour before breakfast. This is the well-known *mistura ferri acidi.* It is unsurpassed as a tonic laxative, and is much used in acne rosacea, erythema multiformæ, urticaria, etc., that is where the patients are robust, and the condition otherwise demands such a combination.   VAN HARLINGEN.

278—℞ Aloin, ... gr. ⅓.
Strychninæ, ... gr. 1/40.
Extract. belladonnæ, . . gr. 1/10.
Extract. cascar. sagrada, . gr. j.—M.
Et ft. pil. No. i.
Sig.: Pill three times a day.

279—℞ Resinæ podophylli, . . gr. ij.
Quiniæ sulphat.,
Ex. aloë Socot., . . āā gr. viij.
Fellis bovini, ... gr. xvj.—M.
Et ft. pil. No. xvi.
Sig.: One or two pills at night.   GOODELL.

280—℞ Pulv. belladonnæ,
Ex. belladonnæ, . . āā gr. ¼.—M.
Et ft. pil. No. i.
Sig.: Take at bedtime.   TROUSSEAU.

281—℞ Mannæ, ... ℥vj.
Magnesiæ,
Sulphur. loti., . . āā ℥iss.
Mellis, ... ℥vj.—M.
Sig.: One or two dessertspoonfuls in milk for an
infant.   FERRAND.

282—℞ Resinæ podophylli, . . gr. ij.-iv.
Ex. nucis vomicæ, . . gr. iv.
Ex. physostig., . . gr. iij.
Ex. belladonnæ, . . gr. iv.—M.
Ft. pil. No. xx.
Sig.: One pill night and morning.   HARE.

283—℞ Aloin., ... gr. vj.
Atropiæ sulphat., . . . gr. ¼.
Strychninæ sulph., . . . gr. j.—M.
Et ft. pil. No. xxx.
Sig.: One pill two or three times a day. (Chronic
form.)   WOOD.

284—℞ Euonymin, ... gr. ij.
Ex. ignatiæ, ... gr. ss.
Ex. belladonna, . . . gr. ⅕.
Piperini, ... gr. j.—M.
Et ft. pil. No. i.
Sig.: One pill three times a day after meals.

285—℞ Podophyllini, ... gr. ¾.
      Alcoholis, ... ℳlxxv.
      Syr. althææ, ... f℥iij.—M.
  Sig.: A dessertspoonful is given daily. (*For infants.*)   Bouchut.

CONVULSIONS.

286—℞ Moschi, ... gr. iij.
      Camphoræ, ... gr. xv.
      Chloral hydrat., . . . gr. viiss.
      Vitelli ovi, ... No. j.
      Aq. destillat., ... f℥iv.—M.
  Sig.: Wash out the rectum with a simple enema and then use the above as an injection.   J. Simon.

287—℞ Mist. assafœtidæ, . . . f℥ij.
  Sig.: Tablespoonful per rectum.   Waring.

288—℞ Ætheris fort., . . . f℥iv.
  Sig.: To be used as an inhalation until the paroxysm is broken.   J. L. Smith.

289—℞ Chloral hydrat., . . . gr. xv.
      Potass. bromid., . . . ʒj.
      Syr. simp., ... f℥v.
      Aq. destillat., ... f℥ij.—M.
  Sig.: Teaspoonful every three hours. (*Convulsions of teething.*)   Kinder-Arzt.

290—Dr. Jacobi first orders a purgative dose of calomel, and then follows in a few hours by—

  ℞ Chloral hydrat., . . . gr. iv.
      Potass. bromid., . . . gr. viij.
      Aquæ,
      Syrupi, ... āā f℥j.—M.
  Sig.: One dose for a child two years old.

CORNS AND CALLOSITIES.

291—℞ Acid. salicylic., ... gr. xxx.
      Ext. cannabis ind., . . . gr. x.
      Collodii, ... f℥iv.—M.
  Sig.: Apply with a brush night and morning.
               Stelwagon.

292—℞ Liq. potassii,
      Tr. iodi, ... āā f℥j.
      Glycerini, ... f℥ss.
      Aquæ, ... f℥j.—M.
  Sig.: Paint the affected parts night and morning.

CORNS AND CALLOSITIES (Continued).

293—℞ Iodi, ... gr. ij.
  Collodii flexil., ... f ℥iij.
  Alcohol., ... f ℥j.
  Potassii iodid., ... gr. ij.—M.
 Sig.: Apply topically.

CROUP, MEMBRANOUS.

294—℞ Hydrarg. chlor. mit., . . gr. ij.
  Sodii bicarb., ... gr. xxiv.
  Pulv. ipecac., ... gr. j.
  Pulv. pepsinæ, . . . gr. xxiv.—M.
 Et ft. chart. No. xii.
 Sig.: One powder every two hours.   STARR.

295—℞ Acid. lactic, ... ℥iiiss.
  Aquæ, ... f℥x.—M.
 Sig.: Use with spray or mop.   MACKENZIE.

296—℞ Tr. ferri chlor., . . . f℥i-iss.
  Potass. chlorat., . . . ℥j.
  Glycerini, ... f℥j.
  Aq. cinnam., . . . ad f℥iv.—M.
 Sig.: Teaspoonful every two hours for a child of
four years.   MEIGS and PEPPER.

297—℞ Pulv. aluminis, . . . ℥iiss.
  Mellis albi, ... ℥x.—M.
 Sig.: Half teaspoonful every hour and insufflations
of powdered alum every four hours.   TROUSSEAU.

CROUP, SPASMODIC.

298—℞ Apomorphiæ hydrochlor., . gr. $\frac{1}{40}$.
 Sig.: Use hypodermically.   DA COSTA.

299—℞ Syr. ipecac., ... f℥iss.
  Tr. opii camph., . . . f℥ij.
  Syr. scillæ, ... f℥j.—M.
  Liq. potass. citrat.,   q. s. ad f℥iij.—M.
 Sig.: Teaspoonful every two hours. (After vomit-
ing has been secured.)   POWELL.

300—℞ Potass. brom.,
  Chloral hydratis, . . āā ℈ij.
  Syr. acaciæ, ... f℥ij.—M.
 Sig.: A teaspoonful or less, according to age.
     ELLIS.

CROUP, SPASMODIC (Continued).

301—℞ Decocti senegæ, . . . f℥iiiss.
   Oxymel. scillæ, . . . fℨij.
   Vini ipecac., ... fℨij.
   Antim. tartar., . . . gr. j.—M.

Sig.: Ten to thirty drops every fifteen minutes to an infant to produce vomiting, or every two hours as an expectorant.   FRENCH HOSPITAL.

302—℞ Tr. belladonnæ, . . . gtt. iv.
   Tr. opii camph., . . . gtt. l.
   Pulv. aluminis, . . . gr. vj.
   Syr. acaciæ, ... ℥ss.
   Aquæ, ... f℥iss.—M.

Sig.: Teaspoonful every two or three hours at six months of age.   MEIGS and PEPPER.

CYSTITIS (See Catarrh).

DEBILITY.

303—℞ Tr. nucis vomicæ, . . . fℨij.
   Elix. calisayæ, . q. s. ad f℥iv.—M.

Sig.: Dessertspoonful three times a day in water.

304—℞ Strychniæ sulphat., . . gr. j.
   Acid. arseniosi, . . . gr. iss.
   Ex. belladonnæ, . . . gr. viij.
   Ferri redacti, ... ℨj.—M.
Et ft. pil. No. xxx.
Sig.: One after each meal.   WOOD.

305—℞ Hyd. chlorid. corros., . . gr. j.
   Elixir calisaya, . . . f℥viij.—M.
Sig.: A teaspoonful before meals for three months.
(In strumous children.)   BLACKWOOD.

306—℞ Tr. cinchonæ,
   Tr. valerinat., . . āā f℥j.
   Tr. cardamomi comp., . . fℨij.
   Aq. menthæ pip., . . . f℥iv.—M.
Sig.: Tablespoonful three times a day.   ELLIS.

307—℞ Ferri lactat.,
   Pulv. glycyrrhizæ, . āā ℨj.
   Mellis, ... q. s.—M.
Et ft. pil. xl.
Sig.: One to six pills daily.   TROUSSEAU.

308—℞ Potass. brom.,
    Ammon. brom., . . āā ℨij.
    Syr. zingiber, . . . fℨj.
    Aquæ, . . . q. s. ad fℨiij.—M.
Sig.: Dessertspoonful every two hours. JOHNSON.

309—℞ Chloral hydrat., . . . ℨss.
    Syr. aurant. cort.,
    Aquæ, ... āā fℨss.—M.
Sig.: To be taken in one dose. LIEBREICH.

DELIRIUM TREMENS.

310—℞ Potass. bromid.,
    Sodii bromid., . . āā gr. xv.
    Chloral hydrat., . . . gr. x.
    Tr. zingiberis, . . . ℳx.
    Tr. capsici, ... ℳv.
    Spt. ammonii arom., . . ℨj.
    Aquæ, ... ℨij.—M.
Sig.: Dose a dessertspoonful. VANDERBILT CLINIC.

311—℞ Potass. brom., . . ℨj.
    Div. in chart. No. viii.
Sig.: One powder in half tumblerful of cold water
every four to six hours. BARTHOLOW.

312—℞ Ex. cannabis indicæ, . . gr. vi–xij.
    Div. in pil. No. xii.
Sig.: One pill every two or three hours till sleep
is procured. PHILLIPS.

313—℞ Sodii brom., ... gr. xv.
    Chloral hydrat., . . . gr. x.
    Syr. aurant. cort.,
    Aquæ, . . āā q. s. ad fℨj.—M.
Sig.: As required. DA COSTA.

314—℞ Liq. morph. sulph. (U. S. P.),
    Ex. valerian. fl., . . āā fℨj.— M.
Sig.: One or two teaspoonfuls as required.
HARTSHORNE.

315—℞ Tr. lupulinæ,
    Syr. amygdalæ, . . āā fℨj.
    Aq. destillat, ... fℨij.—M.
Sig.: Tablespoonful every two hours. HAZARD.

DELIRIUM TREMENS (Continued).

316—℞ Infus. digitalis, . . . f℥iij.

Sig.: Tablespoonful every four hours. (*In anæmic cases with effusion and œdema.*) BARTHOLOW.

317—℞ Sodii brom., ... gr. xv.
Chloral hydrat., . . . gr. x.
Syr. aurant. cort.,
Aquæ, . . āā q. s. ad ft. f℥j.—M.

Sig.: As required. Also to be taken, fluid extract of coca fifteen minims, increased to tolerance. DA COSTA.

DENGUE.

318—℞ Tr. aconiti rad., . . . ♏xxx.
Syr. limonis, ... f℥ss.
Liq. ammon. acetat., q. s. ad f℥iij.—M.

Sig.: Dessertspoonful every three hours. THOMAS.

319—℞ Ex. nucis vomicæ, . . . gr. iv.
Quiniæ sulphat., . . . ℥ss.—M.
Et ft. pil. No. xvi.

Sig.: One pill three times a day. DA COSTA.

DIABETES INSIPIDUS.

320—℞ Codeinæ, . gr. viij.
Glycerinæ,
Aquæ, ... āā f℥j.—M.

Sig.: Half teaspoonful three times a day gradually increased to two teaspoonfuls. PAVY.

321—℞ Tr. opii, ... f℥j.
Tr. ferri chlor., . . . f℥ix.—M.

Sig.: Twenty drops well diluted three times daily. WELLER.

322—℞ Pulv. opii, . . . gr. iv.
Acid. gallici, . . . ℥ij.—M.
Et div. in chart. No. xii.

Sig.: One three or four times daily. H. C. WOOD.

323—℞ Sodii salicylat., . . . ℥iv.
Glycerinæ, ... f℥ij.
Aquæ, . . . q. s. ad f℥iij.—M.

Sig.: Two teaspoonfuls three times daily. DA COSTA.

DIABETES INSIPIDUS (Continued).

324—℞ Ex. ergotæ fl., . . . f℥ij.

Sig.: Teaspoonful three times a day, increased to two teaspoonfuls. . DA COSTA.

DIABETES MELLITUS.

325—℞ Sodii salicylat., . . . ℥iij.
  Liq. potass. arsenitis, . . f℥j.
  Glycerinæ, ... f℥j.
  Aq. cinnam., . . . ad f℥iij.—M.

Sig.: Dessertspoonful three times a day.
           J. C. WILSON.

326—℞ Sodii arsenat., . . gr. j.
  Lithii carbonat., . 3j.
  Codein., . . . gr. iiss.
  Ext. cinchonæ, . . ℥iv.—M.
Divide into 3 cachets.

Sig.: One after breakfast and one after dinner.
           ROBIN.

327—℞ Tr. opii, ... f℥j.
  Tr. ferri chlor., . . . f℥ix.—M.

Sig.: Twenty drops in water three times a day.

328—℞ Iodoform., . . gr. ij.
Div. in pil. No. xii.

Sig.: One pill three times a day after meals.
           LEVI.

329—℞ Ex. ergotæ fl., . . . f℥ij.

Sig. One-half to one teaspoonful three times a day.

DIARRHŒA, CHILDREN.

330—℞ Naphthalin, . . gr. xii–3j.
  Sacch. lact., . . gr. xii–℥ss.—M.
Et ft. chart. No. xii.

Sig.: One powder every three hours. STARR.

331—℞ Pulv. opii, . . . gr. v.
  Bismuth. subnit., . . 3ij.—M.
Et div. in chart. No. xx.

Sig.: One powder every two to four hours for a child of five years. J. L. SMITH.

332—℞ Magnesii sulphat, . . . 3j.
  Tr. opii deod., . . . gtt. xij.
  Syr. simp., ... f℥ss.
  Aq. cinnam., . . q. s. ad f℥iss.—M.

Sig.: Teaspoonful every two hours for a child of one or two years. MEIGS and PEPPER.

DIARRHŒA, CHILDREN (Continued).

333—℞ Bismuth. subcarb., . . ℈ss-℈iss.
Spt. myristicæ, . . . ♏xx.
Spt. vini gal., . . . f℥ij.
Syr. acaciæ, ... f℥iss.
Aq. cinnam., . . q. s. ad f℥iij.—M.
Sig.: (Shake well.) Teaspoonful every two hours.
W. H. BENNETT.

334—℞ Argenti nitrat., . . . gr. j.
Syr. acaciæ, ... f℥ij.
Aq. cinnam., . . q. s. ad f℥iij.—M.
Sig.: Teaspoonful every two hours for a child of two years. STARR.

335—℞ Tr. krameriæ,
Tr. opii camph., . . āā f℥ij.
Mist. cretæ, . . q. s. ad f℥ij.—M.
Sig.: Teaspoonful every two hours for a child of two years.

336—℞ Acid. carbolici, ... gr. ij.
Bismuth. subnit., . . . ℥j.
Syr. acaciæ, ... f℥ss.
Aq. menth. pip., . . ad f℥ij.—M.
Sig.: A half teaspoonful from every two to four hours.

337—℞ Pepsinæ pulv., . . . gr. xxxv.
Bismuth. subnit., . . . ℈j.—M.
Et ft. chart. No. xii.
Sig.: One every two hours. POWELL.

338—℞ Tr. camphoræ, . . . f℥j.
Tr. capsici, ... f℥iss.
Tr. lavandulæ comp., . . f℥j.
Spt. vini gallici, . q. s. ad f℥ij.—M.
Sig.: Teaspoonful every two or three hours. REX.

DIARRHŒA IN ADULTS.

339—℞ Cretæ præp., ... ℈ij.
Tr. catechu, ... f℥ss.
Tr. opii, ... ♏lxxx.
Aq. cinnam., ... f℥viij.—M.
Sig.: Two tablespoonfuls after each stool.
FOTHERGILL.

43

DIARRHŒA IN ADULTS *(Continued)*.

340—℞ Tinct. catechu, ... f℥iv.
 Sodii bicarbonat., . . . ℈iv.
 Spt. ammon. aromat., . . f℥iv.
 Tinct. nucis vomicæ, . . . ℳlxxx.
 Infus. calumbæ, ... f℥viij.—M.
 Sig.: Two tablespoonfuls thrice daily before taking food. YEO.

341—℞ Ex. ergotæ aq., . . . ℈j.
 Ex. nucis vomicæ, . . . gr. v.
 Ex. opii, ... gr. x.—M.
 Et ft. pil. No. xx.
 Sig.: One pill every four to six hours. DA COSTA.

342—℞ Tr. opii camph.,
 Tr. lavandulæ comp., . āā ℥j.
 Spt. vini gall., . . . ℥ij.—M.
 Sig.: Tablespoonful every three hours. STUBBS.

343—℞ Salol, ... ℥ij.
 Bismuthi subnitratis, . . ℥iv.
 Mist. cretæ, . . q. s. ad f℥iij.—M.
 Sig.: One teaspoonful every two hours.

344—℞ Resorcin, ... gr. iss–iij.
 Infus. chamomil., . . . f℥ij.
 Tr. opii, ... gtt. ij.
 Tr. cascarill., ... gtt. xv.—M.
 Sig.: Teaspoonful every two hours. KINDER-ARZT.

345—℞ Potass. brom., . . . ℥iij.
 Tr. opii, ... f℥ij.
 Tr. capsici, ... f℥j.
 Syr. rhei arom., . . . f℥iv.—M.
 Sig.: One teaspoonful as needed.

346—℞ Tr. opii,
 Tr. capsici,
 Spt. camphoræ, . . . āā f℥ss.
 Chloroformi (pur.), . . . f℥ij.
 Alcoholis, . . . q. s. ad f℥iij.—M.
 Sig.: Teaspoonful every four hours.

347—℞ Morphiæ sulphat., . . . gr. 1/12.
 Bismuth. subnit., . . . gr. v.—M.
 Et ft. chart. No. i.
 Sig.: One powder three or four times daily. (*In chronic cases.*) ALONZO CLARK.

44

349—℞ Cupri sulphat.,
    Morphiæ sulphat., . . āā gr. j.
    Quiniæ sulphat., . . . gr. xxiv.—M.
Et div. in capsules No. xii.
Sig.: One capsule three times a day. (*In chronic cases.*)   BARTHOLOW.

350—℞ Pulv. aluminis,
    Pulv. kino, . . ᴠ . āā ℥iss.
    Syr. simp., ... q. s.—M.
Et ft. pil. No. c.
Sig.: Two to ten pills daily.   TROUSSEAU.

351—℞ Creasoti, ... gtt. v.
    Pulv. opii, ... gr. iij.
    Pulv. acaciæ, ... vj.—M.
Et ft. in pil. No. x.
Sig.: One pill every three hours.   BLASIUS.

DIPHTHERIA.

352—℞ Trypsin (Fairchild's), . . ℥j.
    Sodii bicarb., ... gr. xx.
    Aquæ, . . . q. s. ad f℥ij.—M.
Sig.: Apply with atomizer every hour or two as necessary.   KEATING.

353—℞ Ol. eucalypti, ... f℥ij.
    Ol. terebinthinæ, . . . f℥viij.—M.
Sig.: Place in shallow vessel and keep boiling over the stove.   J. LEWIS SMITH.

354—℞ Acid. boric.,
    Sodii borat., . . . āā ℥ss.
    Sodii chlor., ... gr. xx.
    Aquæ, ... Oss.—M.
Sig.: Inject teaspoonful, warm, in each nostril every two hours. (*Nasal form.*)   STARR.

355—℞ Hydrarg. chlor. corros., . . gr. j.
    Spt. vini rect., . . . f℥ij.
    Elix. bismuth. et pepsin, ad f℥iv.—M.
Sig.: Teaspoonful every two hours for a child of six years.   J. LEWIS SMITH.

356—℞ Tr. ferri chlor., . . . f℥-f℥iij.
    Glycerinæ, . . q. s. ad f℥j.—M.
Sig.: Paint tonsils every four hours.   REX.

DIPHTHERIA (Continued).

357—℞ Quiniæ sulphat., . . . gr. xij.
   Potass. chlorat., . . . gr. xlviij.
   Tr. ferri chlor., . . . f3j.
   Syr. zingiber., . . . f℥j.
   Aquæ, . . . q. s. ad f℥iij.—M.

Sig.: Teaspoonful in water every two hours for a child of six to ten years. GOODHART and STARR.

358—℞ Camphoræ, ⁄. . . . 3v.
   Ol. ricini, ... f3iv.
   Alcoholis, ... f3iss.
   Acid. carbolic. (crystals), . ℈iv.
   Acid. tartaric, . . . gr. xvj.—M.

Sig.: For local application.
        LA TRIBUNE MÉDICALE.

359—℞ Pepsinæ, ... 3iss.
   Acid. hydrochlor. dil., . . ℔j.
   Aq. destillat.,
   Glycerinæ, . . . āā f℥ss.—M.

Sig.: Paint throat. (*To remove membrane.*)
        CANADA LANCET.

360—℞ Papain, ... ℥ij.
   Hydronaphthol, . . . gr. iij.
   Acid. hydrochlor. dil., . . gtt. xv.
   Aq. destillat., . . ad f℥xxxij.—M.
Ft. sol.

Sig.: Use carefully and thoroughly, by means of hand atomizer, every half hour on throat, on posterior nares, and pharynx. RICHARDSON.

361—℞ Atropin. sulphat., . . . gr. ⅓.
   Cocain. hydrochlor., . . . gr. v.
   Aq. amygd. amar., . . . f℥iv.—M.

Sig.: One drop for each year of the child's age every hour. To adults, from 10 to 15 drops are given every hour, according to the condition of the patient.

362—℞ Hydrarg. chlor. mit., . . gr. j.
   Sodii bicarb., ... gr. xxiv.
   Pulv. aromat., . . . gr. vj.—M.
Et ft. chart. No. xii.

Sig.: One powder every two hours. STARR.

363—℞ Acid. carbolici, . . gr. x.
   Acid. sulphurosi, . . f3iij.
   Glycerinæ,
   Tr. ferri chlor., . . āā f℥ss.—M.

Sig.: Paint throat frequently. HAZARD

DIPHTHERIA (Continued).

364—℞ Potass. permanganat., . . gr. ij.
Aq. destillat., . . . f℥ij.—M.
Sig.: Teaspoonful every three hours for a child of eight or ten years.   Bartholow.

365—℞ Acid. lactic, ... f℥iiiss.
Aq. destillat., . . . f℥x.—M.
Sig.: Use as a spray or with a mop.
M. Mackenzie.

366—℞ Tr. ferri chlor., . . . f℥ii–iij.
Potass. chlorat., . . . ℨj.
Acid. muriat. dil., . . . gtt. x.
Syr. simp., ... f℥iv.—M.
Sig.: Teaspoonful every hour or two.
J. Lewis Smith.

367—℞ Papayotin, ... ℨj.
Aquæ, ... f℥iv.
Glycerinæ, ... f℥viij.—M.
Sig.: Apply locally to membrane.   Jacobi.

DROPSY.

368—℞ Infus. digitalis, . . . f℥iv.
Sig.: Tablespoonful three times daily.
Bartholow.

369—℞ Pil. scillæ comp.,
Pil. colocynth comp., . āā ℈ij.
Ol. tiglii, ... ♏vj.—M.
Et ft. pil. No. xviii.
Sig.: Three pills twice a week.   Selwyn.

370—℞ Digitalis, ... gr. xij.
Sennæ fol., ... ℥ss.
Aq. bullientis, . . . f℥vj.
Fiat infusum, et adde—
Sodii iodid., ... ℨij.
Sodii phosphat., . . . ℨvj.—M.
Sig.: Tablespoonful every three to six hours. (*In cardiac dropsy.*)   Gerhard.

371—℞ Potass. iodid., . . . ℥ss–j.
Aq. destillat., . . . f℥vj.—M.
Sig.: Tablespoonful three times a day. (*In anasarca with scanty urine.*)   Ringer.

DROPSY (*Continued*).

372—℞ Pulv. jalapæ, . . ℥j.
     Potass. bitart., . . ℥vj.—M.
    Et ft. chart. No. vi.
    Sig.: One powder every three hours. (*In general dropsy due to kidney disease.*) CHAPMAN.

373—℞ Mist. ferri et ammon. acetat. (U. S. P.)
                                f℥vj.
    Sig.: One or two teaspoonfuls four times a day. BASHAM.

374—℞ Pulv. digitalis, . . . gr. xxx.
     Ferri sulph. exsiccat., . . gr. xv.
     Pulv. capsici, . . . gr. xl.
     Pil. aloë et myrrh., . . ℥ij.—M.
    Et ft. pil. No. lx.
    Sig.: One pill twice a day. (*In cardiac dropsy with dyspepsia.*) FOTHERGILL.

375—℞ Pulv. scillæ,
     Pulv. digitalis,
     Caffeine citrat., . . ãã ℥ss.
     Hydrarg. chlor. mit., . . gr. v.—M.
    Et ft. pil. No. xxx.
    Sig.: One pill three times a day. (*In cardiac dropsy.*) WOOD.

DYSENTERY.

376—℞ Pulv. opii, . . . gr. xx.
     Pulv. resinæ, . . . gr. xxx.
     Pulv. acaciæ, . . . gr. xx.
     Aquæ, ... q. s.—M.
    Et ft. pil. No. xxv.
    Sig.: One pill every four hours until relief is obtained. GEER.

377—℞ Cupri sulphat., . . . gr. ss.
     Magnesii sulphat., . . . f℥j.
     Acid. sulphuric. dil., . . f℥j.
     Aquæ, ... f℥iv.—M.
    Sig.: Tablespoonful every four hours. (*In acute form.*) BARTHOLOW.

378—℞ Hydrarg. chlor. mit., . . gr. ij.
     Pulv. opii, ... gr. iv.
     Pulv. ipecac., . . . gr. viij.—M.
    Et div. in chart. No. viii.
    Sig.: One powder every two hours. HAZARD.

DYSENTERY (Continued).

379—℞ Quinin. sulph., ... gr. ij.
    Pulv. ipecac. rad., . . . gr. v.
    Ammon. chlorid., . . . gr. x.
    Tinct. opii, ... ℩xij.
    Aquæ, . . . q. s. ad f℥j.—M.
Sig.: To be given every four hours. (*In acute form.*)

380—℞ Pulv. ipecac. co., . . . gr. vj.
    Bismuth. subcarb., . . ℈j.
    Pulv. aromat., . . . gr. vj.—M.
Et ft. in chart. No. xij.
Sig.: One powder every three hours for a child of three years.   STARR.

381—℞ Strychninæ sulphat., . . gr. ¼.
    Acid. sulphuric. dil., . . f℥ss.
    Morphiæ sulphat., . . . gr. ij.
    Aq. camphoræ, . . . f℥iiiss.—M.
Sig.: Teaspoonful every hour or so, well diluted.
(*Epidemic form.*)   BARTHOLOW.

382—℞ Tr. hamamelis, . . . f℥ss.
    Elix. simp., ... f℥iiiss.
    Syr. simp., ... f℥ss.
    Aq. destillat., ... f℥j.—M.
Sig.: Teaspoonful every two or three hours.
(*Where there is much blood.*)   RINGER.

383—℞ Tr. opii deod.,
    Vini ipecac., .   āā f℥ij.
    Ol. ricini,
    Pulv. acaciæ,
    Syr. simp.,
    Aq. cinnam., . . . āā q. s.
Ft. emulsio, secundum artem ad f℥vj.
Sig.: Tablespoonful every two hours.   GERHARD.

384—℞ Naphthalini, . . . ℥iss.
    Div. in capsules No. xviii.
Sig.: Two capsules every three hours.   HOLT.

DYSMENORRHŒA.

385—℞ Pulv. ipecac., ... gr. iv.
    Ft. in pil. No. xii.
Sig.: One pill every two or three hours.   EMMET.

386—℞ Pulv. camph., . . gr. x.
 Pulv. doveri, . . . gr. xx.
 Ex. hyoscyami, . . gr. x.—M.
Ft. pil. No. x.
Sig.: Two pills every two hours till pain ceases.
CANADA LANCET.

387—℞ Ex. cannab. indicæ, . . gr. ¼.
 Ex. belladonnæ, . . . gr. ¼.
 Ol. theobrom., . . . q. s.—M.
Sig.: This is sufficient for one suppository; five such ones may be made. One suppository may be introduced every evening, commencing the fifth day before the menses. JOURNAL DE MÉDECINE DE PARIS.

388—℞ Phosphori, . . . gr. $\frac{1}{50}$.
 Ferri valerianat.,
 Zinci valerianat.,
 Quininæ sulphat.,
 Ext. aloes, ... āā gr. j.—M.
Sig.: One such pill to be taken three times a day.

389—℞ Tinct. cannabis indicæ, . . ℥x.
 Syr. chloral. hydrat., . . ℥xx.
 Glycerini, ... ℥j.
 Aquæ camphor., . . ad ℥j.—M.
Sig.: Take this dose every three hours, if required.

390—℞ Ex. cannabis indicæ, . . gr. iij.
 Sacch. lact., ... ℥ss—M.
Et ft. chart. No. vi.
Sig.: One powder every two or three hours.
H. C. WOOD.

391—℞ Ext. belladonnæ,
 Ext. stramonii, . . . āā gr. ⅕.
 Ext. hyoscyami, . . . gr. ¼.
 Quininæ sulphatis, . . . gr. ss.—M.
Sig.: Take one such pill thrice daily.

DYSPEPSIA.

392—℞ Strychniæ sulphat., . . gr. j.
 Acid. nitro-muriat. dil., . f℥j.
 Tr. gentian. comp.,
 Tr. cardamom. comp., . āā f℥iss.
 Liq. pepsinæ, . q. s. ad f℥iv.—M.
Sig.: Teaspoonful after each meal. WOOD.

393—℞ Pepsinæ puri, . . . gr. xxx.
    Acid. hydrochlor. dil., . . fℨij.
    Glycerini, ... fℨj.
    Tr. gentianæ comp., q. s. ad fℨiij.—M.
  Sig.: A teaspoonful in water after meals.
                                AULDE.

394—℞ Zinci valerianatis, . . . ℨss.
    Ex. belladonnæ, . . . gr. iij.
    Ex. nucis vomicæ, . . . gr. v.—M.
  Ft. pil. No. xxx.
  Sig.: One pill after each meal. (*In atonic form.*)
                                 PEPPER.

395—℞ Pepsin., ... gr. v.
    Bismuth. subnit., . . . gr. x.
    Strychn. sulph., . . . gr. $\frac{1}{100}$.
    Carbon. ligni, . . . gr. v.
    Thymol, ... gr. $\frac{1}{4}$.—M.
  Et ft. chart. No. i.
  Sig.: Powder after each meal.
                      VANDERBILT CLINIC.

396—℞ Pulv. rhei, ... ℨjss.
    Sodii bicarb., ... ℨss.
    Pulv. ipecac., ... gr. vj.–viij.
    Tr. nucis vomicæ, . . . fℨij.
    Aq. menth. pip., . q. s. ad fℨvj.—M.
  Sig.: Two teaspoonfuls before each meal.

397—℞ Bismuth. subnit., . . . ℈iv.
    Mucil. acaciæ, . . . fℨj.
    Sodii bicarb., . . . ℈iv.
    Infus. calumbæ, . . . fℨviij.—M.
  Sig.: Two tablespoonfuls before each meal.
                           FOTHERGILL.

398—℞ Pepsinæ (Fairchild's), . . gr. xxxvj.
    Carbo. lig., ... gr. xxiv.
    Sodii bicarb., . . . ℨj.—M.
  Et div. in cap. No. xii.
  Sig.: One after each meal.   STARR.

399—℞ Sodii bromid., . . ℨj.
    Pepsin. sacch.,
    Pulv. carbo. lig., . . āā ℨiij.
    Aquæ, ... fℨiv.—M.
  Sig.: Teaspoonful in water three times a day after
    meals. (*Nervous form.*)   HAMMOND.

DYSPEPSIA (Continued).

400—℞ Tr. capsici, ... ℳxvj.
    Tr. nucis vomicæ, . . . f℥ij.
    Tr. gentian. comp., . ad f℥ij.—M.
    Sig.: A teaspoonful in water three times a day.
                                Da Costa.

401—℞ Ex. cascaræ sagrad. fl.,
    Ex. berberis aquifol., . āā f℥j.
    Syr. simp., ... f℥ij.—M.
    Sig.: Teaspoonful three times a day. Bundy.

402—℞ Pepsin. crystallizat., . . ℨj.
    Acid. muriat. dil., . . . f℥ss.
    Glycerinæ, ... f℥j.
    Vini xerici, . . q. s. ad f℥vj.—M.
    Sig.: Tablespoonful after each meal. Gerhard.

403—℞ Acid. nitrohydrochlor. dil., . f℥ss.
    Tr. nucis vom., ... f℥ij.
    Liq. potass. arsenitis, . . gtt. lxxij.
    Ess. pepsin., . . q. s. ad f℥vj.—M.
    Sig.: Dessertspoonful thrice daily after meals.

404—℞ Aq. chloroform., . . . f℥x.
    Aq. destillat., . . . f℥viij.
    Aq. menthæ pip., . . . f℥ij.—M.
    Sig.: A teaspoonful before or after meals. (*Flatu-
lent form.*) Huchard.

EARACHE (See Otitis).

ECTHYMA (See Skin Diseases).

ECZEMA (See Skin Diseases).

EMISSIONS (See Spermatorrhœa).

EMPHYSEMA (See Asthma).

EMPYEMA.

405—℞ Liq. iodi comp., . . . f℥j.
    Aquæ, ... f℥xv.—M.
    Sig.: To wash out the pleural cavity after evacua-
tion. Bartholow.

406—℞ Mist. ferri et ammon. acetat., f℥iv.
    Sig.: One to two teaspoonfuls three or four times
daily with quinia and stimulants. (*In chronic cases.*)
                                Da Costa.

407—℞ Aq. chlorini, ... f℥j.
   Aquæ, ... f℥ix.—M.
 Sig.: To wash out the pleural cavity, after the evacuation of the pus.   RINGER.

ENDOCARDITIS.

408—℞ Tr. aconiti rad., . . . f℥ss.
 Sig.: One drop every hour or two.   RINGER.

409—℞ Lini farinæ,
   Aq. bullientis,   . ad q. s.—M.
  Ft. cataplasma.
 Sig.: Apply over heart as hot as can be borne and renew frequently.   DA COSTA.

410—℞ Tr. digitalis, ... f℥iij.
   Elix. calisayæ, . q. s. ad f℥iij.—M.
 Sig.: Teaspoonful three times a day.   WOOD.

ENTERITIS.

411—℞ Liq. potass. arsenitis, . . gtt. l.
   Tr. opii, ... gtt. cxx.
   Aquæ, ... f℥iij.—M.
 Sig.: Teaspoonful before meals three times a day.
            BARTHOLOW.

412—℞ Ol. ricini,   .   . f℥j.
   Pulv. acaciæ,
   Sacch. alb., . . . āā Ðiss.
   Tr. opii, ... ℳiij.
   Aq. cinnam., ... ℥xj.—M.
 Sig.: Teaspoonful every four hours for a child of one year.   TANNER.

413—℞ Tr. opii deod.,   . . . f℥j.
 Sig.: Ten drops every two or three hours, to the point of tolerance.   DA COSTA.

414—℞ Naphthalini, .   gr. xii–℥j.
   Sacch. lact., .   gr. xii–℥ss.—M.
  Et ft. chart. No. xii.
 Sig.: One powder every three hours. STARR.

415—℞ Bismuth. salicylat.,   . gr. xxiv–lxxij.
   Syr. acaciæ, . . . f℥j.
   Aq. cinnam., . . q. s. ad f℥iij.—M.
 Sig.: Teaspoonful every three hours. POWELL.

ENTERITIS *(Continued).*

416—℞ Pulv. ipecac. comp.,   . ℨj.
   Bismuth. subnit.,   .   . ℥ij.—M.
  Et ft. chart. No. xxiv.

  Sig.: One powder every two to four hours for a child five years old.   J. Lewis Smith.

417—℞ Hydrarg. chlor. mit.,   . gr. j.
   Bismuth. subnit.,   .   . gr. xxxvi-ℨj.—M.
  Et ft. chart. No. xii.

  Sig.: One powder every two hours.   Starr.

EPILEPSY.

418—℞ Lobelinæ hydrobrom.   .   . gr. ½-j.
   Aq. destillat.,   .   .   . fℨiiss.—M.

  Sig.: Teaspoonful three or four times a day.
             Bartholow.

419—℞ Ex. conii fl., ... fℨij.

  Sig.: Fifteen to sixty minims not over three times a day.   Spitzka.

420—℞ Nickel brom.,   .   .   . gr. xvj.
   Aq. destillat.,   .   .   . fℨij.—M.

  Sig.: Teaspoonful several times daily.   Da Costa.

421—℞ Ferri brom., ... gr. iv.
   Potass. brom.,   .   .   . fℨj.
   Syr. simp.,   .   .   . fℨvj.
   Aquæ, ... fℨviij.—M.

  Sig.: Tablespoonful twice daily. *(In anæmic patients.)*   Bartholow.

422—℞ Potass. brom.,
   Ammon. brom.,   .   . āā ℨj.
   Ex. ergotæ fl.,   .   .   . fℨss.
   Aquæ,   .   .   q. s. ad fℨij.—M.

  Sig.: Teaspoonful three times a day, well diluted.
(When maniacal excitement follows the attack, or cerebral congestion or hemorrhage is feared.)   Charles R. Smith.

423—℞ Potassii bromidi,   .   .   . ℨj.
   Sodii bromid.,   .   .   . ℨss.
   Ammonii bromid.,   .   . ℨij.
   Syrup, ... fℨij.
   Aq. gaultheriæ,   .   q. s. ad fℨvj.—M.

  Sig.: A teaspoonful t. d. *(For a child of seven.)*
                Rex.

EPILEPSY *(Continued)*.

424—℞ Potass. brom.,
Sodii brom.,
Ammon. brom.,   āā ℨiij.
Potass. iodid.,
Ammon. iodid., . . āā ℨiss.
Ammon. carbonat., . . ℨj.
Tr. calumbæ, ... f℥iss.
Aquæ, . . . q. s. ad ℥viij.—M.
Sig.: Teaspoonful and a half before each meal and three teaspoonfuls at bedtime.   BROWN-SÉQUARD.

425—℞ Codeinæ, ... ℨj.
Potassii bromidi, . . . ℨij.
Infus. adonidis vernalis, . . f℥iv.—M.
Sig.: Half to one teaspoonful three times a day.

426—℞ Potass. iodid.,
Potass. bromid., . . āā ℨj.
Ammon. bromid., . . . ℨss.
Potass. bicarbonat., . . ϴij.
Infus. calumbæ, . . . f℥vj.—M.
Sig.: Teaspoonful before each meal and thrice the dose at bedtime.   BROWN-SÉQUARD.

427—℞ Antipyrin., ... ℨj.
Ammonii bromid., . . . ℨiiiss.
Strontii bromid., . . . ℨj.
Liq. potassii arsenit., . . . ♏40.
Ex. solani carolinens., . . f℥xss.
Aquæ, . . . q. s. ad f℥vj.—M.
Sig.: A dessertspoonful or more twice daily.

428—℞ Ammon. bromid., . . . ℨvj.
Antipyrin, ... ℨj.
Liq. potass. arsenitis, . . f℥j.
Aq. menthæ pip., . q. s. ad f℥vj.—M.
Sig.: Tablespoonful in water night and morning.   WOOD.

429—℞ Potass. bromid.,
Sodii bromid., . . āā gr. x.
Ammonii bromid., . . . gr. v.
Sodii bicarb., . . . gr. ij.
Liq. potassii arsenit., . . ♏j.
Aquæ, ... ad ℨj.—M.
Sig.: Dose, one teaspoonful.   STARR.

55

EPILEPSY (Continued).

430—R Tr. belladonn., . . . ♏ij.
　　　Sodii bromid., . . . gr. xv.
　　　Chloral hydrat., . . . gr. v.
　　　Aq. menthæ pip., . q. s. ad f3j.—M.
　　Sig.: Dose, one teaspoonful. VANDERBILT CLINIC.

431—R Pulv. sodii borat., . . . 3j.
　　　Syr. aurant. cort., . . . f3j.
　　　Aq. destillat., . q. s. ad f3iv.—M.
　　Sig.: Tablespoonful three times a day.

EPISTAXIS.

432—R Liq. ferri persulphatis, . . f3j.
　　　Aq. destillat., . . . f3iij.—M.
　　Sig.: Inject into nostril. GERHARD.

433—R Ol. erigerontis (Canad.), . f3ij.
　　Sig.: Five to fifteen drops on sugar every four hours, or repeated as required. WILLARD.

434—R Ex. hamamelis fl., . . . f3ij.
　　Sig.: A teaspoonful every one to three hours.
　　　　　　　　　　　　　　　　J. V. SHOEMAKER.

435—R Pulv. aluminis,
　　　Pulv. acid. tannic., . āā 3j.—M.
　　Sig.: Insufflate into the nares anteriorly and posteriorly. SAJOUS.

436—R Antipyrin., . . gr. l.
　　　Acid. tannic., . . gr. j.
　　　Pulv. sacchari, . . gr. x.—M.
　　Sig.: Apply topically. RENDU.

437—R Succi limonis, . . 3ij.
　　Sig.: Inject into nostrils.

438—R Tr. aconit. rad., . . . ♏viij.
　　　Liq. ammon. acetat., . . f3j.—M.
　　Sig.: Teaspoonful every half hour. (In plethoric cases.) THOMAS.

ERYSIPELAS.

439—R Acid. carbolic.,
　　　Tr. iodi,
　　　Alcohol., . . . āā f3j.
　　　Ol. terebinthinæ, . . f3ij.
　　　Glycerin., . . . f3iij.—M.
　　Sig.: Apply with a brush every two hours and cover with aseptic gauze. PRESSE MÉDICALE.

56

ERYSIPELAS (Continued).

440—℞ Tr. ferri chlor.,
Syr. simp., . . . āā f℥j.
Aquæ, . . . q. s. ad f℥iij.—M.
  Sig.: Teaspoonful every two or three hours well diluted.   Charity Hospital, N. Y.

441—℞ Ferri sulphat., . . . ℥j.
Aquæ, ... Oj.—M.
  Sig.: Apply by compresses, and renew every two or three hours.   Velpeau.

442—℞ Acid. tannic., ... ℈ij.
Camphoræ, . . . ℨj.
Æther., ... ℥v.—M.
  Sig.: Paint every hour or two over affected part and adjacent skin.   Spernandino.

443—℞ Ichthyol., ... ℨj.
Lanolini, ... ℨix.—M.
                           Nussbaum.

444—℞ Creolin., ... ℨj.
Iodoformi, ... ℥ss.
Lanolini, ... ℨx.—M.
Ft. unguentum.
  Sig.: Apply with a camel's-hair brush and cover with gutta-percha.   Koch.

445—℞ Argent. nitrat., . . . gr. lxxx.
Aq. destillat., . . . f℥iv.—M.
  Sig.: Paint two or three times all over and a little beyond.   Higginbottom.

446—℞ Plumb. acetat., . . . ℨj.
Tr. opii, ... f℥j.
Aquæ, . . . q. s. ad Oj.—M.
  Sig.: Shake the bottle well, and wet cloths or lint thoroughly with the lotion and apply to the affected parts.   Charity Hospital, N. Y.

447—℞ Aristol., ... gr. xx.
Collodii, ... f℥j.—M.
  Sig.: Apply freely with a camel's-hair brush over and slightly beyond the inflamed area.

ERYTHEMA (See Skin Diseases).

FAVUS (See Skin Diseases).

448—℞ Sapo. mollis. . . . . ℥j.
　　Aquæ, ... f℥iv.
　　Zinci oxidi, ... ℥j.
　　Vaselin., ... ℥ijss.
　　Essent. lavandulæ, . q. s. —M.
　Sig.: Apply topically.

449—℞ Acid. salicylici, . . . gr. xlv.
　　Pulv. amyli, ... ℥v.
　　Pulv. talc, ... ℥xxij.—M.
　Sig.: Dust over the feet. (Used in the German army.)

450—℞ Ol. anethi destillat., . . . Oj.
　　Chloral. hydrat., . . . gr. xxxv.
　　Sodii biborat., . . . gr. xv.—M.
　Sig.: Wash the feet morning and night.
　　　　　　　　　　　　　　　PRACTITIONER.

451—℞ Sodii biborat., . gr. xv.
　　Thymoli, . . gr. viiss.
　　Aq. destillat., . f℥lxxv.—M.
　Sig.: Mouth wash. MAGITOT.

452—℞ Potass. permanganat., . . gr. x-xxx.
　　Aquæ, ... f℥viij.—M.
　Sig.: Apply locally. BARTHOLOW.

453—℞ Powdered rice, . . . ℥ij.
　　Bismuth. subnitrat., . . ℥vij.
　　Potass. permanganat., . . ℥iij.
　　Powdered talc, . . . f℥iss.—M.
　Sig.: To be dusted upon the perspiring parts.
　　　　　　　　　　　　COLL. AND CLIN. REC.

FEVERS—

Catarrhal.

454—℞ Antifebrin, . . . ℥j.
　　Spt. vini gal., . . . f℥ss.
　　Elix. simp., . q. s. ad f℥ij.—M.
　Sig.: Teaspoonful every four hours.
　　　　　　　　　　　　　　HEINZELMANN.

Intermittent

455—℞ Quiniæ sulphat., . . ℈iv.
　　Acid. sulphuric. dil., . q. s. ut ft. sol.
　　Spt. æther. nitro., . . f℥ss.
　　Syr. tolu.,
　　Aquæ, . āā q. s. ad f℥ij.—M.
　Sig.: Teaspoonful three or four times daily.
　　　　　　　　　　　　　　DA COSTA.

456—℞ Quinin. sulph., . . . ℨj.
　　Tinct. ferri chlorid., . . . f℥v.
　　Liq. acid. arsenosi, . . . f℥jss.
　　Potass. chlorat., . . . ℨj
　　Syrup. zingiberis, . q. s. ad f℥iv.—M.
　Sig.: Teaspoonful in water thrice daily. (*Malarial
cachexia.*)

Scarlet.

457—℞ Tr. ferri chlor., . . f℥j.
　　Potass. chlorat., . . gr. xlviij.
　　Glycerinæ, . . . f℥j.
　　Aquæ, . . q. s. ad f℥iij.—M.
　Sig.: Teaspoonful every two hours for a child of
four years.　　　　　　　　　　　　MORRIS.

458—℞ Acid. boracic., . . . ℨss.
　　Potass. chlor., . . . ℨij.
　　Tr. ferri chlor. . . . f℥ij.
　　Glycerinæ,
　　Syr. simp., . . āā f℥j.
　　Aquæ, ... f℥ij.—M.
　Sig.: Teaspoonful every two hours for a child of
five years.　　　　　　　　　J. LEWIS SMITH.

459—℞ Menthol., ... gr. xx.
　　Eucalyptol., . . . ♏x.
　　Paraffin. fluid., ... ℥j.—M.
　Sig.: Spray nares and nasopharynx with atomizer.

460—℞ Acid. carbol., . . . ♏xx.
　　Vaselin., ... ℥j.—M.
　Sig.: Apply to body night and morning.　STARR.

461—℞ Ol. menthæ pip., . . ♏xv.
　　Ol. olivæ, ... f℥iij.—M.
　Sig.: Apply to body night and morning.　STARR.

462—℞ Tr. digitalis, . . . f℥ss.
　　Liq. ammon. acetat., . f℥iss.
　　Spt. æth. nit., . . . f℥ij.
　　Syr. tolu., . . . f℥ss.
　　Aq. cari, . . q. s. ad f℥iij.—M.
　Sig.: Teaspoonful every two hours for a child of
six or eight years.　　GOODHART and STARR.

Spotted (See also Meningitis ; Cerebro-Spinal Meningitis).

464—℞ Morphiæ sulphat., . . gr. ss.
  Acid. sulphur. aromat., . f3j.
  Elix. cinchonæ,   q. s. ad   f℥vj.—M.

Sig.: Teaspoonful every two hours for a child of twelve years.   Meigs and Pepper.

465—℞ Acid. hydrocyanic. dil., . ♏xxx.
  Sodii bicarb., . . . 3j.
  Syr. simp , . . . f℥ss.
  Aquæ, . . q. s. ad   f℥iij.—M.

Sig.: Teaspoonful every three or four hours for vomiting.   Delafield.

Typhoid.

466—℞ Salol., ... 3j.
  Thymol., ... gr. xxxvj.
  Bismuth. subnit., . . . 3ij–3iv.
  Mucil. acaciæ, ... f℥ij.
  Syr. tolutani, ... f℥iv.—M.

Sig.: Tablespoonful thrice daily.

467—℞ Bismuth. subnit., . . 3iij.
  Spt. vini gal., . . . f3vj
  Spt. myristicæ, . . f3ss.
  Syr. acaciæ, . . . f3j.
  Aq. cinnam., . q. s. ad   f℥iij.—M.

Sig.: From one to two teaspoonfuls every three or four hours.   W. H. Bennett.

468—℞ Acid. muriat. dil., . . f3j.
  Syr. rubi idæi, . . . f3vij.
  Aquæ, ... f℥iij.—M.

Sig.: Dessertspoonful every two or three hours.   Gerhard.

Typhus.

469—℞ Quiniæ sulphat., . . Ɖiv.
  Acid. sulphuric. dil., . f3ss.
  Syr. simp., . . . f℥ss.
  Aquæ, . . q. s. ad   f℥ij.—M.

Sig.: Teaspoonful every two hours until temperature is lowered.   Golden.

470—℞ Tr. belladonnæ, . . f℥ss.
  Tr. aconiti rad., . . f3ss.—M.

Sig.: Ten drops every two hours. (*For dry tongue and rapid pulse.*)   Harley.

FEVERS—
Yellow.

471—℞ Pilocarpiæ muriat., . . gr. iij.
    Aq. destillat., . . . f℥ij.—M.
Sig.: ℥x hypodermically.   HEBER SMITH.

472—℞ Hydrarg. chlor. mit.,
    Pulv. jalapæ, . . āā gr. x.—M.
Et ft. pulv. No. i.
Sig.: Use at the onset of the disease.   RUSH.

FISSURE OF ANUS AND NIPPLES.

473—℞ Ex. hydrastis fl., . . f℥j.
Sig.: Apply to fissure.   BARTHOLOW.

474—℞ Acid. carbol., . . . gr. xxiv.
    Aquæ, ... f℥j.—M.
Sig.: Apply several times daily.   PARVIN.

475—℞ Ex. conii, ... ℈iv.
    Ol. ricini, ... f℥iv.
    Lanolin., ... ℥j.—M.
Sig.: Apply topically after each movement of the bowels. (*Fissure of the anus.*)

476—If the fissure is deep and slow to heal, touch with solid stick nitrate of silver.

477—℞ Bismuth. subnit., . . ℥j.
    Ol. ricin., ... f℥ij.—M.
Sig.: Rub in affected parts.   HIRST.

478—℞ Salol, ... ℥j.
    Ætheris, ... f℥j.
    Cocain. hydrochlorat., . gr. ij.
    Collodii, ... f℥v.—M.
Sig.: Apply to the affected part.

479—℞ Acid. boric., . . . gr. xlv.
    Cocain. hydrochlor., . . gr. xv.
    Lanolin, ... ℥j.—M.
Sig.: Apply first to fissure, then apply solid stick of silver nitrate.   L'UNION MÉDICALE.

480—℞ Acid. carbolic., . . . gr. xlviij.
    Tr. iodi, ... f℥ijss.
    Glycerin., ... f℥j.—M.
Sig.: Apply topically. (*Fissure of the tongue.*)

FISTULÆ.

481—℞ Hydrogen peroxide, . . f℥vj.
Sig.: Inject once daily ; dilute if necessary.

482—℞ Cupri sulphat., . . . gr. ii–iv.
Aquæ, . . . f℥iv.—M.
Sig.: Inject once daily.   Sir A. Cooper.

483—℞ Argent. nitrat., . . . gr. ij.
Aq. destillat., . . . f℥viij.—M.
Sig.: Inject once daily. (*Fistula in ano.*)
      Druitt.

484—℞ Tr. iodi., . . . f℈j.
Sig.: Inject once daily.   Waring.

485—Touch with solid stick of argent. nit.

486—℞ Camphor., . . . ℥j.
Salol, ... ℥ss.
Ether, ... f℈j.—M.
Sig.: Use as an injection.   Medical Record.

FLATULENCE (See also Acidity and Dyspepsia).
487—℞ Sodii sulpho-carbolat., . ℈iij.
Syr. zingiber., . . . f℥iss.
Aquæ, . . q. s. ad f℥iv.—M.
Sig.: Dessertspoonful before meals.   Sansom.

488—℞ Tr. nucis vomicæ,
Tr. physostigmatis,
Tr. belladonnæ, . . āā f℈j.—M.
Sig.: Fifteen drops in water two or three times a
day.   Bartholow.

489—℞ Creasotæ, ... gtt. xxiv.
Syr. simp., ... f℥j.
Spt. lavandulæ comp., q. s. ad f℥iij.—M.
Sig.: Teaspoonful in water three times a day after
meals.   Powell.

490—℞ Pulv. calumbæ,
Pulv. zingiber., . āā ℥ss.
Sennæ fol., . . . ℈j.
Aq. bullientis, . . . Oj.
Ft. infusum.
Sig.: Wineglassful three times a day.
     Bartholow.

FLATULENCE (Continued).

491—℞ Pulv. carbol. lig., . . ℨi-ij.
 Div. in capsul. No. xxiv.
 Sig.: Two capsules three times a day.   RINGER.

492—℞ Aq. anisi,
  Liq. calcis, . . . āā fℨss.
  Syr. acaciæ, . . . fℨj.—M.
 Sig.: Add from ten to thirty drops of chloroform
according to age of child, and give a teaspoonful
every two hours.   CONDIE.

493—℞ Ol. cajuputi, . . . fℨss.
  Spt. lavandulæ comp., . fℨss.
  Syr. zingiberis, . . . fℨij.
  Mucil. acaciæ, . . ad fℨij.—M.
 Sig.: Dessertspoonful as required.   HARTSHORNE.

494—℞ Ol. terebinthinæ, . . fℨj.
 Sig.: Three to five drops on sugar.   BARTHOLOW.

FRECKLES, SUNBURN, AND TAN (See Skin Diseases).

FROSTBITE (See also Chilblains).

495—℞ Acid. carbolici, . . . ℨj.
  Tr. iodinii, ... fℨij.
  Acid. tannici, . . . ℨj.
  Cerat. simplicis, . . . ℨiv.—M.
 Sig.: Apply two or three times a day.   MORROW.

496—℞ Lini. camphoræ,
  Lini. saponis comp.,
  Ol. cajuputi, . . āā fℨj.—M.
 Sig.: Apply locally to the unbroken skin.
            BRANDE.

497—℞ Acid. sulphurosi, . fℨiij.
  Glycerinæ,
  Aquæ, . . āā fℨj.—M.
 Sig.: Apply locally.   BARTHOLOW.

498—℞ Iodi., ... Ɵj.
  Potass. iodid., . . . gr. iv.
  Aq. destillat., . . . ℳvj.
  Adipis, ... ℨj.—M.
 Sig.: Apply once daily.   HEBRA.

63

FROSTBITE (*Continued*).

499—℞ Ichthyol.,
Resorcin.,
Acid. tannic., . . . āā ʒj.
Aquæ . . . . . f͠ʒv.—M.
Sig.: Apply with a brush at night. BOECK.

500—℞ Resorcin., ... ʒij.
Mucilag. gummi arabic.,
Aquæ, ... āā f͠ʒij.
Pulv. talc., ... ʒj.—M.
Sig.: Apply topically with a brush. BOECK.

FURUNCLE (*See Carbuncle*).

GALACTORRHŒA.

501—℞ Atropinæ sulphat., . . gr. iv.
Aquæ rosæ, ... f͠ʒj.—M.
Sig.: Apply on lint around the breast and remove
when the throat becomes dry. BARTHOLOW.

502—℞ Potass. iodidi, . . . ʒiij.
Syr. sarsap. comp., . . f͠ʒiss.
Aquæ, . . . q. s. ad f͠ʒiij.—M.
Sig.: Teaspoonful three or four times a day.
HIRST.

GALL-STONES (*See Calculi*).

GANGRENE.

503—℞ Pulv. carbo. lig.,
Micæ panis,
Lactis, . . . āā q. s.—M.
Ft. cataplasma.
Sig.: Apply to correct fetor.

504—℞ Potass. brom., . . ʒij+Ɔij.
Aq. destillat., . . f͠ʒij.
Solve. Dein. adjice—
Bromi, . . . ʒj (by weight).
Aq. destillat., . q. s. ad f͠ʒiv.—M.
Sig.: Apply to slough. (*In hospital gangrene.*)
SMITH.

505—℞ Pulv. acid. salicylici, . . ʒj.
Sig.: Use as a dusting powder. (*To destroy fetor
and change morbid action.*) BARTHOLOW.

506—℞ Brominii, ... ʒj.
Sig.: Apply to slough with glass rod. (*In hospital
gangrene.*) BARTHOLOW.

GANGRENE (Continued).

507—℞ Acid. carbol.,   .   . f℥ij.
        Glyceriuæ, .   .   . f℥viij.—M.
Sig.: Apply ou liut.   LISTER.

GASTRALGIA (See Neuralgia).

GASTRIC ULCER (See Ulcer).

GLAND, ENLARGED LYMPHATIC.

508—℞ Syr. ferri iodid., .   .   . f℥j.
Sig.: Fve to thirty drops, well diluted, after each meal.

509—℞ Ichthyol.,
      Ung. hydrarg.,
      Ung. belladonnæ,   ,   āā ℨj.
      Ung. petrolati,   .   ℥ss.—M.
      Ft. ung.
Sig.: Apply night and morning over affected glands, using friction till absorbed.

510—℞ Tr. iodi., ... f℥j.
Sig.: Paint over enlargements thoroughly and repeat as soon as the dark color commences to disappear.

512—℞ Ichthyol., ... ℨiij.
      Adipis, ... ℨvij.—M.
Sig.: Use as inunction morning and evening.
                              AGNEW.

513—℞ Acidi carbolici,   .   .   . gr. viij.
      Aq. destillat.,   .   .   . f℥j.—M.
Sig.: Inject five to ten minims into the enlarged gland.

514—℞ Potass. iodid.,   .   .   . ℨi–iv.
      Syr. auraut. cor.,   .   . f℥j.
      Aq. cinnamomi, .   . ad f℥iij.—M.
Sig.: Teaspoonful in water three times a day.
                              RINGER.

515—℞ Ungt. plumbi iodidi,   .   . ℥j.
Sig.: Apply locally.   BARTHOLOW.

GLEET (See Gonorrhœa).

GOITRE.

516—℞ Tr. iodinii comp., . . f℥j.
   Sig.: Apply locally with brush ; also five to fifteen minims in water three times a day internally.
BARTHOLOW.

517—℞ Picrotoxin, . . . gr. $\frac{1}{30}$.
     Aq. ex. ergot., . . gr. iiss.—M.
   Ft. pil.
   Sig.: One pill three times a day.   WATKINS.

518—℞ Potass. brom., . . ℥ss.
   Div. in chart. No. xii.
   Sig.: Powder, well diluted, three times a day.
JON. HUTCHINSON.

519—℞ Ungt. hydrarg. iodid. rubr., ℥j.
   Sig.: Rub in a piece the size of a pea and expose to heat.   RINGER.

520—℞ Iodoformi, ... ℨj.
     Adipis, ... ℥j.—M.
   Sig.: Apply locally.

521—℞ Tr. iodinii, ... f℥j.
   Sig.: Inject an hypodermic syringeful into the tumor every week. After three weeks, inject every two weeks until cured.   DUGUET.

GONORRHŒA.

522—℞ Hydrarg. chlor. corros., . gr. iij.
     Sodii chloridi, . . gr. vj.
     Aquæ, ... f℥j.—M.
   Sig.: Add one teaspoonful of the mixture to one pint of hot water and flush urethra thoroughly once or twice a day. (*Males.*)

523—℞ Hydrarg. chlor. corros., . gr. xv.
     Sodii chloridi, . . . gr. xxx.
     Aquæ, ... f℥j.—M.
   Sig.: Add two teaspoonfuls of the mixture to two pints of hot water and flush vagina thoroughly three times a day. (*Females.*)

524—℞ Liq. plumbi subacetat. dil., f℥j.
     Ex. opii aquos, . . . gr. vj.—M.
   Sig.: Use as an injection two to four times daily.
VAN BUREN and KEYES.

525—℞ Alum.,
  Boracis, . . . āā ʒj.
  Quinin. sulphat., . . gr. xv.
  Acid. carbolic.,
  Essentiæ thymi, . . āā gtt. xxx.
  Glycerin., ... fʒij.—M.

Sig.: A tablespoonful to a pint of warm water, and use as a vaginal injection two or three times a day.
             LUTAUD.

526—℞ Zinci sulpho-carbolat., . gr. vj.
  Morph. sulph., . . . gr. iij.
  Aq. destillat., . . . fʒiij.—M.

Sig.: Use as an injection from four to six times a day, after urinating.

527—℞ Zinci sulphatis,
  Acid. tannici, . . āā gr. xv.
  Aq. rosæ, ... fʒvj.—M.

Sig.: A tablespoonful injected two or three times a day.   RICORD.

528—℞ Zinci chloridi, . . . gr. i–ij.
  Aq. destillat., . . . fʒvj.—M.

Sig.: Inject once or twice daily.   LEVIS.

529—℞ Zinci sulphatis, . . . ʒj.
  Aluminis, ... ʒiij.—M.

Sig.: Dissolve a teaspoonful in one pint of water and inject three times a day. (*Females.*) HAZARD.

530—℞ Zinci sulphat., . . . gr. i–iij.
  Liq. plumbi subacetat. dil., fʒj.—M.

Sig.: Shake and inject three to four times daily.
        VAN BUREN and KEYES.

531—℞ Zinci sulphatis, . . . gr. viij.
  Plumbi acetatis, . . . gr. xv.
  Aq. destillat., . . . fʒviij.—M.

Sig.: Use as a urethral injection from two to four times daily.   DA COSTA.

532—℞ Salol,
  Oleores cubebæ,
  Copaibæ, . . . āā ʒj.
  Aluminis, ... ʒiv.
  Pepsinæ sacch., . . . ʒss.
  Ol. gaultheriæ, . . . gtt. x.—M.
Ft. capsul. No. xx.

Sig.: Two every three hours. MACCONNELL.

533—℞ Creasot., . . . ℳx.
    Ex. hamamel. fl.,
    Ex. hydrast. canad., . āā ℳxv.
    Aq. rosæ, ... f℥iv.—M.
Sig.: This should be slightly diluted with warm water before using. (*In chronic form.*) BREIMA.

534—℞ Zinci sulphat., . . . gr. ij.
    Aquæ, ... f℥j.—M.
Sig.: Inject three times a day. AGNEW.

535—℞ Zinci sulphat.,
    Acid. carbolic.,
    Alum. cond., . . . āā gr. xij.
    Aq. destillat., . . . f℥vj.—M.
Sig.: Use locally. (Dilute if painful.) HARE.

536—℞ Acid. boracic., . . . ℨj.
    Hydrarg. bichlor., . . gr. ¼.
    Zinci sulphat., . . . gr. xij.
    Morphiæ sulph., . . . gr. j.
    Aq. destillat., . . . f℥iv.—M.
Sig.: Inject three times a day. SIMES.

537—℞ Hydrarg. chlor. corros., . gr. ii–iv.
    Zinci sulpho-carbolat., . gr. ii–x.
    Acid. boric., . . . ℨj.
    Hydrogen. dioxid., . . f℥j.
    Aquæ, . . q. s. ad f℥viij.—M.
Sig.: Use as injection. WHITE.

538—℞ Zinci sulphatis, . . . gr. vj.
    Tr. opii, ... f℥j.
    Tr. catechu, . . . f℥ij.
    Aq. rosæ, . . . ad f℥ij.—M.
Sig.: Use as an injection three times a day. (*In chronic form.*) WITHERSTINE.

539—℞ Camphoræ, ... gr. c.
    Ex. opii, ... gr. lxxv.
    Alcoholis, ... f℥j.
    Ex. belladonnæ, . . . gr. lxxv.—M.
Et ft. cataplasma.
Sig.: Apply over joint from ten to twelve hours. (*In gonorrhœal rheumatism.*) MED. PROGRESS.

GONORRHŒA (Continued).

540—℞ Hydrarg. salicylat., . . gr. ⅙.
    Aq. destillat., . . . f℥iij.—M.

Sig.: Use as injection three times a day.

SCHRIMMER.

GOUT.

541—℞ Ol. gaultheriæ,
    Ol. olivæ,
    Lini. saponis,
    Tr. aconiti,
    Tr. opii, . . . āā f℥ij.—M.

Sig.: Apply freely and cover with cotton batting.

SATTERLEE.

542—℞ Colchicini, ... gr. j.
    Ex. colocynth. comp., . ℨss.
    Quiniæ sulphat., . . ℨiij.—M.
Et ft. pil. No. lx.

Sig.: One pill every four hours.   BARTHOLOW.

543—℞ Potassii iodidi, ... ℨiv.
    Liniment. saponis,
    Ol. cajuputi,
    Ol. carui, . . . āā f℥ss.
    Spirit. vini rectif., . q. s. ad f℥vij.—M.

Sig.: Apply on lint and cover with protective.

544—℞ Ex. colchici acetici,
    Ex. aloes,
    Pulv. ipecac.,
    Hydrarg. chlor. mitis, . āā gr. j.
    Ex. nucis vomicæ, . . . gr. ¼.—M.

Sig.: One such pill to be taken every four hours
until purgation ensues.   LOOMIS.

545—℞ Tr. stramonii, ... f℥j.
    Tr. colchici, ... f℥iss.
    Tr. guaiaci, ... f℥ij.—M.

Sig.: A teaspoonful three times a day, in milk.

546—℞ Vini sem. colchici, . . f℥ss.
    Potass. iodid., . . . ℨij.
    Liq. potass., . . . f℥ij.
    Tr. zingiberis, . . . f℥iss.—M

Sig.: Teaspoonful twice daily in warm water.

HODGSON.

GOUT *(Continued)*.

547—℞ Tr. iodinii, ... ℥clx.
    Glycerinæ, ... f℥ij.—M.
    Sig.: Teaspoonful three times a day.   GRANVILLE.

548—℞ Veratrinæ, ... ℈j.
    Adipis, ... ℥j.—M.
    Sig.: Apply to painful joint at onset. (*Not when skin is broken.*)   TURNBULL.

549—℞ Ex. colchici acetat., . . gr. ij.
    Pulv. ipecac. comp., . . gr. v.—M.
    Et ft. pil. No. ii.
    Sig.: One night and morning.
                      ST. GEORGE'S HOSPITAL.

550—℞ Potass. carbonat.,
    Potass. nitrat., . . āā ℈iss.
    Aquæ, ... f℥viij.—M.
    Sig.: Tablespoonful three times a day. (*In gouty attacks.*)

551—℞ Potass. iodid., . . . gr. v.
    Potass. bicarb., . . . gr. x.
    Mist. ammoniaci, . . f℥j.—M.
    Et ft. haustus.
    Sig.: To be taken three times a day. FOTHERGILL.

552—℞ Lithii benzoat., ... ℈ij
    Aq. cinnamomi, . . . f℥iiss.—M.
    Sig.: Teaspoonful in a wineglassful of water every four to six hours.   JACCOUD.

553—℞ Paraldehyde, . . . ℥ss.
    Syr. simplicis, . . . f℥iss.—M.
    Sig.: A teaspoonful to a tablespoonful, well diluted, when required. (*For gouty insomnia.*)
                      HODGSON.

554—℞ Potass. brom., . . . gr. xx.
    Tr. hyoscyami, . . . f℥ss.
    Tr. lupuli, ... f℥j.
    Aq. camphoræ, . . f℥j.—M.
    Et ft. haustus.
    Sig.: Take at bedtime. (*For gouty insomnia.*)
                    FOTHERGILL.

GUMS.

555—℞ Glyceriti acidi tannici, . f℥j.
    Sig.: Apply with soft brush. (*For spongy or bleeding gums.*)
                    BARTHOLOW.

GUMS (Continued).

556—℞ Chloral hydrat.,
    Tr. cochleariæ (Ph. P.), aā f℥iss.—M.
  Sig.: Apply to gums with pledgets of cotton, every day or two. (*For gingivitis of pregnancy.*) PINARD.

HÆMATEMESIS.

557—℞ Ergotini, ... gr. xij.
    Aq. destillat., . . . f℥j.—M.
  Sig.: Five to ten minims hypodermically every three hours. RINGER.

558—℞ Liq. ferri subsulphat., . f℥ss.
  Sig.: One or two drops in ice-water frequently.
                             BARTHOLOW.

559—℞ Plumbi acetat., ... ℥ss.
    Hydrarg. chlor. mit., . . gr. v.
    Confection. rosæ, . . q. s.—M.
  Et ft. pil. No. x.
  Sig.: One pill every two to four hours. (*From ulcer.*) ELLIS.

560—℞ Acid. gallici, . . . gr. x.
    Acid. sulphuric. dil., . . ℳx.
    Aquæ, ... f℥j.—M.
  Ft. haustus.
  Sig.: To be repeated in four or six hours if necessary. BRINTON.

561—℞ Tr. hamamelis, . . . f℥ss.
  Sig.: Two to four drops in water every two or three hours. RINGER.

HÆMATURIA.

562—℞ Tr. ferri chlor., . . . ℳxxx.
    Tr. digitalis, . . . ℳxv.
    Aq. menthæ pip., . . f℥iss.—M.
  Sig.: Take one dose every four hours. AITKEN.

563—℞ Acid. gallic., . . . ℥ss.
    Acid. sulphuric. dil.,
    Tr. opii deod., . . aā f℥j.
    Infus. digitalis, . . . f℥iv.—M.
  Sig.: Tablespoonful every four hours. DRUITT.

564—℞ Ex. ergot. fl., . . . f℥ij.
  Sig.: 20 gtt.–℥j every two hours. MORRIS.

565—℞ Tr. hamamelis, . . ♏xxiv.
  Elix. simp.,
  Aquæ, ... āā f℥j.—M.
 Sig.: Teaspoonful every two or three hours.
            RINGER.

HÆMOPTYSIS.

566—℞ Plumbi acetat., . . gr. xx.
  Pulv. digitalis, . . gr. x.
  Pulv. opii, . . . gr. v.—M.
 Et div. in pil. No. xx.
 Sig.: One pill every four hours. BARTHOLOW.

567—℞ Ex. ergotæ fl., . . . f℥j.
  Ol. gaultheriæ, . . . gtt. iv.—M.
 Sig.: Teaspoonful every hour at first; then every
four to six hours.   RINGER.

568—℞ Acid. gallici, . . . f℥ij.
  Acid. sulph. aromat., . . f℥j.
  Glycerinæ, ... f℥j.
  Aq. destillat., . q. s. ad f℥vj.—M.
 Sig.: Teaspoonful at dose; repeat frequently.
            PEPPER.

569—℞ Tr. digitalis, . . . f℥iss.
  Ol. terebinth., . . . f℥iij.
  Ol. menth. pip., . ., . ♏xx.
  Acid. sulph. arom., . . f℥iij.
  Spt. vin. rect., . . . f℥xvj.—M.
 Sig.: Forty to sixty drops, well mixed with sugar,
to which one or more tablespoonfuls of water may be
added every two, three, or four hours, according to
the urgency of hemorrhage.
     CANADA MEDICAL RECORD.

570—℞ Iodoform. . . . gr. vj.
  Acid. tannici, . . gr..viij.—M.
 Et ft. pil. No. vi.
 Sig.: One every two or three hours till relieved.
           CHAUVIN.

571—℞ Pulv. aluminis, . . . ℥j.
  Sacch. alb., . . . ℥ss.
  Pulv. ipecac. comp., . . ℈j.—M.
 Et div. in chart. No. vi.
 Sig.: One powder every two hours. SKODA.

572—℞ Iufus. digitalis, . . . f℥iv.

Sig.: Tablespoonful every hour until the pulse is reduced. BRINTON.

HAIR (See also Alopecia).

573—℞ Sodii biborat., . . . ℨiv.
Aq. ammoniæ, . . . f℥j.
Spt. myrciæ, . . . f℥ij.
Aq. rosæ, . . . f℥xiij.—M.

Sig.: Hair-wash. POTTER.

574—℞ Quiniæ sulphatis, . . gr. x.
Spt. myrciæ, . . . f℥iij.
Glycerinæ, . . . f℥j.
Sodii chloridi, . . ℨij.
Aquæ, . . q. s. ad f℥viij.—M.

Sig.: Use as hair-wash.

575—℞ Barii hydrosulphat., . . gr. x.
Amyli,
Zinic oxidi, . . āā gr. v.
Aquæ, ... q. s.—M.

Sig.: Apply once daily with a camel's-hair pencil.
(*To remove superfluous hair.*) DIETETIC GAZETTE.

576—℞ Ex. jaborandi fl.,
Tr. cantharidis, . . āā f℥ss.
Glycerinæ,
Ol. vaselini, . . āā f℥j.—M.

Sig.: Hair-tonic. For use after fevers. Use at night. BARTHOLOW.

577—℞ Tr. cantharidis, . . . f℥j.
Aceti destillat., . . . f℥iss.
Glycerinæ, . . . f℥iss.
Spt. rosmarini, . . . f℥iss.
Aq. rosæ, . . . ad f℥viij.—M.

Sig. Hair-tonic. Use night and morning.
TILBURY FOX.

578—℞ Liq. hydrogenii peroxidi (10 vol.)
f℥iv.

Sig.: Hair-bleach. Apply with a sponge or soft brush. WILSON.

579—℞ Cocaini muriat., . . . gr. v.
      Aq. destillat., . . . f℥ij.—M.
Sig.: Apply with a camel's-hair brush to the nasal passages.
                                SAJOUS.

580—℞ Zinci valerianat., . . gr. j.
      Pil. assafœtidæ comp., . gr. ij.—M.
Sig.: One or two pills to be taken two or three times daily.
                   SIR MORELL MACKENZIE.

581—℞ Quiniæ muriat., . . . gr. iv–viij.
      Aquæ, ... f℥j.—M.
Sig.: Apply to the nares with a brush or atomizer.
                           BARTHOLOW.

582—℞ Liq. potassii arsenitis,
      Ex. nucis vom. fl.,
      Ex. cinchon. fl. (detannated), āā f℥vj.
      Alcoholis, ... f℥iij.
      Syr. aurantii, . . q. s. ad f℥xvj.—M.
Sig.: One or two teaspoonfuls three times daily, with or after meals.
                           HALL.

583—℞ Menthol., ... gr. xx.
      Ol. amyg. dulcis, . . . f℥ij.
      Acid. carbolici, . . . ℳx.
      Cocain. hydrochlor., . . gr. vj.
      Ung. zinci oxidi, . . . ℥ss.—M.
Sig.: Apply thoroughly to the nostrils on cotton attached to a probe.
                        MED. RECORD.

584—℞ Pulv. boracis, . . . gr. xx.
      Pulv. capsici, . . . gr. xv.
      Ammon. carbonatis., . . gr. x.—M.
Make a *fine* powder and place in a two ounce bottle.
Sig.: Shake the bottle well and inhale the powder that rises.
                           GRANVILLE.

585—℞ Syr. acid. hydriodici, . . f℥iv.
Sig.: Teaspoonful every two hours.
                           JUDKINS.

HEADACHE.

586—℞ Caffeini citrat.,
      Ammon. carb., . . āā Ðj.
      Elix. guaranæ, . . . f℥j.—M.
Sig.: Teaspoonful every hour until the pain is relieved.
                           HURD.

587—℞ Ammonii chloridi,   .   .   gr. iss.
      Morphinæ acetat.,   .   .   gr. $\frac{1}{8}$.
      Caffeinæ citrat.,   .   .   .   gr. $\frac{1}{20}$.
      Spt. ammoniæ arom.,   .   .   ♏ⅰ̷.
      Aq. menthæ pip.,   .   .   ʒss.
      Elix. guaranæ,   .   q. s. ad   ʒj.—M.
   Sig.: Dose, one teaspoonful.

588—℞ Tr. belladonnæ,   .   .   .   fʒss.
   Sig.: Six drops every three hours. (*Congestive headache.*)   RINGER.

589—℞ Sodii arseniat.,   .   .   .   gr. $\frac{1}{12}$.
      Ex. cannabis indicæ,   .   .   gr. $\frac{1}{6}$.
      Ex. belladonnæ,   .   .   gr. $\frac{1}{8}$.—M.
   Et ft. pil. No. i.
   Sig.: Pill twice daily.   LITTLE.

590—℞ Caffeinæ citrat.,   .   •   .   gr. xl.
      Sodii bromid.,   .   .   .   ʒiv.
      Antipyrin, ...   ʒij.—M.
   Et ft. in chart. No. xx.
   Sig.: One powder in water as needed.   HARE.

591—℞ Ex. cannabis indicæ,   .   .   gr. $\frac{1}{6}$.
      Acid. arsenosi,   .   .   .   gr. $\frac{1}{50}$.
      Ferri pulv.,   .   .   .   gr. j.—M.
   Sig.: One such pill three times a day, increasing if necessary to two, or even three, pills a day.

Or

592—℞ Ex. cannabis indicæ,   .   .   gr. $\frac{1}{6}$.
      Pulv. digitalis,   .   .   .   gr. ss.
      Ferri lactatis,   .   .   .   gr. ij.—M.
   Sig.: One such pill three times a day after meals.

593—℞ Antipyrin,   .   .   •   .   ʒij.
      Aq. destillat.,   .   .   .   fʒiss.
      Tr. cardam. comp.,   .   .   fʒss.
      Syr. aurant. cort.,   .   .   fʒj.—M.
   Sig.: Dessertspoonful every hour until relieved.
                                ENGEL.

594—℞ Caffeinæ citrat.,   .   .   .   gr. xviij.
      Phenacetin,   .   •   .   gr. xxxvj.
      Sacch. alb.,   .   .   .   gr. xviij.—M.
   Et ft. chart. No. xviii.
   Sig.: One powder every hour or two until relieved.

HEADACHE (Continued).

595—℞ Tr. nucis vomicæ, . . f℥ss.

Sig.: One drop in a little water frequently. (*Bilious headache with nausea.*)   RINGER.

596—℞ Zinci phosphidi, . . gr. iij.
Ex. nucis vomicæ, . gr. x.—M.
Et ft. in pil. No. xxx.

Sig.: One pill after each meal.   BARKER.

597—℞ Potass. citratis, . . .- Ɉj.
Spt. juniperi, . . . fℨj.
Spt. æther. nitro., . . m̥xx.
Infus. scoparii, . . . f℥j.—M.

Sig.: To be taken three times a day. (*Urœmic form.*)   DAY.

598—℞ Potass. acetat., . . . ℨvj.
Infus. digitalis, . . . f℥vj.—M.

Sig.: Tablespoonful every three hours. (*Urœmic headache*).   A. A. SMITH.

HEART DISEASE.

599—℞ Pulv. digitalis, . . . gr. xxx.
Ferri sulph. exsiccat., . . gr. xv.
Pulv. capsici, . . . gr. xl.
Pil. aloe et myrrhæ, . . ℨij.—M.
Et ft. pil. No. lx.

Sig.: One pill night and morning. (*Chronic heart trouble, with constipation.*)   FOTHERGILL.

600—℞ Tr. strophanthi (1-20), . f℥j.

Sig.: Five to fifteen drops three times daily. (*In fatty heart and valvular disease.*)   FRASER.

601—℞ Ex. ergotæ fl., . . . f℥iiiss.
Tr. digitalis, . . . f℥ss.—M.

Sig.: Teaspoonful three times a day. (*Enlarged heart without valvular lesion.*)   BARTHOLOW.

602—℞ Ferri redacti,
Pulv. digitalis,
Quiniæ sulphat., . . āā Ɉj.
Pulv. scillæ, . . . gr. x.—M.
Et ft. pil. No. xx.

Sig.: One pill three or four times a day. (*In fatty heart, dilatation of cavities, and mitral regurgitation.*)   BARTHOLOW.

603—℞ Tr. digitalis, . . . f℥ij.

Sig.: Ten drops three times a day. (*In irritable heart with palpitation.*) DA COSTA.

604—℞ Tr. veratri viridis. . . f℥ss.

Sig.: Five drops three times daily. (*In hypertrophy.*) BARTHOLOW.

605—℞ Tr. digitalis, . . . f℥ij.
Tr. belladonnæ, . . . f℥j.
Tr. cardamom. comp., . . f℥ij.
Elix. simplicis, . . . f℥j.—M.

Sig.: Teaspoonful in water after meals. (*In hypertrophy.*) DA COSTA.

606—℞ Tr. digitalis, . . . f℥ij.
Spt. chloroform., . . . f℥v.
Infus. buchu, . . . f℥xij.—M.

Sig.: Two tablespoonfuls in wineglassful of water three times a day. (*In simple cardiac debility.*) FOTHERGILL.

607—℞ Potass. iodid., . . . gr. v.
Ex. digitalis fl., . . . ♏ij.
Ex. convallariæ majalis fl., . ♏xx.—M.

Sig.: For a dose repeated after each meal. (*Dilated heart.*) DELAFIELD.

608—℞ Tr. aconiti, ... gtt. j.
Tr. verat. viridis, . . gtt. iij.
Syr. zingiberis, . . . gtt. vij.—M.

Sig.: This dose t. d. (*In hypertrophy.*) DA COSTA.

609—℞ Pulv. digitalis,
Pulv. ferri,
Quiniæ sulphat., . . ℥ss.—M.
Et ft. in pil. No. xxx.

Sig.: One pill three times a day. (*In palpitation due to anæmia and chlorosis.*) GERHARD.

610—℞ Potass. iodid., . . . ℥j.
Potass. bicarbon., . . ℥iij.
Infus. buchu, . . . f℥xij.—M.

Sig.: Two tablespoonfuls three or four times daily. (*In hypertrophy.*) FOTHERGILL.

611—℞ Camphoræ, ... ℥j.
Ol. olivæ, ... f℥x.—M.

Sig.: Inject two syringefuls (about 5 cu. cm.) into each arm. (*In cardiac failure.*) WEST.

HEART DISEASE (Continued).

612—℞ Sol. nitro-glycerin. (1 per ct.), f℥j.

Sig.: Two to four drops three times daily for two weeks; then use the iodides. (*For atheromatous condition of the heart.*)   HUCHARD.

613—℞ Tr. nucis vomicæ,   .   ♏xxiv.
      Tr. digitalis,   .   .   f℥j.
      Ex. cascaræ sagrad. fl.,
      Ex. berberis aquefol.,
      Elix. simplex.,   .   āā   f℥j.—M.

Sig.: Teaspoonful in water three times a day. (*When constipation exists.*)   VAN WINKLE.

614—℞ Ex. convallariæ majalis fl., . f℥j.

Sig.: Five drops every four hours. (*In aortic and mitral insufficiency.*)   SEE.

HEMICRANIA (See Headache).

HEMIPLEGIA (See Paralysis).

HEMORRHAGE.

615—℞ Morphiæ sulphat.,   .   gr. ⅙.
      Ergotinæ,   .   .   gr. iij.—M.

Sig. Use hypodermically.   GROSS.

616—℞ Ergotinæ,   .   .   .   gr. xvj.
      Syr. aurant. fl.,   .   .   f℥j.
      Aquæ,   .   .   .   f℥iij.—M.

Sig.: Tablespoonful every three hours. BONJEAN.

617—℞ Acid. gallici,   .   .   .   ℨj.
      Glycerinæ, .   .   .   f℥ss.
      Aq. destillat.,   .   .   f℥vj.—M.

Sig.: Two tablespoonfuls three times a day.
      FARQUHARSON.

618—℞ Acid. tannici,   .   .   .   gr. xx.
      Glycerinæ, .   .   .   f℥ij.
      Aq. destillat.,   .   q. s. ad   f℥viij.—M.

Sig.: Use in atomizer frequently.   HARE.

Avoid using Monsel's solution and tannic acid on same patient=Ink.

619—℞ Acid. acetici dil.,   .   .   ℥iv.

Sig.: Apply locally. (*For cuts, leech-bites, etc.*)
      RINGER.

620—℞ Plumbi acetat., . . gr. xx.
  Pulv. digitalis, . . gr. x.
  Pulv. opii, . . . gr. v.
Ft. pil. No. x.
Sig.: One pill every four hours.   BARTHOLOW.
Use opium or morphine to quiet patient.

621—℞ Aluminis, . • . . gr. vj.
  Aq. destillat., . . . f℥iij.—M.
Sig.: Use in an atomizer frequently.   HARE.

622—℞ Morphiæ sulphat., . . gr. iij.
  Tr. damianæ,
  Tr. rhois glab., . . āā f℥ij.—M.
Sig.: Teaspoonful every four hours. (*In hemorrhage
from kidney or bladder.*)   J. H. HAMMOND.

623—℞ Potass. carbonat., . . ℨij.
  Saponis, ... ℨi-ij.
  Alcoholis, ... f℥iij.—M.
Sig. Use as styptic, especially for operations about
the face.   JOS. PANCOAST.

624—℞ Ol. terebinth., . . . f℥iij.
  Ex. digitalis fl., . . . f℥j.
  Mucil. acaciæ, . . . f℥ss.
  Aq. menthæ pip., . . f℥j—M.
Sig.: Teaspoonful every three hours. (*In passive
hemorrhages.*)   BARTHOLOW.

625—℞ Argenti nitrat. fusæ, . . q. s.
Sig.: Wipe the wound dry and apply locally.
  RINGER.

626—℞ Infus. digitalis, . . f℥ij.
  Ex. ergotæ fl.,
  Tr. krameriæ, . . āā f℥j.—M.
Sig. Tablespoonful as required.   BARTHOLOW.

HEMORRHOIDS.

627—℞ Iodoform., ... ℨii–iv.
  Adipis benzoat., . . . ℨj.—M.
Sig.: Apply locally after washing.

628—℞ Ex. hamamelis fl., . . f℥iv.
Sig.: Inject some into the rectum and apply pledgets of lint soaked in this solution.   HARE.

HEMORRHOIDS (*Continued*).

629—℞ Cocain. hydrochlor., . . gr. ij.
Ex. belladonnæ, . . . ʒj.
Acid. tannici, . . . ℥ij.
Ungt. petrolati, . . . ℥j.—M.
Sig.: Apply night and morning. ALRICH.

630—℞ Ex. opii, ... gr. x.
Pulv. stramonii, . . ʒj.
Pulv. tabaci, . . . ʒss.
Ungt. simplicis, . . . ℥ss.—M.
Sig.: Use locally. SHOEMAKER.

631—℞ Ext. hamamelis fl., . . . f℥j.
Ext. hydrastis fl. . . . f℥iv.
Tr. benzoin. comp., . . . f℥iv.
Tr. belladonnæ, ... f℥j.
Ol. olivæ carbolat. (5%), q. s. ad f℥iij.—M.
Sig.: Apply frequently.
MEDICAL AND SURGICAL REPORTER.

632—℞ Atropiæ sulph., . . . gr. j.
Tr. ferri chlor., . . . gtt. xxx.
Vaseline, ... ℥j.—M.
Sig.: Apply locally. (*For internal hemorrhoids.*)
LAPLACE.

633—℞ Glycer. acid. salicylic.,
Glycer. acid. boraci., . āā f℥iv.
Acid. carbolic., . . . f℥iij.—M.
Sig.: Inject five to ten minims into each tumor.
SHUFFORD.

634—R Ferri subsulph., ... gr. iij.
Plumb. acet., ... gr. j.
Mass. hydrarg., . . . gr. ss.
Ol. theobrom., ... q. s.—M.
Ft. suppos. j.
Sig.: Introduce one morning and evening.
HORWITZ.

635—℞ Cocainæ muriat., . . gr. xx.
Morphinæ sulph., . . gr. v.
Atropiæ sulph., . . . gr. iv.
Pulv. tannin., . . . gr. xx.
Vaseline, ... ℥j.
Ol. rosæ, ... q. s.—M.
Sig.: Apply after each evacuation of bowels. Of course contents of bowels should be kept in soluble condition. MEDICAL MIRROR.

HEMORRHOIDS *(Continued).*

636—℞ Acid. gallici, . . gr. x.
    Ex. opii,
    Ex. belladonnæ, . . . ãã gr. iv.
    Ungt. simplicis, . . . ʒiv.—M.
    Sig.: Apply night and morning.   HARE.

637—℞ Chrysarobin., . . . gr. xij.
    Iodoform., ... gr. ivss.
    Ext. belladonnæ, . . gr. ix.
    Vaselin., ... ʒvjɟ.—M.
    Sig.: Apply topically.   (*External hemorrhoids.*)

638—℞ Chrysarobin., ... gr. jɟ.
    Iodoform., ... gr. ₁₀³·
    Ext. belladonnæ, . . . gr. ⅙.
    Ol. theobrom., ... gr. xxx.—M.
    Sig.: Introduce such a suppository into the bowel.
    (*For internal hemorrhoids.*)

639—℞ Pulv. opii, . . . ʒj.
    Cocain. hydrochlorat., . gr. x.
    Acid. tannic., . . . gr. vj.
    Hydrarg. chlorid. mitis, . gr. xxx.
    Ung. belladonnæ,
    Lanolin., ... ãã ʒss.--M.
    Sig.: Apply three times a day.

640—℞ Ol. amygdalæ dulcis, . . fʒij.
    Zinci oxidi, . . . ʒj.
    Bismuthi subnitrat., . . ʒj.
    Adipis benzoinat., . . ʒvj.—M.
    Ft. unguent.
    Sig.: Apply topically.

641—℞ Potass. bromid., . . . ʒiij.
    Glycerinæ, ... fʒiss.—M.
    Sig.: Apply locally to ease pain.   RINGER.

642—℞ Pulv. teucrii scordii, . . ʒij.
    Ungt. petrolei, . . . ʒj.—M.
    Sig.: Apply after each action of bowels.
        R. B. CRUICE.

643—℞ Hydrarg. chlor. mit., . . ʒij.
    Ungt. petrolei, . . . ʒj.—M.
    Sig.: Apply twice daily.   BARTLETT.

81

HEPATITIS *(See Catarrh and Biliousness).*

HERPES *(See Skin Diseases).*

HICCOUGH.

644—℞ Hydrarg. chlor. mit., . . **gr. j.**
 Sacch. lact., . . . **ℨss.—M.**
Et ft. chart. No. xii.
Sig.: One powder every hour. (*In obstinate cases*
with extreme debility.)   GERHARD.

645—℞ Pilocarpinæ muriat., . . **gr. ₃¹₈.**
 Aquæ, ... **m̃x.—M.**
Sig.: Inject hypodermically.   ORTILLE.

646—℞ Zinci valerianat., . . **gr. ix.**
 Ex. belladonnæ, . . . **gr. iij.—M.**
Et ft. pil. No. xij.
Sig.: One every six hours as required.   DANET.

647—℞ Apomorphiæ muriat., . . **gr. ₁¹₀.**
 Aquæ, ... **m̃x.—M.**
Sig.: Inject hypodermically.   RINGER.

HOOPING-COUGH *(See Whooping-Cough).*

HYDROCEPHALUS.

648—℞ Potass. iodid., . . . **ℨss–j.**
 Syr. aurant. cort., . . **fℨj.**
 Aquæ, ... ad **fℨiv.—M.**
Sig.: Teaspoonful every two hours for an infant of
six months.   J. LEWIS SMITH.

649—℞ Ungt. hydrarg., . . . **ℨj.**
Sig.: Rub into scalp and take—

650—℞ Potass. iodid., . . . **gr. xij.**
 Aq. menth. pip., . . . **fℨss.—M.**
Sig.: Teaspoonful three times a day.   HAZARD.

651—℞ Ol. tiglii, ... **m̃ij.**
 Mucil. acaciæ, . . . **fℨij.**
 Aquæ, ... **fℨj.—M.**
Sig.: Take the fourth part every four hours. (*To*
remove fluid from ventricles.)   DUNGLISON.

652—℞ Collodii cum cantharidis, . **fℨiv.**
 Sig.: Paint the back of neck every few days.
       HARTSHORNE.

HYDROCEPHALUS (Continued).

653—℞ Ungt. hydrarg. biniodid., . ℥i–iv.
    Cerati simp., . . . ℥j.—M.

Sig.: Rub into scalp every four hours. (Use in connection with the iodide of potassium.) CHRISTIE.

654—℞ Pulv. digitalis,
    Hydrarg. chlor. mit.,
    Pulv. ipecac., . . āā gr. ij.
    Sacch. alb., ... gr. x.—M.
Et ft. chart. No. xii.

Sig.: One powder every three or four hours. (*In subacute form.*) CONDIE.

HYDROTHORAX (See Dropsy).

HYPOCHONDRIA.

655—℞ Auri chloridi, . . . gr. i–iss.
    Ex. gentian., . . . gr. xv.—M.
Et ft. pil. No. xxx.

Sig.: One pill three times a day. (*In anæmic cases.*)
    BARTHOLOW.

656—℞ Potass. bromid., . . . ℥ss.
Div. in chart. No. xii.

Sig.: One powder well diluted three times a day.
    RINGER.

657—℞ Liq. potass. arsenitis, . . ♏xl.
    Tr. opii, ... f℥ss–j.
    Aq. menthæ pip., . ad f℥iiss.—M.

Sig.: Teaspoonful three times a day. (*In old people with gloomy fancies.*) LEMARE-PICQUOT.

658—℞ Mist. assafœtidæ, . . . f℥iv.

Sig.: One to two tablespoonfuls three or four times a day. BARTHOLOW.

659—℞ Spt. lavandulæ comp., . f℥ss.
    Spt. ammon. aromat., . . f℥ij.
    Mist. assafœtidæ, . . . f℥vss.—M.

Sig.: From one to three tablespoonfuls three times a day. AINSLIE.

660—℞ Tr. opii deodorat., . . f℥ss.

Sig.: Five to ten drops three times a day.
    KRAFFT-EBING.

661—℞ Zinci valerianat.,   . .   gr. xxiv.
    Div. in pil. No. xii.
    Sig.: One pill four times a day and the following
at night :—

662—℞ Chloral hydrat., .   . gr. x.
    Sodii bromid.,   .   . gr. xx.—M.
    Et ft. chart. No. i.
    Sig.: Take at bedtime.   Da Costa.

663—℞ Pulv. camphoræ,
    Ex. eucalypti,   . . āā gr. xij.—M.
    Et ft. pil. No. xii.
    Sig.: One pill every three hours.   Bartholow.

664—℞ Tr. opii deod.,   . . . f℥iss.
    Tr. castorei,   . . . f℥iiss.
    Tr. valerianat. ammon.,
    Spt. æther. comp.,   . āā f℥vj.—M.
    Sig.: Teaspoonful in water every two hours. (*For
laughing hysterics.*)   Gerhard.

665—℞ Ext. sumbul.,
    Ferri sulphat. exsic., . . āā gr. xx.
    Pulv. asafœtidæ,   . . gr. xl.
    Acid. arsenosi, . . . gr. ss.—M.
    Ft. pilulæ No. xx.
    Sig.: One or two pills thrice daily.   Goodell.

667—℞ Tr. opii, ... f℥j.
    Tr. nucis vomicæ,   . . f℥ij.—M.
    Sig.: Three drops in water three times a day. (*For
weight on the head, flushings, and hot and cold perspira-
tions.*)   Ringer.

668—℞ Ex. conii fl.,
    Ex. hyoscyami fl.,   . āā ♏vij.
    Chloral hydratis,   . . gr. x.
    Aquæ,   . . . ad f℥j.—M.
    Ft. haustus.
    Sig.: To be taken at a single dose and repeated as
required.   Madigan.

669—℞ Ex. salicis nigræ,
    Elix. simp.,   . . āā f℥j.—M.
    Sig.: Teaspoonful three times a day.
                         Hutchinson.

HYSTERIA (Continued).

670—℞ Ammon. bromidi, . . ℨij.
Spt. ammon. aromat., . fℨj.
Aquæ, ... fℨiv.—M.

Sig.: Dessertspoonful well diluted three times a day.   HARTSHORNE.

ICHTHYOSIS (See Skin Diseases).

IMPETIGO (See Skin Diseases).

IMPOTENCE.

671—℞ Zinci phosphidi, . . . gr. ij.
Confect. rosæ, . . . Əj.—M.
Ft. massa et div. in pil. No. xxiv.
Sig.: One to three pills thrice daily.

BARTHOLOW.

672—℞ Tr. cantharidis, . . gtt. vj.
Tr. ferri chlor., . . gtt. xv–xx.—M.
Sig.: Take thrice daily well diluted. H. C. WOOD.

673—℞ Ferri arsenitis, . . . gr. v.
Ergotini (aq. ext.), . . ℨss.—M.
Ft. pil. No. xxx.
Sig.: One night and morning.   BARTHOLOW.

674—℞ Ex. cannabis indicæ,
Ex. nucis vomicæ, . ãã gr. xv.
Ex. ergotæ aquosi, . . ℨj.—M.
Et ft. pil. No. xxx.
Sig.: One pill morning and evening.   DA COSTA.

675—℞ Tr. sanguinariæ, . . fℨiij.
Ex. stillingiæ fl., . . fℨv.—M.
Sig.: Fifteen or twenty drops in water three times a day.   BARTHOLOW.

676—℞ Pulv. sanguinariæ, . . gr. ij.
Ex. ergotæ, . . . Əj.—M.
Et ft. pil. No. xx.
Sig.: One pill three times a day.   S. O. POTTER.

677—℞ Ex. vanillæ fl., . . . fℨj.
Sig.: Teaspoonful at bedtime.   GERHARD.

85

INCONTINENCE OF URINE.

678—℞ Atropinæ sulphat.,   .   . gr. j.
      Aquæ, ... f℥j.—M.

Sig.: Four to eight drops in water. (*For children.*)

BARTHOLOW.

679—℞ Ext. rhus aromat. fl., .   .   . f℥ss.
      Ext. ergot. fl.,   .   .   . f℥vj.
      Ext. belladonnæ fl.,   .   . f℥ss.
      Potassii bromid.,   .   . ℥iss.
      Sodii bromid., .   .   . ℥iss.
      Strychnin. sulphat., .   . gr. ¼.
      Syr. aurantii cort.,   . q. s. ad f℥iv.—M.

Sig.: A teaspoonful for a child five or six years old.

681—℞ Strychniæ sulphat.,   .   . gr. j.
      Acid. acetic.,   .   . gtt. ij.
      Sacch. alb.,   .   . ℥ij.
      Aquæ,   .   .   . f℥ij.—M.

Sig.: Fifteen to thirty drops for a child of six to twelve years. MAGENDIE.

682—℞ Sodii benzoatis,
      Sodii salicylatis,   .   āā gr. xx.
      Ex. belladonnæ fl.,   .   . gtt. ij.
      Aq. cinnamomi,   .   . f℥ijss.—M.

Sig.: A teaspoonful four or five times daily.

WHITE.

INDIGESTION (See Dyspepsia).

INFLAMMATION—

Fever Mixtures.

683—℞ Potass. bromid.,   .   . ℈iv.
      Tr. belladonnæ,   .   . ♏xxxij.
      Tr. aconit. rad.,   .   . gtt. viij.
      Spt. ætheris nit.,   .   . f℥iij.
      Mist. potass. cit.,   q. s. ad f℥viij.—M.

Sig.: One tablespoonful every two to three hours. Keep in a cool place. WHITE.

684—℞ Morph. acetat.,   .   . gr. j.
      Sacchar. alb., .   .   . ℥ij.
      Spt. ætheris nit.,   .   . f℥ij.
      Liq. ammonii acet., .   . f℥iv.
      Aq. camphoræ,   q. s. ad f℥viij.—M.

Sig.: One tablespoonful every two to three hours.

ASHHURST.

INFLAMMATION—

Fever Mixtures (Continued).

685—℞ Morph. acetat.,   · · gr. ⅔.
     Tr. aconit.,   · · · ℥x.
     Spt. ætheris nit.,   · · f℥iij.
     Mist. potass. cit.,   q. s. ad   f℥vj.—M.

Sig.: Two teaspoonfuls every one to two hours.

Laxatives.

686—℞ Hydrarg. chlor. mit.,   · gr. iij.
     Sodii bicarb., · · · ℨj.—M.
Ft. pulv. No. xxiv.

Sig.: One powder every hour.

687—℞ Hydrarg. chlor. mit.,   · gr. iv.
     Sodii bicarb., · · · ℨj.
     Pepsinæ, · · · ℨss.—M.
Ft. pulv. No. xxiv.

Sig.: One powder every hour.

688—Add ℨij of Rochelle salts to the white paper of a Seidlitz powder, take it and follow it every two hours by ℨij of Rochelle salts until bowels move.   GOODELL.

689—℞ Syr. rhei aromat.,   · · f℥ss.
     Aquæ, · · · f℥ij.
     Magnesii sulph.,   q. s. ad   sat. sol.—M.

Sig.: A teaspoonful every hour or two until bowels move.

690—℞ Hydrarg. chlor. mit.,   · gr. j.
     Sacch. lactis, · · · ℨj.—M.
Ft. pulv. No. xii.

Sig.: One powder every one to three hours. (*For children.*)

691—℞ Pulv. glycyrrhizæ comp.,   ℥ss.

Sig.: One teaspoonful in water. Repeat every two hours if necessary.

INFLUENZA (See Catarrh and Hay Fever).

INGROWING TOE-NAIL.

692—℞ Liq. potassæ, · · · f℥ij.
     Aquæ, · · · · f℥j.—M.

Sig.: Apply with pledgets of cotton-wool.
                            NORTON.

INGROWING TOE-NAIL (Continued).

693—℞ Acid. tannic., . . . ℨj.
  Aquæ, ... f℥vj.—M.
 Sig.: Paint soft parts twice daily.   MIALL.

694—℞ Pulv. plumbi acetat., . . ℨj.
  Tr. opii, ... f℥j.
  Aquæ, . . . ad f℥viij —M.
 Sig.: Shake well and apply constantly until the inflammation is reduced; then separate the granulating surface from the nail and insert a small pledget of cotton; then use :—

695—℞ Argenti nitrat., . . . gr. xxx.
  Aquæ, ... f℥ij.—M.
 Sig.: Apply two or three times daily with a brush.
           DAVIDSON.

INSOMNIA.

696—℞ Antipyrin, ... ℨi-ij.
  Syr. aurant. cort., . . f℥j.
  Aq. cinnam., . . ad f℥iij.—M.
 Sig.: Tablespoonful every hour or two till effective.
           WILLIAMS.

697—℞ Methylal, ... ℨj.
  Syr. aurant. flor., . ad f℥iv.—M.
 Sig.: A tablespoonful at bedtime.   RICHARDSON.

698—℞ Antimonii et potass. tartrat., gr. i-ij.
  Morphiæ sulphat., . . gr. iss.
  Aq. laurocerasi, . . . f℥j.—M.
 Sig.: Teaspoonful every two, three, or four hours as required. (*In the wakefulness of fevers.*)
           BARTHOLOW.

699—℞ Atropiæ sulphat., . . gr. ¼.
  Morphiæ sulphat., . . gr. xij.
  Acid. acetic., . . . gtt. x.
  Aquæ, ... f℥iij.—M.
 Sig.: Teaspoonful once or twice daily. (*In cases of depression and low temperature.*)   GERHARD.

700—℞ Sulphonal, ... gr. xxx.
  Syrupi, ... f℥ij.
  Mucilag. acaciæ, . . . f℥ij.
  Aquæ, . . q. s. ad f℥j.—M.
 Sig.: Half to all of this at one dose, as may be required.   HARE.

701—℞ Narceinæ, ... gr. viij.
    Confect. rosæ, . . . gr. xv.—M.
  Et ft. pil. No. xxiv.
  Sig.: One to three pills at bedtime.   LABORDE.

702—℞ Ex. piscidiæ erythrin. fl., . f℥j.
    Syr. simp., . . . f℥j.
    Aq. aurant. flor., . ad f℥iv.—M.
  Sig.: From one to four teaspoonfuls at bedtime.
            PAYNE.

703—℞ Antikamniæ, . . . ℨij.
  Div. in chart. No. xii.
  Sig.: Take one powder at bedtime.   POWELL.

704—℞ Potass. bromid., . . . ℨiv.
    Chloral hydrat., . . . ℨij.
    Syr. prun. virg., . . . f℥j.
    Aquæ, ... ad f℥iij.—M.
  Sig.: Dessertspoonful in a wineglassful of water at
bedtime.

INTERMITTENT FEVER (See Fever).

INTERTRIGO (See Skin Diseases).

INTESTINAL CATARRH (See Catarrh).

INTESTINAL PARASITES (See Worms).

ITCH (See Skin Diseases.)

INTUSSUSCEPTION.

705—℞ Sodii bicarb., . . . Ɔii–iij.
    Aquæ, ... f℥vj.—M.
  Sig.: Inject into the rectum and follow at once
with—

706—℞ Acid. tartaric. pulv., . gr. xxxv–xlviij.
    Aquæ, . . . f℥iv.—M.
  Sig.: Inject immediately into the bowels after the
preceding.   BARTHOLOW.

707—℞ Ex. belladonnæ, . . . gr. iv.
    Aq. ferventis, . . . Oj.—M.
  Sig.: Inject into the rectum.   WARING.

INTUSSUSCEPTION *(Continued).*

708—℞ Tabaci, ... ʒj.
　　　Aq. bullientis, . . . Oj.
　　Macera per sextum horæ partem, et cola.
　　Sig.: Inject one-quarter or one-half, and repeat in
　　half an hour if necessary, carefully watching its
　　effect. GUY'S HOSPITAL.

709—℞ Lobeliæ, ... ʒss.
　　　Aq. bullientis, . . . Oj.—M.
　　Ft. infusum.
　　Sig.: Inject one-fourth or one-half, and repeat if
　　permissible. BARTHOLOW.

IRITIS.

710—℞ Atropinæ sulphatis, . . gr. ij.
　　　Aq. destillat., . . . fʒss.—M.
　　Sig.: One drop into each eye twice daily, continu-
　　ing for a week. KEYSER.

711—℞ Atropinæ sulphatis, . . gr. i–iij.
　　　Morphinæ sulphatis, . . gr. iv.
　　　Zinci sulphatis, . . . gr. ii–viij.
　　　Aquæ destillat., . . . fʒj.—M.
　　Sig.: Apply as a lotion. BARTHOLOW.

712—℞ Scopolinæ, ... gr. j.
　　　Aq. destillat., . . . fʒj.—M.
　　Sig.: One to three drops into the eye two or three
　　times daily. DUNN.

713—℞ Emplast. cantharidis, . . 1 in. ✕ 1 in.
　　Sig.: Apply behind the ear, and poultice when
　　blistered. HARTSHORNE.

714—℞ Hydrarg. chlor. corros., . gr. j.
　　　Potass. iodid., . . . ʒj.
　　　Tr. calumbæ, . . . fʒij.
　　　Aquæ, ... ad fʒvj.—M.
　　Sig.: A dessertspoonful in a wineglassful of water
　　two or three times a day. LAWSON.

715—℞ Ol. terebinthinæ, . . . fʒj.
　　　Mucil. acaciæ, q. s. ut ft. emul.
　　　Syr. simp., ... fʒj.
　　　Aq. menthæ pip., . . fʒiv.—M.
　　Sig.: Dessertspoonful in water three times a day.
　　　　　　　　　　　　　　　　　　　　HOGG.

IRITIS (Continued).

716—℞ Duboisiæ sulphat., . . gr. j.
   Aq. destillat., . . . f℥j.—M.
 Sig.: One drop into the eye once or twice daily.
             TWEEDY.

717—℞ Hydrarg. chlor. mit., . gr. x.
   Ex. glycyrrhizæ, . . q. s.—M.
 Et ft. pil. No. xx.
 Sig.: Two pills twice a day.   NIEMEYER.

JAUNDICE (See Biliousness, Catarrh, etc.).

JOINTS, DISEASES OF (See Synovitis).

KERATITIS, PHLYCTENULAR.

718—℞ Atropinæ sulphat., . . gr. ii–iv.
   Aq. destillat., . . . f℥j.—M.
 Sig.: One or two drops in each eye two or three
times a day.   BARTHOLOW.

719—℞ Hydrarg. chlor. corros., . gr. j.
   Aq. destillat., . . . f℥iv.—M.
 Sig.: Use as an eye-bath. GRANDMONT.

720—℞ Duboisiæ sulphat., . . gr. j.
   Aq. rosæ, ... f℥j.—M.
 Sig. One or two drops in the eye two or three
times a day.   THOMPSON.

KIDNEYS, DISEASES OF (See Albuminuria, Nephritis).

LABOR.

721—℞ Potass. bromid., . . . ℨss.
   Chloral hydrat., . . . ℈iss.
   Syr. aurant. cort., . . f℥ss.
   Aquæ, . . q. s. ad f℥ij.—M.
 Sig.: Dose, one-half of the above. (In false labor.)
            GERHARD.

722—℞ Tr. opii deod., . . gtt. xlv.
   Tr. lactucarii,
   Syr. papaveris, . . aa f℥iij.
   Aq. aurant. flor., . . f℥iss.—M.
 Sig.: Dose, the one-third part. (In protracted labor,
due to irregular, tetanic pains.) VELPEAU.

LABOR (Continued).

723—℞ Quiniæ bisulphat.,   . gr. x.
Ft. chart. No. i.
Sig.: One dose. (*In atony of the womb.*) GERHARD.

724—℞ Chloral hydrat., .   . ℨij.
Syr. aurant. cort.,   . fℨj.
Aq. aurant. flor.,   . fℨiv.—M.
Sig.: Tablespoonful every twenty minutes for three doses. PLAYFAIR.

725—℞ Chloroformi,   . . . fℨiv.
Sig.: Let patient inhale, but not to complete anæs-
thesia. SIMPSON.

726—℞ Amyl nitritis,   . . . fℨj.
Sig.: Three to five drops to be inhaled from a
handkerchief. (*In hour-glass contraction of the uterus.*)
BARNES.

727—℞ Tr. nucis vomicæ,   . . fℨj.
Ex. ergotæ fl.,   . . . fℨvj.
Elix. simp.,   . . ad fℨvj.—M.
Sig.: A teaspoonful in a wineglassful of water
every three hours. (*In retained placenta.*)
LOMBE ATTHILL.

728—℞ Morphiæ sulphat.,   . . gr. ij.
Aq. camphoræ,   . . . fℨij.—M.
Sig.: Teaspoonful every three or four hours as
required. (*For after-pains.*) WITHERSTINE.

729—℞ Morphiæ sulphat.,   . gr. i-ij.
Ol. theobromæ, .   . ℨij.—M.
Et ft. suppos. No. iv.
Sig.: One as required. (*In precipitate labor.*)
LEISHMAN.

730—℞ Quiniæ sulphat.,   . . ℈ij.
Acid. sulphuric. aromat., q. s. ut ft. sol.
Syr. zingiberis,   . . . fℨj.
Aquæ,   . . . ad fℨij.—M.
Sig.: A tablespoonful at once, and afterwards a
dessertspoonful every four hours. (*In atony of the*
uterus.) RINGER.

LARYNGISMUS STRIDULUS.

731—℞ Syr. ipecac.,   . . . fℨij.
Sig.: Teaspoonful every ten or fifteen minutes until
free emesis occurs. BARTHOLOW.

732—℞ Chloral hydrat., . . . gr. v–xv.
   Syr. simp.,
   Aq. cinnam., . . aa ℨss.—M.
  Sig.: One dose. (*To arrest impending attack.*)
                           BARTHOLOW.

733—℞ Potass. citrat., . . . ℨj.
   Syr. ipecac., . . . fℨij.
   Tr. opii deod., . . . gtt. xij.
   Syr. simp., ... fℨij.
   Aquæ, ... f℥iss.—M.
  Sig.: Teaspoonful every two hours for a child of two years.   MEIGS and PEPPER.

734—℞ Tr. aconiti rad., . . . fℨss.
  Sig.: One drop in a teaspoonful of water every hour for three or four doses ; then every two hours.
                           RINGER.

735—℞ Potass. bromid.,
   Sodii bromid., . . aa ℨj.
   Chloral hydrat., . . gr. xlviij.
   Syr. simp., . . . f℥j.
   Aq. cinnam., . q. s. ad f℥iij.—M.
  Sig.: Teaspoonful every half hour or hour as required.   POWELL.

736—℞ Tr. moschi, ... fℨss.
   Tr. belladonnæ, . . . ♏xv.
   Aq. lauro-cerasi, . . . fℨiij.
   Syr. aurantii, ... f℥j.
   Aq. lactucarii, ... f℥iv.—M.
  Sig.: A tablespoonful twice a day.

LARYNGITIS.

737—℞ Tr. aconiti rad., . . . fℨss.
  Sig.: One drop every hour, in water. Best results when following a dose of castor oil. When it has existed several days give—

738—℞ Tr. aconiti, ... gtt. xij.
   Sodii bromid. . . . . ℨij.
   Syr. lactucarii, . . . f℥j.
   Aquæ, . . . q. s. ad f℥iij.—M.
  Sig.: A teaspoonful every four hours. (*Acute form.*)

739—℞ Tr. pulsatillæ, . . . fℨj.
   Syr. ipecac., . . . f℥j.
   Liq. potass. citrat., . . fℨv.—M.
  Sig.: Tablespoonful every three hours. GERHARD.

740—℞ Argenti nitrat., . . . gr. lx.
    Aquæ, ... f℥j.—M.
Sig.: Apply locally on cotton ; then immediately apply the following :—

741—℞ Cocaine muriat. (10 per cent. sol.),
                              f℥j.
Sig.: Apply locally to the larynx. (*Chronic form.*)
                                   SEILER.

742—℞ Hydrarg. cyanidi, . . gr. ij.
    Sacch. lact., . . . gr. xv.
    Mucil. acaciæ, . . . q. s.—M.
Et div. in pil. No. xx.
Sig.: One pill twice daily. (*Syphilitic form.*)
                               M. MACKENZIE.

743—℞ Potassii permanganitis, . gr. ij.
    Aq. destillat., . . . f℥ij.—M.
Sig.: Use with an atomizer several times daily.
(*Fœtid chronic form.*)   SAJOUS.

744—℞ Hydrarg. chlor. corros., . gr. i–ij.
    Aquæ, ... f℥ij.—M.
Sig.: Inhale from an atomizer several times a day.
(*In syphilitic form.*)   DEMARQUAY.

745—℞ Acid. benzoic., . . gr. ss.
    Sodii biborat., . . gr. iss.
    Acaciæ, . . . q. s.—M.
Et ft. trochiscum No. i.
Sig.: One every hour. (*In acute laryngitis.*)
                                SAJOUS.

746—℞ Iodol, ... ℥j.
Sig.: Insufflate a small portion once a day, or several times a week. (*In tuberculous laryngitis.*)
                                LUBLINSKI

747—℞ Menthol, ... gr. xxv–c.
    Ol. olivæ, ... f℥j —M.
Sig.: Apply locally to the ulcerations. (*In tuberculous laryngitis.*)   ROSENBERG.

748—℞ Acid. carbolici, . . . ♏xv–♏lxxx.
    Acid. lactici, . . . ℨss–ℨiv.
    Glycerini pur., . . . f℥v.—M.
Sig.: Apply topically after anesthetizing the larynx with a 10 per cent. solution of cocain.

LEAD-POISONING (See Colic).

LEPRA (See Skin Diseases).

LEUCOCYTHÆMIA.

749—℞ Sodii arsenitis, . . . gr. j.
Div. in pil. No. xl.
Sig.: One pill three times a day. And:—

750—℞ Iodi, ... ℈j.
Ol. bergami, . . . gtt. j.
Lanolin, ... ℥j.—M.
Sig.: Rub over the spleen at night. DA COSTA.

751—℞ Quiniæ sulphat., . . . ℥j.
Ferri sulphat. exsiccat., . ℥iss.—M.
Et ft. pil. No. xxx.
Sig.: Four or five pills daily. BARTHOLOW.

752—℞ Ol. eucalypti, . . . gtt. c.
Piperini,
Ceræ albæ, . . āā ℥j.
Pulv. althææ, . . ℥ij.—M.
Et ft. pil. No. c.
Sig.: Three to five pills three times a day.
MOSLER.

753—℞ Acid. arseniosi, . . gr. j.
Pil. ferri carbonatis,
Quinidiæ sulphat., . āā ℥j.—M.
Et ft. pil. No. xl.
Sig.: Two pills three times a day. DA COSTA.

LEUCORRHŒA.

754—℞ Sodii bicarb., . . . ℥j.
Tr. belladonnæ, . . . f℥ij.
Aquæ, ... Oj.—M.
Sig.: Use as a vaginal wash. RINGER.

755—℞ Creolin, ... gtt. xxx.
Ex. hydrastis fl., . . f℥iss.—M.
Sig.: Two teaspoonfuls in a pint of warm water,
to be used for one vaginal injection.
JOURNAL DE MÉDECINE, PARIS.

756—℞ Potass. chlorat., . . . ℥ij.
Sig.: A teaspoonful to a pint of warm water, as a
vaginal injection. (In simple cases.) PARVIN.

95

757—℞ Acid. boracic., . . . ℥vj.
Aq. ferventes, . . . Oj.—M.

Sig.: Use as a vaginal injection. RINGER.

758—℞ Sulpho-calcine, . . . ℥vj.
Glycerinæ, ... f℥j.
Menthol, ... gr. xx.—M.

Sig.: Tablespoonful in a quart of hot water, used twice a day as a vaginal injection. DIXON.

759—℞ Acid. salicylic,
Acid. thymic, . . āā ℨss.
Ess. amber, ... gtt. xx.
Alcoholis, 90°, . . . f℥viss.
Cologne, ... f℥iss.
Aq. destillat., . . . f℥ix.—M.

Sig. A tablespoonful of this mixture is put into about a quart of water, and it is used as an injection three or four times daily, in order to suppress the fœtidity of the discharge. PRESSE MÉDICALE BELGE.

760—℞ Liq. sodæ chlorinat., . . f℥ij.
Aquæ, ... f℥xx.—M.

Sig.: Use as an injection once or twice daily.
TROUSSEAU.

761—℞ Acid. tannic., . . . ℥iv.
Glycerinæ, ... f℥xvj.—M.

Sig.: Tablespoonful to a quart of tepid water as a vaginal injection night and morning.
T. GAILLARD THOMAS.

762—℞ Potass. chlorat., . . . ℨiij.
Tr. opii, ... f℥iiss.
Aq. picis, ... f℥ix.—M.

Sig.: From one to two tablespoonfuls to a quart of hot water as an injection twice daily. CHÉRON.

763—℞ Creasoti, ... ♏xij.
Mucil. tragacanth., . . ℥ij.
Aquæ ferventis, . . . f℥xiv.—M.

Sig.: After washing out the vagina with warm water use the injection. MACKENZIE.

764—℞ Pulv. catechu,
Aluminis, . . . āā ℨj.
Ol. theobrom., . . . q. s.—M.

Et ft. suppos. vaginalis No. vi.
Sig.: Use one night and morning. HAZARD.

LEUCORRHŒA *(Continued)*.

765—℞ Iodoformi, ... ʒj.
Acid. tannic., . . . ʒj.—M.

Sig.: Pack a sufficient quantity in the dry state
around the cervix uteri. BARTHOLOW.

766—℞ Potass. permanganitis, . gr. xx.
Aquæ, ... Oj.—M.

Sig.: Inject a small quantity several times a day.
(*In fœtid discharges.*) GIRWOOD.

767—℞ Ex. yerbæ santæ fl.,
Ex. pinus canaden. fl.,
Ex. hamamelis fl., . āā fʒiv.
Glycerinæ, . . q. s. ad fʒv.—M.

Sig.: Teaspoonful four times a day. BIXBY.

768—℞ Zinci sulphatis,
Aluminis sulphatis, . āā ʒiss.
Glycerinæ, ... fʒvj.—M.

Sig.: Tablespoonful to a quart of hot water, as an
injection. T. GAILLARD THOMAS.

LICE.

769—℞ Sodii hyposulphitis, . . ʒij.
Acid. sulphurosi dil., . . fʒiv.
Aquæ, . . . q. s. ad fʒxvi.—M.

Sig.: Apply once daily. (*Head lice.*) STARTIN.

770—℞ Hydrarg. chlor. corros., . gr. iv.
Spt. vini rectificat., . . fʒvj.
Ammon. muriat., . . ʒss.
Aq. rosæ, . . q. s. ad fʒvj.—M.

Sig.: For scabies and tinea versicolor.
TILBURY FOX.

771—℞ Sulphur. sublim., . . . ʒij.
Potassii subcarbonat., . . ʒj.
Adipis simplicis, . . . ʒvij.—M.

Sig.: Apply night and morning. (*For scabies.*)

772—℞ β naphthol, ... gr. xl.
Sulph. præcip., ... gr. lxxx.
Styracis,
Pulv. rad. pyrethri, . . āā ʒss.
Adipis, ... ʒiss.—M.

Sig.: Rub into affected areas once daily for three
days. (*For scabies.*)

LICE (Continued).

773—℞ Hydrarg. oleat., . . . gr. v.
    Acid. oleici, ... gr. xcv.
    Ætheris, ... gtt. xij.—M.
    Sig.: Apply twice, twenty-four hours apart.
                        JOHN MARSHALL.

774—℞ Acid. carbolic., . . . f℥i–ij.
    Glycerinæ, ... f℥j.
    Aquæ, ... f℥viij.—M.
    Sig.: Apply as a wash. (*To destroy lice or relieve pruritus.*)   HARTSHORNE.

775—℞ Ol. rosmarini, . . . f℥ss.
    Ol. olivæ, ... f℥iss.—M.
    Sig.: Apply once daily.   RINGER.

LICHEN (See Skin Diseases).

LIVER, DISEASES OF (See Biliousness, Colic, Catarrh).

LOCOMOTOR ATAXIA.

776—℞ Argent. nitrat., . . gr. x.
    Confect. rosæ, . . Ɗj.—M.
    Et ft. pil. No. xl.
    Sig.: One or two pills three times a day. Cease giving after a few weeks, to prevent argyria.
                        DA COSTA.

777—℞ Strychniæ sulph., . . gr. iss.
    Syr. hypophos., . . f℥xij.—M.
    Sig.: Teaspoonful in water three times a day. (*When the system is saturated with silver.*)   DA COSTA.

778—℞ Ex. physostigmat., . . gr. x.
    Pulv. zingiberis, . . . Ɗj.—M.
    Et ft. pil. No. xii.
    Sig.: One pill three times a day.   RINGER.

779—℞ Antipyrin, ... ℥j.
    Syr. zingiber., . . . f℥j.
    Aquæ, ... ad f℥iv.—M.
    Sig.: A teaspoonful every one to four hours for three to six doses. (*In lightning pains.*)
                      GERMAIN SÉE.

LUMBAGO.

780—℞ Methyl chloridi, . . . ℥ss.
    Sig.: Use locally, applying carefully.   DEBOVE.

781—℞ Potass. iodid., . . . ℨij.
Vini colchici sem., . . f℥j.
Syr. zingiber., . . . f℥iss.
Aquæ, . . . q. s. ad f℥iv.—M.
Sig.: Dessertspoonful every three hours.

GERHARD.

782—℞ Potass. iodid.,
Potass. carbonat., . ãã ℨj.
Tr. aconiti rad., . . . f℥ij.
Aquæ, ... f℥x.—M.
Sig.: Use locally every three hours. (*Mark poison.*)

ERICHSEN.

783—℞ Ex. cimicifugæ fl.,
Syr. acaciæ, . . . ãã f℥ss.
Aq. amygdalæ amar., . . f℥iij.—M.
Sig.: Teaspoonful every three hours. BARTLETT.

784—℞ Atropinæ sulphatis, . . gr. j.
Morphinæ sulphatis, . . gr. xvj.
Aq. destillat., . . . f℥j.—M.
Sig.: Five minims injected deeply into muscles of the back.

785—℞ Antipyrin, ... ℨj.
Syr. tolutani, . . . f℥j.
Aq. menthæ pip., q. s. ad f℥iv.—M.
Sig.: A teaspoonful every one to four hours for three to six doses. GERMAIN SÉE.

786—℞ Tr. iodi., ... f℥ij.
Tr. aconitii rad., . . f℥iij.
Chloroformi, . . . f℥iv.
Liniment. sapon. comp., .
q. s. ad f℥iij.—M.
Sig.: Apply every few hours locally.

BELLEVUE HOSPITAL, N. Y.

787—℞ Potass. iodidi, . . . ℨss.
Tr. opii deodorat., . . f℥ij.
Spts. lavandulæ comp., . f℥j.
Spts. æth. nit., . . . f℥ss.
Aq. destillat., . . . f℥xij.—M.
Sig.: Take two tablespoonfuls twice daily.

BRODIE.

788—℞ Chloroformi, . . . f℥ij.—M.
Sig.: Twenty minims injected deeply in region of pain.

LUMBAGO (*Continued*).

789—℞ Sodii salicylat., ... ℥ss.
    Potassii iodid., ... ℨij.
    Syr. sarsaparillæ comp., . . f℥iss.
    Aquæ, ... q. s. f℥iij.—M.
    Sig.: A teaspoonful in water thrice daily, after
meals.   S. SOLIS-COHEN.

LUPUS.

790—℞ Hydrargyri oleatis (2½–5 per
    cent.), ... ℨj.
    Acidi salicylici, . . . gr. x-xv.
    Ichthyolis, ... ♏xv.
    Ol. lavandulæ, vel
    Ol. citronellæ, . . . q. s.—M.
    Sig.: Rub in ten minutes in the morning and
twenty minutes in the evening. MR. H. G. BROOKE.

791—℞ Zinci chloridi, . . . ℨj.
    Morph. sulph., . . . gr. ss.
    Pulv. acaciæ, . . . ℨiij.
    Sig.: Make into a paste by adding a few drops of
water or alcohol and spread a thin layer over and
just beyond the ulcer. Use carefully. AGNEW.

792—℞ Ichthyol., ... ℨj.
    Adipis benzoat., . . . ℨv.—M.
    Sig.: Apply over affected part. HARE.

793—℞ Tr. iodi., ... fℨij.
    Sig.: Paint around the growth; apply to retard
its spread over the surface also.

794—℞ Liq. hydrargyri nit., . . fℨj.
    Sig.: Use with a glass rod until growth is on a
level with the skin; use carefully, protecting surrounding parts with lard or oil. MARTIN.

795—℞ Acidi pyrogallici, . . ℨj.
    Cerati simplicis, . . . ℨix.—M.
    Sig.: Apply locally. (*For lupus of eyelids and skin.*)
            KAPOSI.

796—℞ Resorcin, ... ℨiiss.
    Vaselini, ... ℨiv.—M.
    Sig.: Apply locally. BERTARELLI.

LUPUS (Continued).

797—℞ Acid. chromici,   . . gr. c.
    Aquæ, ... f℥j.—M.
  Sig.: Apply locally.   BARTHOLOW.

798—℞ Acid. arseniosi,   . . . ℈j.
    Hydrarg. sulphuret. rub., . ℨj.
    Ungt. simplicis, . . . ℥j.—M.
  Sig.: Spread thickly on cloth, and apply to the
patch for two or three days, until the lupus nodules
and points are blackish and destroyed.   HEDRA.

799—℞ Acid. lactic puri, .   . . f℥j.
  Sig.: Soak a pledget of absorbent cotton and apply
to the ulcer. Cover with oiled silk and bandage.
Protect normal tissue with grease.   WICHMANN.

800—℞ Sat. sol. cocaini muriat.,   . f℥ij.
  Sig.: Apply locally.   FOWLER.

MALARIA (See Fever).

MAMMARY INFLAMMATION (See also Abscesses).

801—℞ Morph. sulph., . . . gr. x.
    Hydrarg. oleat., . . . ℨss.
    Acidi oleici, . . . ℥ixss.—M.
  Sig.: Anoint three times a day.   MARSHALL.

802—℞ Ex. belladonnæ, . . . ℨj.
    Liq. plumbi subacetat. dil., . Oj.—M.
  Sig.: Use as a lotion.   GRAEFE.

803—A tablespoonful of granular effervescent citrate
   of magnesia in water, followed by ten grains
   of quinine if there · be fever. (In incipient
   mammitis.)   STARR.

804—℞ Cerati resinæ co., . . ℨj.
    Olei olivæ, . . . ℨi–ij.—M.
  Ft. ungt.
  Sig.: Apply, spread generously on a soft rag.
(When suppuration is threatened.)   WITHERSTINE.

805—℞ Hydrarg. chlor. mit.,
    Pulv. jalapæ, . . āā gr. x.—M.
  Et ft. chart. No. i.
  Sig.: Take at once. (Brisk purge for incipient mas-
titis.)   RUSH.

806—℞ Atropinæ sulphat.,   . . gr. viij.
       Aq. rosæ, ... f℥ij.—M.
  Sig.: Apply locally, but discontinue in case of dilatation of pupils or dryness of throat.   STARR.

807—℞ Lini camphoræ, . . . f℥viij.
  Sig.: Apply locally. (*In incipient mastitis.*)
                                     PARRY.

808—℞ Pulv. camphoræ, . . . ℥j.
  Sig.: Dampen two pads of oakum and mix with the camphor, and apply under a tight body.
                                GERUARD.

809—℞ Tr. belladonnæ, . . . f℥ij.
       Lini saponis camphorat., . f℥viij.—M.
  Sig.: Use locally.   NELIGAN.

810—℞ Ammon. carbonat., . . ℥j.
       Aquæ, ... Oj.—M.
  Sig.: Apply locally.   STARR.

811—℞ Ungt. belladonnæ, . . ℥j.
       Pulv. camphoræ, . . . ℥j.—M.
  Sig.: Apply locally, supporting the breast with a bandage.   WITHERSTINE.

MANIA, ACUTE.

812—℞ Ex. gelsemii fl., . . . f℥iv–viij.
       Syr. limonis, . . . f℥j.
       Aquæ, ... ad f ℥iij.—M.
  Sig.: Teaspoonful two or three times a day; increase the dose until the pupils dilate and eyelids droop.   BARTHOLOW.

813—℞ Paraldehyde, . . . f℥ss.
  Sig.: Thirty to fifty minims in water by the rectum.   RINGER.

814—℞ Hyoscyami sulphat., . . gr. j.
       Aquæ, ... f℥xij.—M.
  Sig.: Five to twelve minims hypodermically.
       WARD'S ISLAND INSANE ASYLUM, N. Y.

815—℞ Potass. bromid., . . . gr. xxv.
       Tr. hyoscyami, . . . f℥ss.
       Spt. chloroform., . . . ♏x.
       Aquæ, . . . q. s. ad f℥iss.—M.
  Sig.: Take at once.   TYLER SMITH.

816—℞ Potass. bromid., . . . ℨj.
  Tr. cannabis indicæ, . . fℨj.
  Syr. simp., ... fℨij.
  Aquæ, . . . q. s. ad fℨiv.—M.

Sig.: Tablespoonful, well diluted, three times a day. (*In periodical and senile mania.*) CLOUSTON.

817—℞ Chloral hydrat., . . . gr. xxv.
  Tr. cardamom. comp., . . fℨss.
  Syr. simp., ... fℨij.
  Infus. caryophylli, q. s. ad fℨiss.—M.

Sig.: Take at once and repeat dose in an hour if necessary. PRIESTLEY.

818—℞ Coninæ, ... gr. ij.
  Spt. rectif., ... fℨss.
  Aquæ, . . q. s. ad fℨss.—M.

Sig.: Dose, a teaspoonful. FRONMUELLER

819—℞ Methylal, ... ℨij.
  Syr. aurant. cort., . . fℨij.
  Aquæ, . . . ad fℨiv.—M.

Sig.: From a teaspoonful to a tablespoonful, to be repeated if necessary.

820—℞ Ex. conii fl.,
  Ex. hyoscyami fl., . āā ℳvij.
  Chloral hydrat., . . . gr. x.
  Aquæ, ... fℨij.—M.

Sig.: To be taken at one dose, and repeated if necessary. MADIGAN.

MANIA, CHRONIC.

821—℞ Caffeinæ citrat., . . . ℨss.
  Syr. acid. citrici, . . fℨss.
  Aquæ, ... fℨiss.—M.

Sig.: Teaspoonful three or four times a day.
  BARTHOLOW.

822—℞ Tr. ferri chlor.,
  Tr. nucis vomicæ, . āā fℨj.
  Aquæ, . . q. s. ad fℨvj.—M.

Sig.: Teaspoonful three times a day, after meals.
  WARD'S ISLAND INSANE ASYLUM, N. Y.

823—℞ Tr. ferri chlor., . . . fℨij.
  Spt. æther. nitro., . . fℨss.
  Infus. quassiæ, . q. s. ad fℨvj.—M.

Sig.: Tablespoonful three times a day. TUKE.

MANIA, CHRONIC (Continued).

824—℞ Ex. ergotæ fl., . . . f℥iss.
Syr. aurant. cort., . . f℥j.
Aquæ, . . . ad f℥vj.—M.

Sig.: Tablespoonful in water three or four times a
day. CRICHTON BROWNE.

825—℞ Tr. ferri chlor., . . . f℥ij.
Syr. zingiber., . . . f℥j.
Aquæ, . . . ad f℥viij.—M.

Sig.: Tablespoonful three or four times a day. (In
anæmic cases.) BUCKNILL.

MANIA, PUERPERAL.

826—℞ Ex. cimicifugæ fl., . . f℥iss.
Mucil. acaciæ, . . . f℥j.
Aquæ, ... f℥iiiss.—M.

Sig.: Tablespoonful every three hours. RINGER.

827—℞ Potass. bromid., . . . ℨij.
Chloral hydrat., . . ℥ss.
Syr. aurant. cort., . . f℥j.
Aq. fœniculi, . q. s. ad f℥vj.—M.

Sig.: Tablespoonful every two hours. QUAIN.

MARASMUS.

828—℞ Emul. ol. morrhuæ et lactophos. calcis, . . . f℥iij.

Sig.: From one-half to one teaspoonful three times
a day. STARR.

829—℞ Syr. ferri iodid., . . f℥j.

Sig.: Three to five drops in water three times a
day, after meals. EUSTACE SMITH.

830—℞ Tr. cinchonæ comp.,
Tr. gentian. comp., . āā f℥j.—M.

Sig.: Fifteen drops to a teaspoonful in water, three
times a day. J. LEWIS SMITH.

831—℞ Syr. ferri iodid., . . . f℥ij.
Maltini, ... f℥iij.—M.

Sig.: From one-half to a teaspoonful three times a
day. POWELL.

MARASMUS (Continued).

832—℞ Pepsinæ sacch., . . . ℨj.
Div. in chart. No. xii.
Sig.: One powder after each feeding. BARTHEZ.

833—℞ Ol. morrhuæ, . . f℥ij.
Sig.: One teaspoonful for inunction.
WITHERSTINE.

834—℞ Pepsinæ pulv., . . . gr. xij.
Sodii bicarb., . . . gr. xxiv.
Pulv. aromat., . . . gr. iij.—M.
Et ft. chart. No. xii.
Sig.: One powder after each feeding. POWELL.

MEASLES (See Fever).

MELANCHOLIA (See also Hypochondria).

835—℞ Camphoræ,
Ex. hyoscyami, . . āā ℈iss.—M.
Et ft. pil. No. xl.
Sig.: Two pills three times a day. GOOCH.

836—℞ Moschi opt., . . . ℨiij.
Tr. castorei, . . . f℥iss.
Syr. zingiber., . . . f℥j.
Aquæ, . . q. s. ad f℥vj.—M.
Sig.: Dessertspoonful three or four times a day.
E. J. CLARK.

837—℞ Tr. ferri chlor.,
Syr. simp., . . āā f℥j.—M.
Sig.: Twenty or thirty drops, well diluted, three
times a day. BARTHOLOW.

838—℞ Zinci valerianat.,
Ferri valerianat.,
Quiniæ valerianat., . āā ℈j.—M.
Et ft. pil. No. xx.
Sig.: One pill three times daily. WITHERSTINE.

839—℞ Potass. bromid., . . . ℨij.
Tr. calumbæ, . . . f℥iij.
Spt. ammon. aromat., . f℥ij.
Aq. cinnam., . . . f℥iij.
Aquæ, . . q. s. ad f℥viij.—M.
Sig.: Wineglassful two or three times a day.
LAWRENCE.

840—℞ Sodii brom.,
 Chloral hydrat., . . āā ʒj.
 Syr. auraut. cort., . . fʒj.
 Aquæ, . . q. s. ad f℥iij.—M.
 Sig.: Dessertspoonful well diluted every hour until
excitement abates.   HERMANN.

841—℞ Tr. opii deod.,
 Ex. gelsemii fl., . . āā fʒj.
 Syr. limonis, . . . fʒij.
 Aq. fœniculi, . . . f℥iss.—M.
 Sig.: Teaspoonful every two hours.   BARTHOLOW.

842—℞ Hydrarg. chlor. mit., . . gr. iij.
 Sacch. lact., . . . ʒss.—M.
 Et ft. chart. No. xii.
 Sig.: One powder every two hours.   GERHARD.

843—℞ Morphiæ sulphat., . . gr. ij.
 Aquæ, ... fʒj.—M.
 Sig.: Five minims hypodermically every three to
five hours. (*In cerebro-spinal form.*)   LEYDEN.

844—℞ Tr. aconiti rad., . . . fʒij.
 Tr. opii deod., . . . fʒv.—M.
 Sig.: Seven drops in water every two hours during
the stage of excitement. (*Cerebro-spinal form.*)
           BARTHOLOW.

845—℞ Hydrarg. chlor. mit.,
 Pulv. jalapæ,
 Sacch. alb., . . āā ʒj.—M.
 Et div. in chart. No. v.
 Sig.: A powder every hour until free purgation
occurs. (*In cerebro-spinal meningitis.*)   KOHERT.

846—℞ Pulv. opii, ... gr. ij.
 Pulv. acaciæ, . . . gr. iv.
 Sacch. alb., . . . gr. xv.—M.
 Div. in chart. No. x.
 Sig.: One every hour until narcotism is produced.
   GAZETTE MÉDICALE DE MONTRÉAL.

847—℞ Potass. bromid., . . . ℥ss.
 Syr. simp., ... f℥ss.
 Aquæ, ... f℥j.—M.
 Sig.: Teaspoonful well diluted every two hours.
(*In after remaining convulsions.*)   RINGER.

MENINGITIS (Continued).

848—℞ Tr. aconit. rad., . . . ♏xlviij.
Tr. opii deod., . . . f℥ij.
Syr. simp., ... f℥vj.
Aquæ, . . q. s. ad f℥ij.—M.
Sig.: Teaspoonful every two hours in water.
(*Before effusion has taken place*)   GERHARD.

849—℞ Acid. tannici, . . . ℨj.
Div. in capsulas No. xx
Sig.: One capsule every three hours, with ice to
the head. (*In simple meningitis.*)   LARDIER.

MENINGITIS, CEREBRO-SPINAL (See Meningitis).

MENORRHAGIA.

850—℞ Ex. ergotæ, ... ℨiss.
Acid. salicylic., . . . gr. viij.
Aq. cinnam., . . . f℥vj.
Syr. cort. aurant. amar.,
Spt. juniperi, . . āā f℥ss.—M.
Sig.: Tablespoonful three times a day.
                ROKITANSKY.

851—℞ Ex. geranii maculat. fl., . f℥iv.
Sig.: Teaspoonful every hour for a few doses; then
every three or four hours.   SHOEMAKER.

852—℞ Ergot. dialysat., . . . f℥x.
Glycerinæ, ... f℥v.
Acid. salicylic., . . . gr. xxx.
Aq. destillat., . . . f℥iiss.—M.
Sig.: Inject into the rectum once a day a teaspoon-
ful of this mixture diluted with three teaspoonfuls
of water. AMERICAN PRACTITIONER AND NEWS.

853—℞ Ex. ipecac. fl.,
Ex. digitalis fl., . . āā f℥ij.
Ex. ergotæ fl., . . . f℥ss.—M.
Sig.: One-half to one teaspoonful at a dose, as re-
quired.   BARTHOLOW.

854—℞ Acid. gallici, . . . ℨss.
Acid. sulphuric. dil.,
Tr. opii deod., . . āā f℥j.
Infus. rosæ comp., . . f℥iv.—M.
Sig.: Tablespoonful every four hours or oftener.
                BARTHOLOW.

MENORRHAGIA *(Continued).*

855—℞ Tr. sabinæ, ... f℥ss.

Sig.: Five to ten drops in water every half to three hours. Phillips.

856—℞ Tr. ferri chlor., . . . f℥iss.
Acid. phosphoric. dil., . . f℥iiss.
Syr. limonis, . q. s. ad f℥iv.—M.

Sig.: Dessertspoonful three times a day, well diluted. *(In anæmic cases.)* Gerhard.

857—℞ Ex. gossypii fl.,
Syr. simp., . . . āā f℥j.—M.

Sig.: Teaspoonful every four hours. Parvin.

858—℞ Acid. gallici, . . . gr. xv.
Acid. sulphuric. aromat., . ♏xv.
Tr. cinnam., . . . f℥ij.
Aquæ, ... f℥ij.—M.

Sig.: One dose. Take every four hours until bleeding ceases. *(In profuse bleeding.)* Hazard.

859—℞ Acid. gallici, . . . gr. ij.
Ex. maticæ, . . . gr. j.
Ex. opii, ... gr. ss.—M.
Et ft. pil. No. i.

Sig.: Take three or four pills during the day.
Tilt.

860—℞ Tr. hamamelis, . . . f℥ij.

Sig.: One-half to one teaspoonful three times a day. Ringer.

861—℞ Ex. Rhois aromat. fl., . . f℥j.

Sig.: Fifteen to sixty minims three times a day.
Unna.

MERCURIALISM *(See Ptyalism).*

METRITIS.

862—℞ Tr. aconit. rad., . . . gtt. xvj.
Ex. gelsemii fl., . . . f℥j.
Ex. ergotæ fl., . . ad f℥j.—M.

Sig.: Teaspoonful every two to six hours. *(Also in uterine tumor.)* Bartholow.

863—℞ Tr. iodinii comp., . . f℥j.—M.

Sig.: Use on a probe wrapped with absorbent cotton once or twice a week and place a glycerin tampon against the cervix. In the interval let patient use hot water as a vaginal injection twice a day. T. G. Thomas.

MIGRAINE (See Headache and Neuralgia).

MITRAL DISEASE (See Heart Disease).

MORNING SICKNESS (See also Vomiting).

864—℞ Vini ipecac.,   . . . f℥j.
    Sig.: One drop every hour with the following :—

865—℞ Pepsinæ sacch.,   . . . ℨj.
    Div. in chart. No. xii.
    Sig.: One powder every two hours.   BAER.

866—℞ Cocaini hydrochlor.,   . . gr. j.
    Aquæ, ... f℥j.—M.
    Sig.: Teaspoonful three times daily before meals.
                              PARVIN.

867—℞ Tr. nucis vomicæ,   . . f℥ss.
    Sig.: One drop every hour or two in water.
                              RINGER.

868—℞ Liq. calcis,
    Aq. cinnam.,   . . āā f℥ij.—M.
    Sig.: Dessertspoonful in ice-water when required.
                              STARR.

869—℞ Cerii oxalat.,   . . gr. xxiv.
    Ex. hyoscyami, . . gr. xxxvj.—M.
    Et ft. pil. No. xii.
    Sig. One pill twice a day.   GOODELL.

870—℞ Bismuth. subnit.,   . . ℨij.
    Div. in pulv. No. xii.
    Sig.: A powder three times a day before meals.
                              CAZEAUX.

871—℞ Tr. cantharidis,
    Tr. ferri chlor., . . āā f℥j.—M.
    Sig.: Twenty-five drops, well diluted, three times
  a day.   HIGGINS.

872—℞ Cerii oxalat.,
    Bismuth. subcarb.,
    Pepsinæ,   . . . āā ℨj.—M
    Et ft. pil. No. xxiv.
    Sig.: Two pills three times a day.   WHITE.

873—℞ Cupri sulphat.,   . . . gr. ij.
    Aquæ, ... f℥ss.—M.
    Sig.: Six drops three times a day.   BARTHOLOW.

MUMPS (*See also* **Fever**).

874—℞ Ichthyol.,
  Plumbi iodidi, . . . āā gr. xlv.
  Ammon. chloridi, . . . gr. xxx.
  Adipis, ... ℥j.—M.
 Sig.: Apply twice a day.

875—℞ Tr. belladonnæ,
  Tr. opii,
  Ætheris, . . . āā f℥j.
  Liniment. saponis, . . f℥iij.—M.
 Sig.: Use locally.   HAZARD.

876—℞ Magnesii sulph., . . . ℥iv.
  Aq. puræ, ... f℥iv.
  Antimonii et potass. tart., . gr. j.
  Spt. æth. nit., . . . f℥iij.
  Sacch. alb., . . . f℥vj.—M.
 Sig.: Teaspoonful every three hours, after the bowels have been well moved. Flaxseed poultices locally.   CONDIE.

MYALGIA.

877—℞ Ungt. iodi. comp.,
  Ungt. belladonnæ, . āā ℥j.—M.
 Sig.: Rub in twice a day and apply heat.

878—℞ Liniment. chloroformi, . f℥iij.
  Tr. iodinii,
  Tr. aconit. rad., . . āā f℥ij.
  Tr. opii, . . . f℥ss.—M.
 Sig.: Use externally.

879—℞ Ammon. chlor., . . ℥j.
  Ex. cimicifugæ, . . f℥ij.
  Syr. acaciæ,
  Aq. laurocerasi, . āā f℥j.—M.
 Sig.: Teaspoonful three or four times a day.
        ANSTIE.

880—℞ Ex. xanthoxyli fl., . . f℥j.
 Sig.: From fifteen minims to two drachms.
        BARTHOLOW.

NÆVUS.

881—℞ Creasoti, . . . f℥ss.
 Sig.: Paint the parts daily.   WARING.

882—Electrolysis, or galvano-cautery is useful.

NÆVUS (Continued).

883—℞ Acid. chromici, . . . **gr. c.**
    Aquæ, ... **f℥j.—M.**
  Sig.: Apply locally.   BARTHOLOW.

NECROSIS (See Caries).

NEPHRITIS (See also Albuminuria).

884—℞ Tr. ferri chlor., . . . **f℥iij.**
    Acid. acetici dil., . . **f℥iss.**
    Syr. simp., ... **f℥ss.**
    Liq. ammon. acetat., q. s. ad **f℥iv.—M.**
  Sig.: Dessertspoonful every three or four hours.
                        BASHAM.

885—℞ Pulv. jalapæ comp., . . **℥j.**
    Div. in chart. No. xii.
  Sig.: One powder every four hours until catharsis
occurs. To be given after the patient has been rolled
in blankets wrung out of hot water. (*In acute
nephritis.*)   FOTHERGILL.

886—℞ Potass. bitartratis, . . **℥ij.**
    Aq. ferventis, . . . **Oij.**
    Corticis limonis,
    Sacch., . . . āā q. s. ad concilian-
                         dum gustum.
  Sig.: Use *ad libitum.*   JOY.

887—℞ Tr. ferri chlor., . . . **♏x.**
    Syr. limonis, . . . **♏j.**
    Aquæ, ... **f℥ij.—M.**
  Sig.: Take three times daily in a wineglassful of
water.   DA COSTA.

888—℞ Potass. tartratis, . . **℥j.**
    Potass. nitratis, . . . **℥ss.**
    Mannæ opt., . . . **℥j.**
    Decoct. taraxaci, . . **f℥vj.—M.**
  Sig.: Tablespoonful every hour or two.   PHŒBUS.

889—℞ Sodii iodid., . . . **gr. xv.**
    Sodii phosphatis, . . **gr. xxx.**
    Sodii chlor., . . . **gr. xc.—M.**
  Sig.: Dissolve in water, and give in the course of
the twenty-four hours, either alone or in milk.
                      SEMMOLA.

890—℞ Pulv. scillæ,
 Pulv. digitalis, .   āā gr. ⅓.
 Ex. gentian., .   . gr. j.—M.
Et ft. pil. No. i.
Sig.: One pill three times a day.   STEWART.

891—℞ Camphoræ, ... gr. v.
 Lanolini,
 Ungt. belladonnæ, . āā ʒss.—M.
Sig.: Apply to the abdomen. (*For tympany occurring in chronic Bright's disease, and due to peritoneal congestion.*)   DA COSTA.

892—℞ Sodii phosphatis,
 Sodii chloridi,
 Sodii iodid., . . āā Ʒij.
 Sodii bromid., . . . Ʒj.
 Aquæ, ... fʒxiiss.—M.
Sig.: Tablespoonful four times a day in milk.
Used with the following :—

893—℞ Acid. tannic.,
 Ex. cinchonæ, . gr. xxx.
 Fuchsin, . . gr. xv.—M.
Et ft. pil. No. xx.
Sig.: One pill morning and evening. (*In chronic cases.*)   MONIN.

894—℞ Infus. digitalis, . . . fʒiss.
 Spt. æther. nitros., . ad fʒvj.
 Syr. simp., ... fʒss.
 Aquæ, . . . ad fʒvj.—M.
Sig.: Tablespoonful three times a day.   STEWART.

895—℞ Tr. ferri chlor., . . . fʒj.
 Acid. acetic. dil., . . fʒiss.
 Liq. ammon. acetat., . . fʒx.
 Elix. aurant., . . . fʒv.
 Syr. simp., ... fʒj.
 Aquæ, . . q. s. ad fʒvj.—M.
Sig.: Tablespoonful three or four times a day for a child of four years.   STARK.

896—℞ Potass. acetat., . . . ʒss.
 Infus. digitalis, . . . fʒvj.—M.
Sig.: Teaspoonful every four hours for a child of five years, used with the following :—

NEPHRITIS (*Continued*).

897—℞ Tr. grindeliæ robustæ, . . f℥j.
Tr. convallariæ maj., . . f℥iiss.
Tr. scillæ, ... f℥ji.—M.
Sig.: Fifteen drops thrice daily. HUCHARD.

898—℞ Ex. jaborandi fl., . . f℥j.
Elix. simp.,
Syr. simpl., . . aa f℥ss.—M.
Sig.: One to two teaspoonfuls. (*With uræmia.*)
BARTHOLOW.

899—℞ Ex. jaborandi fl., . . f℥j.
Sig.: Five to ten minims every hour or half hour,
until free diaphoresis occurs. (*In acute nephritis.*)
DA COSTA.

NEURALGIA.

900—℞ Quiniæ sulphat., . . ℨj.
Morphiæ sulphat.,
Acid. arseniosi, . . aa gr. iss.
Ex. aconiti, . . . gr. xv.
Strychniæ sulph., . . gr. j.—M.
Et ft. pil. No. xxx.
Sig.: One pill three times a day. S. D. GROSS.

'01—℞ Ext. actææ racemosæ fl., . . f℥jss.
Ext. gelsemii fl., . . . f℥jss.
Ext. valerianæ fl., . . . f℥j.—M.
Sig.: A teaspoonful every four hours. (*Tic doulou-
reux.*)

902—℞ Menthol, ... gr. xxiiss.
Cocaini muriat., . . gr. viiss.
Chloral hydrat., . . gr. ivss.
Vaselini, ... ℨiiss—M.
Sig.: Apply to the painful part and cover with
court-plaster. GALEZOWSKI.

903—℞ Menthol, ... f℥j.
Lini. saponis co., . . f℥ij.—M.
Sig.: Use locally. WITHERSTINE.

904—℞ Aconitiæ, ... gr. iss.
Spt. vini rect., . . . q. s.
Adipis præp., . . . ℨij.—M.
Sig.: To be rubbed in three times daily.
BROCKES.

113

NEURALGIA (Continued).

905—℞ Chloral hydrat.,
Pulv. camphoræ, . āā ℥iv.—M.
Sig.: Apply with a camel's-hair brush.
GEORGE BIRD.

906—℞ Ferri carbonat., . . . ℥ij.
Quiniæ sulphat., . . gr. vj.
Ex. opii, ... gr. ¾.
Syr. simp., . . . q. s.—M.
Et ft. pil. No. xvi.
Sig.: Eight pills during the day. JOLLY.

907—℞ Methyl chlor. pur., . . f℥j.
Sig.: Apply with brush to the painful parts.
DEBOVE.

908—℞ Sol. nitro-glycerin (1 per cent.),
℥ss.
Sig.: One or two drops on the tongue every four
to six hours. TRUSSEWITECH.

909—℞ Aconitiæ, ... gr. iv.
Veratriæ, ... gr. xv.
Glycerinæ, ... ℥ij.
Cerati, ... ℥vj.—M.
Sig.: To be rubbed over the parts. Do not apply
to any abrasion of the skin. DA COSTA.

910—℞ Pil. phenacetini (Bayer), . gr. ij.
Sig.: Two pills three times a day. POWELL.

911—℞ Arsenic. iodid., . . gr. j.
Ex. belladonnæ,
Morphinæ valerianat., āā gr. viij.
Ex. gentian. pulv., . . gr. v.
Ex. aconiti fl. rad., . . gtt. v.—M.
Et ft. pil. No. lx.
Sig.: One to three pills in twenty-four hours.
COVERT.

912—℞ Tr. cannabis indicæ, . . ♏xv.
Spt. vini rect., . . . ♏xlv.—M.
Ft. haustus.
Sig.: To be mixed with water at the time of taking.
DONOVAN.

913—℞ Antipyrin, ... ℥iss.
Aquæ, ... f℥v.—M.
Sig.: Twenty-five minims hypodermically every
three or four hours till relieved. WITHERSTINE.

114

914—℞ Acid. arsenosi, . . . gr. iv.
  Strychninæ sulph., . . . gr. iij.
  Ext. belladonnæ, . . . gr. xxiv.
  Quininæ sulph., . . . ℥j.
  Pil. ferri carbonat., . . . ℥v.—M.
Ft. pilulæ No. cxx.
Sig.: One after each meal.

915—℞ Ex. hyoscyami,
  Pulv. valerianat. rad.,
  Zinci oxidi, . . āā gr. j.—M.
Et ft. pil. No. i.
Sig.: A pill twice a day.   DAY.

916—℞ Ichthyol., ... gr. xv.
  Ung. hydrarg., ... gr. xv.
  Chloroformi,
  Spt. camphoræ, . . āā fℨiss.—M.
Sig.: Apply topically.   EULENBURG.

917—℞ Ferri sulphat. exsiccat.,
  Potass. carbonatis, . āā gr. ccl.—M.
Et ft. pil. No. c.
Sig.: Begin with three a day and increase to six.
        J. E. GARRETSON.

918—℞ Ex. belladonnæ, . . . ℥iss.
  Tr. opii, ... ♏xl.
  Chloroform., . . . fℨj.—M.
Sig.: Apply locally.   HAZARD.

919—℞ Veratrinæ,
  Morphinæ sulphat., . āā gr. x.
  Adipis, ... ℥j.—M.
Sig.: Rub in three times daily.   KENNARD.

920—℞ Camphoræ, ... ℥iss.
  Chloroform., . . . fℨss.
  Ol. olivæ, ... fℨij.—M.
Sig.: Apply frequently.   HAZARD.

921—℞ Ex. cocæ fl., . . . fℨj.
  Syr. aurant. flor., . . fℨv.
  Aquæ, ... ad fℨij.—M.
Sig.: A teaspoonful every hour until relieved.
(*For gastralgia.*)   D'ARDENNE.

NEURALGIA *(Continued)*.

922—℞ Menthol, ... gr. xxx.
　　Cocaini hydrochlorat. crystal, gr. vj.
　　Alcohol., . . q. s. ad f℥j.—M.
　Sig.: Use locally. PALMER.

NEURASTHENIA.

923—℞ Ext. sumbul.,
　　Ferri sulphat. exsic., . . āā gr. xx.
　　Pulv. asafœtidæ, . . . gr. xl.
　　Acid. arsenosi, ... gr. ss.—M.
　Ft. pil. No. xx.
　Sig.: One or two thrice a day. GOODELL.

924—℞ Asafœtidæ, ... ℨj.
　　Acid. arsenosi, ... gr. ss.
　　Strychnin. sulph., . . . gr. ss.
　　Ext. sumbul., ... ℨss.
　　Ferri subcarb., . . . ℈ij.
　　Quinin. valerianat., . . ℈j.—M.
　Ft. capsulæ No. xxiv.
　Sig.: One after each meal.

925—℞ Quinin. bisulphat., . . ℈j.
　　Ferri subcarb., . . . ℨj.
　　Strychnin. sulphat., . . gr. ss.
　　Ext. damianæ, . . . ℈j.
　　Ext. cinchonæ, . . . ℈ij.—M.
　Ft. capsulæ No. xx.
　Sig.: One after each meal.

NIPPLES, SORE *(See Fissures)*.
OBESITY.

926—℞ Ext. glandulæ thyreoideæ desiccat., ℈j.
　　Div. in chart. vel tabellæ, No. xx.
　Sig.: From one to five daily.

ŒDEMA *(See Dropsy)*.
ONYCHIA.

928—℞ Pulv. plumbi nitrat., . . ℥ss.
　Sig.: Dust on diseased tissue night and morning.
　　　　　　　　SCOTT and McCORMACK.

929—Use hot flaxseed poultices for three or four days,
　　before each renewal of the poultice thor-
　　oughly washing with—
　　℞ Tr. iodi.,
　　　Tr. belladonnæ,
　　　Tr. opii, . . . āā f℥ij.—M.
　Sig.: Then dust with iodoform and dress antisep-
　tically. AGNEW.

ONYCHIA *(Continued)*.

930—In the early stages a couple of leeches above the nail will have a good effect.   AGNEW.

931—℞ Acid. arseniosi, .   .   . gr. j.
      Glycerol. amyli, .   .   . f℥j.—M.
Sig.: Apply with a soft rag.   AGNEW.

932—℞ Ungt. hydrarg., .   .   . ℥ss.
Sig.: Apply for ten minutes every hour, applying poultices at other times.   RINGER.

933—℞ Ol. terebinthinæ,   .   . f℥ij.
Sig.: Apply a pledget of lint wet with the solution.   RINGER.

OPHTHALMIA *(See also Conjunctivitis)*.

934—℞ Pulv. aluminis, .   .   . gr. x.
      Aq. rosæ, ... f℥iij.—M.
Sig.: Apply three times a day.   BRANDE.

935—℞ Hydrarg. chlor. mit., .   . ℨij.
Sig.: Evert the lid and dust over once or twice daily.   BARTHOLOW.

936—℞ Argenti nitratis, .   .   . gr. iv.
      Aq. destillat., .   .   . f℥j.—M.
Sig.: One drop in the eye every five or six hours (*In catarrhal ophthalmia and superficial ulceration.*)   MACKENZIE.

937—℞ Hydrarg. chloridi corros., . gr. j.
      Aq. destillat., .   .   . f℥ix.—M.
Sig.: Use locally. (*In gonorrhœal ophthalmia.*)   ELLIS.

938—℞ Acid. boracic., .   .   . gr. xvj.
      Acid. salicylici, .   .   . gr. ij.
      Glycerinæ, ... ℳxl.
      Aq. bullientis, .   q. s. ad f℥j.—M.
Sig.: Instil into eye, after cauterizing trachoma follicle with the thermo-cautery. (*In trachoma.*)   ARMAIGNAC.

939—℞ Hydrarg. oxidi flav., .   . gr. v.
      Zinci sulphatis, .   .   . gr. x.
      Adipis, ... ℥j.—M.
Sig.: Apply to the everted eyelids and on the free border of the lids. (*In chronic scrofulous form.*)   DUPUYTREN.

OPHTHALMIA (*Continued*).

940—℞ Iodoform., ... ℥ss.
   Sacch. lactis, . . . ℥iij.—M.
   Sig.: Evert the lids and dust over. (*In granular form.*) WITHERSTINE.

941—℞ Cocain. sulphat., . . gr. iv.
   Atropinæ sulphat., . . gr. ss.
   Vaselini, ... ℈v.—M.
   Sig.: To be applied with a camel's-hair brush.
   LEAHY.

942—℞ Hydrarg. oxidi rubri, . . gr. vj.
   Plumbi subacetat. cryst., . gr. iij.
   Vaselini, ... ℥v.—M.
   Sig.: Apply to the free border of the eyelids once daily. (*In chronic blepharitis.*) PARINAUD.

943—℞ Argenti nitrat., . . . gr. ii–x.
   Liq. plumbi subacetat., . ♏x–xx.
   Cerat. cetacii, . . . ℥j.—M.
   Sig.: A piece the size of a pin's head to be put within the eyelids and repeated according to the degree of inflammation produced. (*In opacity of the cornea.*) GUTHRIE.

OPIUM-HABIT.

944—℞ Zinci oxidi, . . . ℥ss.
   Div. in pil. No. xxx.
   Sig.: One pill once daily, increasing to tolerance. (*For vomiting and diarrhœa.*) DA COSTA.

945—℞ Tr. nucis vomicæ, . . gtt. xij.
   Acid. phosphoric. dil., . gtt. xx.
   Syr. pruni virg., . . f℥ss.—M.
   Sig.: To be taken twice daily. WITHERSTINE.

946—℞ Tr. capsici, ... f℥iv.
   Potass. bromid., . . . ℥iv.
   Spt. ammon. aromat., . . f℥iiiss.
   Aq. camphoræ, . . ad f℥vj.—M.
   Sig.: Dessertspoonful several times daily for the depression. RINGER.

947—℞ Strychninæ sulph., . . gr. ss.
   Tr. belladonnæ,
   Tr. capsici, . . āā f℥iij.—M.
   Sig.: Ten drops in water every three hours, increasing three drops daily. POTTER.

OPIUM-HABIT *(Continued).*

948—℞ Acid. phosphoric. dil., . 13x.
Tr. lupulini, . . . f3xx.—M.
Sig.: Dessertspoonful in a wineglass of water every
four hours, one hour before food. FLEMING.

949—℞ Tr. cannabis indicæ, . . ℔xl–lx.
Spt. ætheris, . . . f3j.
Aquæ, . . q. s. ad f3j.—M.
Sig : One dose, if insomnia is very protracted.
FLEMING.

950—℞ Zinci valerianat., . gr. xxiv.
Quiniæ sulphat., . gr. xij.
Ex. lupuli (B. P.), . q. s.—M.
Et ft. pil. No. xii.
Sig.: One pill morning and evening, every second
day, alternating with some form of iron. FLEMING.

ORCHITIS.

951—℞ Keep the testicles elevated.

952—℞ Strap with adhesive strips.
Sig.: First envelop scrotum in thick layer of cotton; over this rubber-dam; then use an ordinary
suspensory that is close fitting.
HORAND-LANGLEBERT.

953—℞ Iodi., ... gr. iv.
Lanolin, ... 3j.—M.
Sig.: Apply locally after acute symptoms are past.
MARTIN.

954—℞ Ungt. hydrarg.,
Ungt. belladonnæ, . āā 3ss.—M.
Sig.: Apply locally morning and evening.
MARTIN.

955—℞ Guaiacol., . . . 3ij.
Lanolini,
Resorcin., ... aa 3iij.—M.
Sig.: Apply topically. (*For gonorrheal epididymitis.*)

956—℞ Tr. aconiti, ... ℔j.
Morphiæ sulphat., . . gr. $\frac{1}{20}$.
Antimonii et potassii tart., . gr. $\frac{1}{12}$.
Magnesii sulphatis, . . gr. xj.—M.
Sig.: Give at one dose, and repeat thrice daily or
oftener if required. (*Have testicle strapped.*)
PHILADELPHIA HOSPITAL.

119

ORCHITIS *(Continued).*

957—R Tr. iodi, ... f3ij.

Sig.: Paint affected parts after acute symptoms are over.

958—R Ammon. chloridi, . 3ij.
Spt. vini rectificat.,
Aquæ, . . . aā f3ij.—M.

Sig.: Saturate thin cloths and apply frequently, allowing the fluid to evaporate. BARTHOLOW.

959—R Morphinæ sulphat., . . . gr. xvj.
Hydrarg. oleatis (10%), . . 3ij.—M.

Sig.: Apply twice daily. (*To remove induration.*)
MARSHALL.

960—R Tr. pulsatillæ, . . gtt. xxiv–xlviij.
Syr. zingiber., . . f3j.
Aquæ, . q. s. ad f3iij.—M.

Sig.: Teaspoonful every hour or two. STURGIS.

OTITIS AND OTORRHŒA.

961—R Tr. aconiti rad., . . . f3iss.
Glycerinæ, ... f3iss.—M.

Sig.: To be warmed and dropped into the ear. (*In earache.*) GERHARD.

962—R Potassii iodid., . . . gr. xx.
Tr. iodi, ... f3iij.
Alcohol.,
Glycerin., ... aā f3iv.
Iodoform., ... gr. xx.—M.

Sig.: Inject a small quantity into the auditory canal. (*In chronic form.*)

963—R Chloral camphorat., . . gr. v.
Glycerinæ, ... gr. xxx.
Ol. amygdal. dulc., . . gr. x.—M.

Sig.: Apply a little on absorbent cotton and place in ear. (*In earache.*) JOURN. DE MÉDECINE.

964—R Acid. carbol.,
Zinci sulphat.,
Plumbi acetat., . . aā gr. x.
Aq. destillat., . . . f3viij.—M.

Sig.: Inject twice a day. (*When discharge is offensive.*) HAZARD.

965—R Glyceriti acid. tannic., . f3j.

Sig.: Fill meatus and plug with cotton. (*In chronic form.*) RINGER.

966—℞ Liq. hydrogenii peroxidi (10 vol.),
　　　　　　　　　　　　　　　　　　　　℥iv.

Sig.: Syringe the ear carefully with one part solu
tion to two of water, and when cleansed drop in a few
drops of the above solution.　　　C. H. BURNETT.

967—℞ Ungt. hydrarg. nitrat. rub.,　℥ss.

Sig.: Apply a small quantity to the affected skin.
(*In chronic inflammation of external meatus.*)
　　　　　　　　　　　　　　　　　　　　BARTHOLOW.

968—℞ Acid. carbol.,　　．　　．　　．　f℈j.
　　　Glycerinæ, .　　．　　．　　．　f℈ix.—M.

Sig.: Drop a few drops into the ear two or three
times daily, after cleansing.　　　HARTMANN.

969—℞ Pulv. iodoform., .　　．　　．　℈ij.

Sig.: Insufflate into the ear, after thoroughly
cleansing and drying it. (*In chronic cases when discharge is slight.*)　　　　　　　　　BEZOLD.

OXALURIA.

970—℞ Acid. hydrochlor. dil.,　．　f℥ss.
　　　Tr. ferri chlor.,　．　　．　．　f℥ij.
　　　Syr. simp.,　.　　．　　．　f℥iss.
　　　Aquæ,　　．　　．　　．　f℥iij.—M.

Sig.: Tablespoonful three times a day through a
glass-tube. (*With anæmia and nervous atony.*)
　　　　　　　　　　　　　　　　　　　　HAZARD.

971—℞ Glyceriti pepsinæ,　　．　．　f℥iss.
　　　Acid. lactic.,　　．　．　ad　f℥ij.—M.

Sig.: Teaspoonful after meals three times a day.
　　　　　　　　　　　　　　　　　　　　BARTHOLOW.

OZŒNA.

972—℞ Ex. hydrastis fl.,　　．　．　f℥ij.

Sig.: Five minims in water three times a day.

973—℞ Ex. hydrastis fl.,　　．　．　f℈j.
　　　Aquæ,　　．　　．　　．　．　Oj.—M.

Sig.: Use for syringing the nares.　BARTHOLOW.

974—℞ Sodii biborat.,
　　　Ammon. chloridi,　．　āā　℈j.
　　　Potass. permanganat.,　．　gr. x.—M.

Sig.: To be dissolved in one pint of water, and
used with a syringe three times a day.　SAJOUS.

OZŒNA (Continued).

975—℞ Hydrarg. chlor. mit., . . gr. xv.
    Sacch. alb., . . . ℨiv.—M.
    Sig.: For insufflation.   Trousseau.

976—℞ Plumbi nitrat., . . . ℈ij.
    Aquæ, ... f℥iv.—M.
    Sig.: Inject into nostril night and morning.
                                      Stillé.

977—℞ Potass. permanganat., . ℨss.
    Tr. myrrhæ, . . . f℥ij.
    Aquæ, ... Oj.—M.
    Sig.: Use as a douche three times a day.
                                      Hazard.

978—℞ Tr. iodi, ... f℥iv.
    Acidi carbol., . . . f℥i–ij.—M.
    Sig.: Use on sponge in a wide-mouthed bottle as
inhalation.   Potter.

979—℞ Creolin, ... gtt. v.
    Aquæ, ... Oj.—M.
    Sig.: For douching the nose.   Lichtwitz.

980—℞ Pulv. saloli,
    Pulv. talc, . . . āā ℨij.—M.
    Sig.: Insufflate the nose every two hours.
                                        Georgi.

981—℞ Acid. carbol., . . . ♏xx.
    Aq. calcis, ... Oj.—M.
    Sig.: Use as a wash or spray.   Potter.

982—℞ Sodii carbonatis,
    Sodii borat., . . āā ℨij.
    Liq. sodæ chloratæ, . . f℥ss.–ij.
    Glycerinæ, ... f℥j.
    Aquæ, . . q. s. ad f℥vj.—M.
    Sig.: Use as a spray.   Thornton.

983—℞ Bromi, ... ℨss.
    Alcoholis, ... f℥iv.—M.
    Sig.: Place in wide-mouthed bottle. Hold in the
and and snuff the vapor well into the nose.
                                       Bartholow.

PAIN (See Neuralgia, Myalgia, etc.).

PALPITATION (See Heart Disease).

984—℞ Hyoscyam. sulph.,   . .   gr. ss.
      Aquæ, ...   f℥vj.—M.

Sig.: Five minims hypodermically once daily or by the stomach twice daily. (*In paralysis agitans.*)
                                  Séguin.

985—℞ Strychniæ sulph.,   . .   gr. ij.
      Aquæ, ...   ℥c.—M.

Sig.: Two to four minims hypodermically every second day or daily. (*In all forms of paralysis except cerebral and spinal paralysis.*)   Barwell.

986—℞ Ammon. iodid.,   . . .   ℨj.
      Ammon. carbonat.,   .   ℨij.
      Liq. ammon. acetat.,   .   f℥vj.—M.

Sig.: Tablespoonful three times a day. (*To absorb thrombi in incipient hemiplegic paralysis due to endarteritis deformans.*)   Bartholow.

987—℞ Phosphori, ...   gr. ij.
      Alcoholis absolut.,   . .   fℨxxij.
      Tr. vanillæ,   . . .   f℥ss.
      Ol. aurant. cort.,   . .   ℥xij.
      Alcoholis absolut.,   q. s. ad   f℥iij.—M.

Sig.: Twenty to forty minims two or three times a day. (*In cerebral softening and hysterical paralysis.*)
                                  Hammond.

988—℞ Strychniæ sulph.,   . .   gr. ij.
      Aq. destillat.,   . .   fℨj.—M.

Sig.: One to five minims hypodermically. (*In infantile paralysis, etc.*)   Bartholow.

989—℞ Ex. physostigmatis,   .   gr. j.
      Ex. gentian,   . .   Əj.—M.
      Et div. in pil. No. xxx.

Sig.: One pill every two hours. (*In general paralysis of the insane.*)   Crichton Browne.

990—℞ Strychniæ sulphat.,   . .   gr. j.
      Acid. arseniosi,   . . .   gr. ij.
      Ex. belladonnæ, . .   gr. v.
      Quiniæ sulphat.,
      Pil. ferri carbonat.,   .   āā   Əij.
      Ex. taraxaci,   . .   Əj.—M.
      Et ft. pil. No. xl.

Sig.: One pill three times a day. (*In paralysis agitans.*)   S. W. Gross.

PARALYSIS *(Continued).*

991—℞ Eserinæ, ... gr. ij.
    Aquæ, ... f℥j.—M.
   Sig.: Instil into the eye. (*In ocular spasm and paralysis.*)   WHARTON JONES.

992—℞ Ex. buchu fl.,
    Ex. uvæ ursi, . . āā f℥ij.
    Syr. acaciæ, . . . f℥ss.
    Aq. menthæ viridis, . . f℥j.—M.
   Sig.: Dessertspoonful every three hours. HAZARD.

PARTURITION *(See Labor).*

PEDICULI *(See Lice).*

PEMPHIGUS *(See Skin Diseases).*

PERICARDITIS *(See also Heart Disease).*

993—℞ Hydrarg. chlor. mit.,
    Pulv. ipecac., . . āā gr. vj.
    Potass. nitrat., . . . ℨiss.—M.
   Et div. in chart. No. xii.
   Sig.: Powder every three hours. HARTSHORNE.

994—℞ Antimonii et potass. tart., . gr. iv.
    Tr. opii, ... f℥j.
    Aq. camphoræ, . . . f℥viij.—M.
   Sig.: Tablespoonful every two hours. (*In acute form.*)   GRAVES.

995—℞ Tr. veratri viridis, . . f℥ss.—M.
   Sig.: From three to five drops. (*To reduce heart's action.*)   HAZARD.

996—℞ Tr. aconiti rad., . . . f℥ss.—M.
   Sig.: Half a drop to a drop in a little water every fifteen minutes for two hours; then every hour or two.   RINGER.

PERIOSTITIS *(NODES).*

997—℞ Iodini, ... gr. ss.
    Potass. iodid., . . . ℨss.
    Syr. zingiberis, . . . f℥j.
    Aquæ, ... f℥viij.—M.
   Sig.: Two tablespoonfuls three times a day.
          TYRELL.

PERIOSTITIS (Continued).

998—℞ Potass. iodid., . . . ℨij.
   Ammon. iodid., . . . ℨj.
   Tr. cinchonæ comp., . . f℥iij.—M.
 Sig.: A teaspoonful well diluted with water after
 eating.   VAN BUREN and KEYES.

999—℞ Iodi.,
   Terebinthinæ canaden., āā ℨj.
 · Collodii, ... f℥iv.—M.
 Sig.: Apply with a brush.   SHINN.

1000—℞ Cadmii iodid., . . . ℨss.
   Ætheris, ... ℳxl
   Terre simul. et adde—
   Adipis, ... ℨj.—M.
 Sig.: Use locally.   GARROD.

1001—℞ Sodii iodid., . . . ℨj.—M.
   Decoct. sarsaparillæ comp., f℥viij.—M.
 Sig.: One-sixth part three times a day. TANNER.

1002—℞ Potass. iodid., . . . ℈j.
   Syr. aurant. cort., . . f℥j.
   Aq. aurant. flor., . . f℥v.—M.
 Sig.: Tablespoonful twice daily in hop tea.
          LISFRANC.

1003—℞ Cadmii iodid., . . . ℨj.
   Adipis preparat., . . ℥j.
   Liniment. aconiti, . . f℥ij.—M.
 Sig.: Use locally.   TANNER.

1004—℞ Hydrarg. biniodidi, . . gr. vij.
   Potass. iodid., . . . ℈j.
   Adipis, ... ℥j.—M.
 Sig.: Use locally.   HILDRETH.

1005—℞ Zinci iodidi, . . . ℨj.
   Adipis, . . . ℥j.—M.
 Sig.: Apply twice a day. HOOPER.

1006—℞ Morphiæ, ... gr. viij.
   Hydrarg. oleat. (10 per cent.
   ad 20 per cent.), . . ℥j.—M.
 Sig.: Apply with a brush. MARSHALL.

1007—℞ Tr. aconitii rad., . . f℥ij.
           Tr. opii deod., . . . f℥vj.—M.
Sig.: Eight drops in water every hour or two.
                             BARTHOLOW.

1008—℞ Magnesii sulphat., . ℥iss.
Div. in pulv. No. xii.
Sig.: A powder in hot peppermint water every hour until the bowels are freely opened. (*Use in beginning of attack.*)   MUNDE.

1009—℞ Morph. sulph., . . . gr. iv.
           Aq. destillat., . . . f℥ij.—M.
Sig.: Ten to fifteen minims as required, hypodermically, to control the vomiting.   TAIT.

1010—℞ Tr. aconiti fol., . . . f℥v.
           Ex. veratri viridis fl., . f℥j.—M.
Sig.: Twelve drops in water every two hours. (*Where opium is inadmissible.*)   ELLIS.

1011—℞ Acid. tannici, . . . gr. iii-clxxx.
           Glycerinæ, . . . q.s.ad.ft.sol.
Sig.: To be taken in divided doses during the day. (*In localized peritonitis*))   DEBOUÉ.

1012—℞ Tr. opii, ... ♏xvj.
           Syr. zingiberis, . . . f℥j.
           Aquæ, . . q. s. ad f℥ij.—M.
Sig.: Teaspoonful every two hours for a child of five years.   STARR.

1013—℞ Pulv. opii, . . . gr. i-ij.
           Sacch. lact., . . . gr. xij.—M.
Et ft. in chart. No. xii.
Sig.: One powder every two hours for a child.
                  GOODHART and STARR.

1014—℞ Potass. iodid., . . . ℥ii-iv.
           Ferri pyrophos., . . gr. xlviij.
           Tr. lavandulæ comp., . f℥ss.
           Aquæ, . . q. s. ad f℥iij.—M.
Sig.: Teaspoonful every six hours.   HUGHES.

PERTUSSIS (See Whooping-Cough).

PHAGEDENA.

1015—℞ Acid. salicylic., . . ℥ss.
Sig. Dust over the slough.   BARTHOLOW.

PHAGEDENA (Continued).

1016—℞ Acid. nitric. dil.,   .   . ℥x.
    Ex. opii, ... gr. v.
    Aquæ,   .   .   .   f℥j.—M.
   Sig.: Locally. *(In sloughing, incised wounds.)*
            ERICHSEN.

1017—℞ Saloli, ... gr. v–l.
    Amyli,   .   .   . ℥j.—M.
   Sig.: Dust over locally.   SEIFERT.

1018—℞ Iodoform.,   .   . ℥iiss.
    Thymoli,   .   .   . ℥v.
    Sacch. lact.,   .   . gr. ij.—M.
   Sig.: Dust over sores.   HOWARD.

1019—℞ Hydrarg. chlor. corros.,   . gr. j.
    Iodoformi,
    Ferri redacti,   . āā ℈j.—M.
   Et ft. pil. No. xx.
   Sig.: One pill three times a day. *(In sloughing
phagedena.)*   BARTHOLOW.

PHARYNGITIS.

1020—℞ Cocaine muriat.,   . gr. x.
    Aquæ,   .   .   . f℥ss.—M.
   Sig.: Use locally.   SAJOUS.

1021—℞ Zinci sulphat.,   .   .   . ℥j.
    Aquæ,   .   .   . f℥j.—M.
   Sig.: Use locally.   MORRIS.

1022—℞ Pilocarpinæ muriat.,   . gr. ij.
    Aquæ,
    Glycerinæ,   .   . āā f℥j.—M.
   Sig.: Teaspoonful three times a day. *(In dry
pharyngitis.)*   SAJOUS.

1023—℞ Tr. ferri chlor.,   .   . f℥iij.
    Potass. chlorat.,   .   . ℥j.
    Syr. zingiber.,   .   . f℥ij.
    Aquæ,   .   . q. s. ad f℥iij.—M.
   Sig.: Teaspoonful every two hours.   STARR.

1024—℞ Ex. ergotæ aq.,   .   .   . gr. xx.
    Tr. iodini,   .   .   . f℥j.
    Glycerinæ,   .   .   . f℥j.—M.
   Sig.: Use locally with camel's-hair brush.
            HAZARD.

PHARYNGITIS *(Continued).*

1025—℞ Tr. guaiaci ammon., f℥j.

Sig.: A teaspoonful in a half-glassful of milk, used as a gargle and swallowed every three hours. (*In rheumatic subjects.*) SAJOUS.

1026—℞ Ex. rhois glab. fl.,
Ex. hydrast. canaden. fl., āā f℥j.
Potass. chlorat., . . ℨiss.
Aquæ, . . q. s. ad f℥vj.—M.

Sig.: Use tablespoonful in water as gargle.
WOOD.

1027—℞ Sodii borat., . . . ℈j.
Acid. boric., . . . ℈ij.
Acid. salicylic., . . gr. x.
Essent. thymi sat., . . Oij.—M.

Sig.: To be used as a gargle.

1028—℞ Tr. myrrhæ,
Aceti, . . . āā f℥ij.
Mellis, ... ℨj.
Infus. serpentariæ, . . Oiss.—M.

Sig.: Use as a gargle. FOTHERGILL.

1029—℞ Argenti nitrat., . . gr. xl.
Aquæ, ... f℥j.—M.

Sig.: Apply to the throat after cleansing it. (*In chronic cases.*) SAJOUS.

PHLEGMASIA DOLENS.

1030—℞ Ex. hamamelis fl., . f℥j.
Elix. simp.,
Syr. simp., . . āā f℥ss.—M.

Sig.: One to two teaspoonfuls three or four times a day. PRESTON.

1031—℞ Pulv. lini,
Aq. bullientis, . . . q. s.
Ft. cataplasma.

Sig.: Sprinkle with laudanum and apply locally.
LEISHMAN.

1032—℞ Ex. belladonnæ fl., . . f℥j.
Tr. opii, ... f℥j
Tr. iodini, . . . f℥j.
Ol. olivæ, ... f℥viij.—M.

Sig.: Apply as warm as can be borne by the leg and bandage. SMITH.

PHLEGMON *(See Carbuncle)*.

PHTHISIS *(See also Bronchitis, Diarrhœa, Sweating, and Hœmoptysis)*.

1033—℞ Codeinæ sulphat., . . gr. ⅕.
    Acid. hydrocyanic. dil., . ℳ ij.
    Syr. tolu., ... f℥j.—M.
Sig.: Take four times a day. DA COSTA.

1034—℞ Ex. ergotæ fl., . . . f℥j.
Sig.: Twenty drops three times a day. *(To relieve diarrhœa and night sweats.)* HODGSON.

1035—℞ Quiniæ sulphat., . . gr. j.
    Pulv. digitalis, . . . gr. ss.
    Pulv. opii, . . . gr. ¼.
    Pulv. ipecac., . . . gr. ¼.—M.
Sig.: One pill three or four times a day. *(For fever.)* NIEMEYER.

1036—℞ Tr. benzoin. comp., . . f℥j.
    Aq. bullientis, . . . Oss.—M.
Sig.: Inhale twice daily. RINGER.

1037—℞ Morphiæ sulphat., . . gr. j.
    Acid. muriat. dil., . . ℳ v.
    Acid. hydrocyanic. dil., . ℳ xxx.
    Syr. scillæ,
    Aquæ, . . . āā f℥j.—M.
Sig.: Teaspoonful when the cough is troublesome. THOMPSON.

1038—℞ Acid. camphoric., . . gr. xx.
Sig.: Give dry on tongue for night-sweats. HARE.

1039—℞ Thallin., . . . gr. xxx.
    Div. in pil. No. xx.
Sig.: A pill three times a day.

1040—℞ Pulv. catechu, . . . gr. xxxvj.
    Syr. krameriæ, . . . f℥j.
    Tr. cinnamomi, . . . gtt. x.
    Vini rubri, ... f℥iij.—M.
Sig.: A tablespoonful three or four times daily. *(For diarrhea.)*

1041—℞ Creasoti, ... ℳ vj.
    Glycerinæ, . . . f℥j.
    Spt. frument., . . . f℥ij.
Sig.: Tablespoonful three times a day. BENEDICT.

1042—℞ Iodoformi, ... gr. xxiv.
  Creasoti (Morson's) . . ℆iv.
  Ol. eucalypti, . . . ℆viij.
  Chloroformi, . . . ℆xlviij.
  Alcoholis,
  Ætheris, . āā q. s. ad f℥ss.—M.
  Sig.: Five to twenty drops to be used in inhaler every three hours.   WILLIAM PERRY WATSON.

1043—℞ Cupri acetat., . . . gr. ij.
  Sodii carbonatis, . . gr. xij.—M.
  Et ft. pil. No. xii.
  Sig.: One pill night and morning on an empty stomach.   LUTON.

1044—℞ Terebene, ... ℥iv.
  Pulv. acaciæ, . . . ℥iij.
  Syr. zingiberis, . . . f℥viiss.
  Aquæ, ... f℥xv.—M.
  Sig.: Teaspoonful three times a day. (*Relieves dyspnœa and flatulence.*)   VIGIER.

1045—℞ Creasoti, ... ℆xxxij.
  Tr. capsici, . . . f℥iss.
  Mucil. acaciæ, . . . f℥iiss.
  Aquæ, ... f℥ij.—M.
  Sig.: Teaspoonful, well diluted, after meals.
     ROOSEVELT HOSPITAL.

1046—℞ Pilocarpinæ muriat., . . gr. iij.
  Aq. destillat., . . . f℥ij.—M.
  Sig.: Five minims three times daily hypoder-mically. (*In paroxysmal dyspnœa of phthisis.*) RIESS.

1047—℞ Plumbi acet., . . . gr. x.
  Ext. gentianæ, . . . q. s.—M.
  Ft. chart. No. xii.
  Sig.: From 3 to 5 powders daily. (*For night-sweats.*)

1048—℞ Creasoti, ... ℆xv.
  Tr. gentian, . . . ℆xij.
  Spt. vin. rect., . . . f℥vj.
  Vini xerici, . . . f℥vj.—M.
  Sig.: Tablespoonful three times a day. FRANTZEL

1049—℞ Bismuth. subnit., . . ℥ij.
  Div. in chart. No. xii.
  Sig.: One powder every four hours. (*In diarrhœa.*)
     THOMPSON.

1050—℞ Ammon. carb., . . . gr. v.
       Ammon. iodid., . . . gr. v-x.
       Syr. tolu., ... f℥ij.
       Syr. prun. virg., . . f℥ij.—M.

Sig.: Take a dose every five hours, alternating with—

1051—℞ Liq. potass. arseuitis, . ♏v.
       Mass. ferri carb., . . gr. v.
       Vini xerici, . . . f℥j.
       Aq. destillat., . q. s. ad f℥iss.—M.

Sig.: For one dose.   Hughes.

1052—℞ Chloral hydrat., . . ℨiij.
       Syr. tolu., ... f℥j.
       Aquæ, . . q. s. ad f℥iij.—M.

Sig.: Tablespoonful at bedtime. (To procure sleep.)
       Walsh.

1053—℞ Atropinæ sulphat., . . gr. j.
       Morphiæ sulphat., . . gr. viij.
       Acid. sulphuric. arom., . f℥ij.
       Aq. menthæ pip., q. s. ad f℥j.—M.

Sig.: Five drops every three hours at night. (For night-sweats.)   William Perry Watson.

1054—℞ Terpinol,
       Sodii benzoatis, . . āā gr. xv.—M.
       Et div. in capsulas No. x.

Sig.: A capsule every hour or two. (To diminish the expectoration and remove its odor.)   Rabow.

1055—℞ Ol. delphinidæ (porpoise oil), Oss.

Sig.: A teaspoonful to a tablespoonful after meals.
       West.

1056—℞ Sodii tellurat., . . . gr. ij-iij.
       Alcohol. (90 %), . . . f℥ij.—M.

Sig.: A teaspoonful night and morning in a little sugar and water. (For night-sweats.)

1057—℞ Balsam. Peruviani, . . gr. lxxv.
       Olei morrhuæ, . . f℥iiss.
       Pulv. acaciæ, . . . gr. lxxv.
       Aq. destillat., . . . f℥iiss.
       Syr. aurantii, . . . f℥v.—M.
       Ft. emulsio.

Sig.: Teaspoonful every two hours.   Schmey.

PILES *(See Hemorrhoids).*

PITYRIASIS *(See Skin Diseases).*

PLEURISY.

1058—℞ Tr. opii deod., . . . f℥vj.
    Tr. aconiti rad., . . f℥ij.—M.
Sig.: Eight drops in water every hour or two. (*In acute stage before effusion.*) BARTHOLOW.

1059—℞ Potass. acetat., . . . ℥vss.
    Spt. æther. nit., . . f℥ij.
    Aquæ, . . . ad f℥viij.—M.
Sig.: Tablespoonful every three or four hours. (*In pleuritic effusion.*) HARTSHORNE.

1060—℞ Potass. acetat., . . . gr. xv.
    Spt. æther. nitro., . . f℥ss.
    Vini ipecac., . . . gtt. iij.
    Sy. tolu., ... f℥ss.—M.
Sig.: Take four times daily. (*In subacute pleurisy.*) DA COSTA.

1061—℞ Morphiæ sulphat., . gr. ¼.
    Quiniæ sulphat., . gr. xv.—M.
Et div. in chart. No. i.
Sig.: Take at once. (*To abort an incipient pleurisy.*) BARTHOLOW.

1062—℞ Tr. iodinii, . . . f℥ss.
    Potass. iodid., . . ℥ij.
    Aquæ, ... f℥ij.—M.
Sig.: Apply on the affected side of chest. NIEMEYER.

1063—℞ Morphiæ acetat., . . gr. ss.
    Potass. acetat., . . . ℥ss.
    Tr. veratri viridis, . . ♏xxiv.
    Syr. tolu., ... f℥ss.
    Liq. potass. citrat., . . f℥iiss.—M.
Sig.: Dessertspoonful every three hours. (*In dry pleurisy.*) DA COSTA.

1064—℞ Syr. ferri iodid., . . f℥iiss.
    Potass. iodid., . . . ℥j, Эj.
    Syr. sarsaparillæ comp., . ℥j.
    Aquæ, . . q. s. ad ℥ij.—M.
Sig.: Teaspoonful four times daily, in water. ANDERS.

1065—℞ Ex. jaborandi fl., . . ℨj.

Sig.: Take at once, in a cup of hot water.

1066—℞ Sodii citrat.,
Sodii acetat.,
Sodii salicylat., . . āā ℨij.
Aq. menth. pip., q. s. ad f℥v.—M.

Sig.: Tablespoonful every two to four hours. Hot flannels to chest, sprinkled with laudanum, and a towel pinned tightly around body ; dry diet ; rest in bed ; flannel underclothing and night-dress.

WAUGH.

1067—℞ Potass. iodid., . . . ℨiv.
Aquæ, ... f℥vj.—M.

Sig.: One teaspoonful in milk every four hours with the following :—

1068—℞ Tr. iodinii comp., . . f℥iij.

Sig.: Divide the surface of the affected part into three sections, and paint one section each day. (*For chronic pleuritic effusion.*) BARTHOLOW.

1069—℞ Collodii cum cantharidi, . f℥ss.

Sig.: Apply with a brush over a small area, heat quickly, and repeat. (*In pleuritic effusion.*) RINGER.

1070—℞ Tr. iodinii, . . . f℥j.
Potass. iodid., . . . ℥ss.
Camphoræ, . . . ℨij.
Spt. rect., ... f℥x.—M.

Sig.: Apply locally. STARR.

1071—℞ Potass. acetat., . . . gr. xxx.
Infus. digitalis, . . . ℨij.—M.

Sig.: Take every three or four hours. (*For effusion.*) HUGUES.

1072—The treatment should consist of rest in bed, animal broths, and milk. The following febrifuge mixture should be given to a child four years of age :—

℞ Spt. ætheris nitrosi, . . gtt. xx.
Liq. ammon. acet., . . f℥ss.
Chloroformi, . . . gtt. ij.
Aq. menthæ vir., q. s. ad ℨj.—M.

Sig.: One dose. Take every two hours.

PLEURISY *(Continued).*

1073—℞ Mist. ferri et ammon.,
    Acetat., ... f℥vj.—M.
  Sig.: Teaspoonful to tablespoonful. *(In the second stage.)*   POTTER.

1074—℞ Pulv. sinapis,   .   .   . ℥ss.
    Pulv. lini,   .   .   . ℥viij.
    Aq. bullientis,   .   .   . q. s.—M.
Et ft. cataplasma.
  Sig.: Make the poultice wet and place it between two pieces of muslin, covered with oiled silk, and renew when beginning to cool. *(In pleurisy of children.)*   J. LEWIS SMITH.

1075—℞ Magnesii sulphat.,   .   . ℥vi–viij.
Div. in chart. No. viii.
  Sig.: A powder in two tablespoonfuls of water before food, and no fluids for some time afterwards. *(In pleuritic effusion.)*   HAY.

1076—℞ Acid. tannic.,   .   . gr. xxx.
Div. in pil. No. xv.
  Sig.: Four to eight pills daily; one-half in the morning, the remainder in the evening. *(In purulent pleurisy.)*   DUBOUÉ.

1077—℞ Tr. opii deodorat.,   .   . gtt. xx.
    Tr. digitalis,   .   .   . gtt. xvj.
    Syr. pruni virg.,   .   . f℥j.
    Aquæ, ... f℥iss.—M.
  Sig.: Teaspoonful every three hours for a child of two years. *(For first stage.)*   J. LEWIS SMITH.

1078—℞ Potass. acetat.,   .   .   . ℥ij.
    Infus. digitalis,   .   . ℥iij.—M.
  Sig.: Teaspoonful every three hours. *(To remove effusion.)*   J. L. SMITH.

PLEURODYNIA *(See Neuralgia).*

PNEUMONIA.

1079—℞ Tr. veratri viridis,   .   . ♏xl.
    Spt. æther. nitros.,   .   . f℥vj.
    Liq. potass. citrat.,   .   . f℥ivss.
    Syr. zingiber.,   .   . ad f℥vj.—M.
  Sig. Tablespoonful every three hours. *(In the early stage.)*   DA COSTA.

1080—℞ Potass. iodi., . . . ℥j.
    Ammon. chlor., . . ℥iss.
    Mist. glycyrrhizæ comp., f℥vj.—M.

Sig.: Tablespoonful four times a day, to promote absorption. DA COSTA.

1081—℞ Pulv. digitalis, . . gr. vj.
    Quiniæ sulphat., . . gr. xij.
    Ex. opii,
    Ex. ipecac., . . āā gr. iij.—M.
Et ft. pil. No. xii.

Sig.: One pill three times a day with the preceding mixture. DA COSTA.

1082—℞ Thallin sulphat., . . gr. xxxij.
    Aq. aurant. flor., . . f℥j.—M.

Sig.: Teaspoonful every three hours till the fever declines. OSLER.

1083—℞ Tr. aconiti rad., . . f℥ij.
    Tr. opii, ... f℥iij.—M.

Sig.: Thirteen drops at once, followed by five drops every hour or two. (*In stage of congestion*)
    BARTHOLOW.

1084—℞ Ammon. carbonat., . . gr. v.
    Ammon. iodidi, . . gr. v–x.
    Mucil. acaciæ, . . . q. s.
    Syr. glycyrrh., . . . f℥j–ij.
    Syr. pruni virg., q. s. ad f℥ii–iv.—M.

Sig.: At one dose every three hours. HUGHES.

1085—℞ Quininæ sulph., . . gr. ij.
    Pulv. digitalis, . . . gr. j.—M.
Et ft. pil. No. i.

Sig.: Every four hours. (*In pleuro-pneumonia.*)
    DA COSTA.

1086—℞ Tr. ipecac. comp. (Squibb), gtt. xxxij.
    Tr. aconiti rad., . . gtt. xvj.
    Syr. tolu.,
    Aquæ, . . . āā f℥j.—M.

Sig.: Teaspoonful every three hours for a child of five years. (*In the congestive stage.*) J. L. SMITH.

1087—℞ Sodii iodid., . . . ℥iss.
    Morphinæ sulphat., . . gr. ss.
    Elix. aromat , . . . f℥ij.—M.

Sig.: Teaspoonful three times a day, with blisters over the apex. (*In catarrhal pneumonia.*) DA COSTA.

PNEUMONIA (Continued).

1088—℞ Ammon. carbonat., . . gr. xl.
Infus. serpentariæ, . . f℥iv.—M.
Sig.: Teaspoonful every three hours. (*As a stimulant about the crisis.*) BARTHOLOW.

1089—℞ Ammon. iodid., . . gr. xl.
Spt. ammon. aromat., . f℥ij.
Elix. aromat., . . . f℥j.
Aquæ, . . q. s. ad f℥viij.—M.
Sig.: One-eighth thrice daily. (*In syphilitic lobar pneumonia.*)

1090—℞ Ammonii salicylat.,
Ammonii carb., ãã gr. v.
Spt. ætheris nit., . ℔xv.
Ex. cocæ fl.,
Glycerinæ, . . ãã f℥j.
Liq. ammonii acetat., q. s. ad f℥ss.—M.
Sig.: Give at one dose every three or four hours.
S. S. COHEN.

1091—℞ Quininæ bisulph., . . Əj.
Ol. theobromæ, . . . ℥j.—M.
Et div. in supposit. No. iv.
Sig.: One every eight hours.
Also paint the back of the chest with iodine, and envelop in flaxseed jacket. Internally, give digitalis or ergot, in small doses. (*In infantile pneumonia.*)
WAUGH.

1092—℞ Antipyrin, . . . gr. v.
Quinin. hydrochlorat., . gr. ij.
Camphor. monobrom., . gr. ss.—M.
Sig.: In capsule, as needed. (*For fever.*)
WOODBURY.

1093—℞ Morphiæ sulphat , . ; gr. j.
Syr. ipecac., . . . f℥ss.
Syr. tolu., . . . f℥iiiss.—M.
Sig.: Teaspoonful every three hours to a child of five years. (*In the stage of hepatization.*)
J. LEWIS SMITH.

1094—℞ Acid. salicylici, . ℥ij.
Div. in chart. No. vi.
Sig.: One powder every two hours until four or five are taken. (*To abort an impending attack.*)
SILVERTHORN.

PNEUMONIA *(Continued).*

1095—℞ Acid. sulph. aromat., . ♏iij.
    Tr. opii deodorat., . . ♏v.
    Syr. prun. virg., q. s. ad f℥j.—M.
  Sig.: Take at one dose for cough.   WOODBURY.

1096—℞ Ex. cascaræ sagrad. fl.,
    Tr. cardamom. comp.,
    Syr. aurant. cor., . āā ♏xx.—M.
  Sig.: Take at one dose as a laxative. WOODBURY.

1097—℞ Ex. veratri viridis fl., . f℥j.
  Sig.: Four to six minims every hour until the
pulse falls to sixty-five or seventy.   STROUD.

POLYURIA *(See Diabetes Insipidus).*

PRIAPISM *(See Nymphomania).*

PRICKLY HEAT *(See Skin Diseases).*

PROSTATITIS.

1098—℞ Ex. opii aquos, . . gr. viij.
    Ex. hyoscyami, . gr. iv.—M.
    Ft. suppos. No. viii.
  Sig.: Insert one into the rectum and repeat when
necessary.   MARTIN.

1099—℞ Iodoformi,
    Ext. hyoscyamus, . . āā gr. ss.
    Ol. theobromæ, . . . gr. xlv.—M.
  Sig.: Use as a suppository.

1100—℞ Liq. potassæ, . . f℥ii-iv.
    Ex. hyoscyami, . Ɔj-iv.
    Syr. aurant. cort.,
    Aq. cinnam., . . āā f℥iij.—M.
  Sig.: A tablespoonful in a wineglass of water every
eight hours.   VAN BUREN and KEYES.

1101—℞ Potass. bicarbonat., . . ℥iv.
    Ex. hyoscyami fl., . . f℥ij.
    Syr. simp., . . . f℥ij.
    Aquæ, . . q. s. ad f℥vj.—M.
  Sig.: A dessertspoonful every two to four hours.
    MARTIN.

1102—℞ Tr. cantharidis,   .   .   f℥ss.

Sig.: One to five drops in water three times a day.

RINGER.

1103—℞ Ergotinæ,
Pil. hydrargyri pulv.,   āā ℈j.
Saloli, ... ℥iij.—M.

Et divide in capsulas No. xx.

Sig.: Take one capsule thrice a day.   *(Enlarged prostate.)*

GERHARD.

1104—℞ Iodoform., .   .   . ℥ss.
Ol. theobromæ,
Ceræ flavæ,   .   . āā ℥j.—M.
Et ft. suppos. No. v.

Sig.: One night and morning. *(In chronic enlarge-ment.)*

MARTIN.

1105—℞ Leeches to the perineum.

1106—℞ Ex. opii aquos, .   . gr. viij.
Ex. belladonnæ,   . gr. ij.—M.
Ft. suppos. No. viii.

Sig.: Introduce one into the rectum and repeat on return of pain.

1107—Very hot or very cold water injected into the rectum, against the prostate, through a two-way rectal tube, from two to four quarts at a time, three or four times a day.

1108—℞ Carbonis animalis,   .   . gr. iij.
Ammon. chlor.,   .   . ℈j.
Ex. conii, ... gr. ij.
Pulv. glycyrrhizæ,   .   . q. s.—M.
Ft. bolus.

Sig.: One three times a day. *(In swelled and scir-rhous prostate.)*

MAGENDIE.

PROSTATORRHŒA.

1109—℞ Potass. citratis,   .   . ℥ss–j.
Spt. limonis,   .   .   . f℥ss.
Syr. simp.,   .   .   . f℥ij.
Aquæ, ... f℥j.—M.

Sig.: Dessertspoonful, largely diluted with water, three times a day.   VAN BUREN and KEYES.

PROSTATORRHŒA *(Continued).*

1110—℞ Tr. nucis vomicæ, . . f℥j.
    Tr. ferri chlor., . . . f℥iij.—M.
  Sig.: Twenty drops, well diluted, three times a day. GROSS.

1111—℞ Potass. bromid., . . f℥iij.
    Syr. limonis, . . . ℥iss.
    Aquæ, . . q. s. ad f℥iij.—M.
  Sig.: Dessertspoonful when necessary. GROSS

1112—℞ Tr. ferri chlor., . . . f℥vj.
    Tr. cantharidis, . . f℥ij.—M.
  Sig.: Fifteen drops in water three times a day.
                           BARTHOLOW.

1113—℞ Ex. hydrastis fl., . . f℥j.
  Sig.: Twenty drops in water three times a day.
                           BARTHOLOW.

PRURIGO—PRURITIS *(See also Skin Diseases).*

1114—℞ Morph. sulphatis, . . gr. vj.
    Sodii borat., . . . ℥iv.
    Aq. camphoræ, . . . f℥vj.—M.
  Sig.: Wash the parts first with castile soap and warm water and apply the above twice a day.
                           BAER.

1115—℞ Hydrarg. chlor. corros., . gr. j.
    Pulv. aluminis, . . . ℈j.
    Pulv. amyli, . . . ℥iss.
    Aquæ, ... f℥vj.—M.
  Sig.: Apply locally. GOODELL.

1116—℞ Hydrarg. chlor. corros., . gr. ij.
    Acid. hydrochloric., . . gtt. x.
    Aquæ, ... f℥viij.—M.
  Sig.: Apply locally, lukewarm. *(For pruritus ani and vulvæ.)* LAPLACE.

1117—℞ Chloral camph.,
    Bismuth. subnit., . āā ℥ij.
    Aq. rosæ, . . . ad f℥iv.—M.
  Sig.: Apply to the parts.

1118—℞ Argenti nitratis, . . gr. xx.
    Aquæ, ... f℥j.—M.
  Sig.: Paint over the affected parts. *(In pruritus vulvæ.)* BARTHOLOW.

PRURIGO (*Continued*).

1119—℞ Acid. hydrocyanic. dil.,
   Tr. opii, . . . āā f℥ij. ⸲
   Potass. carb., . . . ℥ij.
   Aq. rosæ, . . āā f℥iv.—M.
Sig.: Apply to the parts.   REYNOLDS.

1120—℞ Menthol, . . .   gr. xxiv.
   Spt. vini rectif., . . f℥j.—M.
Sig.: Use locally.

1121—℞ Naphthol., . .   gr. ccxxv.
   Saponis viridis, . . ℥xiiss.
   Cretæ præp., . . ℥iiss.
   Adipis, . . . ℥cxxv.—M.
Sig.: Apply to the parts and then powder them
with starch.   KAPOSI.

1122—℞ Acid. carbol., .   gr. vj.
   Aquæ, . . f℥j.—M.
Sig.: Use locally.   HEATH.

1123—℞ Pulv. camphoræ, . gr. xxx.
   Zinci oxid.,
   Bismuthi,
   Talc., . . . āā ℥j.—M.
Sig.: Apply with absorbent cotton. (*Pruritus ani.*)

1124—℞ Acid. hydrocyanic. dil., . f℥ij.
   Sodii borat., . . . ℥j.
   Aq. rosæ, . . . f℥viij.—M.
Sig.: Use locally.   Fox.

1125—℞ Chloral., . . .   gr. v.
   Cocain. hydrochlorat., .   gr. x.
   Aq. lauro-cerasi, . . f℥j.
   Aq. destillat., . . f℥j.—M.
Sig.: Apply topically. (*Pruritus of urticaria.*)
      JOURN. DE MÉD. DE PARIS.

1127—℞ Liq. carbonis deterg., . f℥ij.
   Aquæ, .   q. s. ad Oj.—M.
Sig.: Apply as a lotion.

1128—℞ Acid. carbolic., .   . gtt. v-xx.
   Adipis benzoin.,
   Ungt. petrol., . . āā ℥ij.—M.
Sig.: Apply as an ointment.

1129—℞ Chloroformi, . . . ♏x–xx.
Adipis benzoin., . . ℨij.—M.
Sig.: Apply as an ointment.

1130—℞ Aluminii nitratis, . . gr. vj.
Aq. destillat., . . . fℨj.—M.
Sig.: Apply with a soft sponge.   GILL.

1131—℞ Acid. acetic., . . . fℨj.
Glycerinæ, . . . fℨiij.—M.
Sig.: Apply locally.   GOODELL.

1132—℞ Chloral hydrat.,
Pulv. camphoræ, . āā ℨj.
Vaselini, ... ℨx.—M.
Sig.: Use twice a day. (*In hemiplegic prurigo.*)
      KOEBNER.

1133—℞ Cocaini muriat., . . gr. v.
Lanolin, ... ℨj.—M.
Sig.: Apply locally after washing with warm
water. (*In pruritus ani.*)   BESNIER.

1134—℞ Ex. nucis vomicæ,
Ex. belladonnæ, . . āā gr. iv.—M.
Et ft. pil. No. xvi.
Sig.: One pill night and morning. (*In senile pru-
ritus.*)

1135—℞ Sodii hyposulphitis, . . ℨviiss.
Acid. carbolic., . . . gr. lxxv.
Glycerinæ, . . . fℨiv.
Aquæ, ... fℨviiss.—M.
Sig.: Bathe with cold water and apply the above
three times a day or oftener. (*For pruritus ani.*)
      JOHNSTON.

1136—℞ Sodii bicarb., . . . ℨxvj.
Sig.: Put the above in bath of warm water and
bathe two or three times a week until relieved.
      HOWARD.

1137—℞ Menthol., ... ℨj.
Cerat. simplicis, . . . ℨij.
Olei amygdalæ dulcis, . . fℨj.
Acid. carbolic., . . . ℨj.
Pulv. zinci oxid., . . . ℨij.—M.
Sig.: Apply morning, noon, and night.   KELSEY.

PRURIGO (Continued).

1138—℞ Menthol, . . . gr. xv–xxx.
      Lanolin, . . . ℥j.—M.
   Sig.: Apply locally.

PSORIASIS (See Skin Diseases).

PTYALISM (SALIVATION).

1139—℞ Potass. iodid., . . . ℥ij.
      Aquæ, ... f℥ij.—M.
   Sig.: Half teaspoonful, well diluted, three times a
day.   HAMMOND.

1140—℞ Liq. plumbi subacetat., . f℥j.
      Aquæ, ... f℥viij.—M.
   Sig.: Use as a mouth-wash.   GROSS.

1141—℞ Tr. myrrhæ, . . . f℥j.
      Aquæ, . . . f℥vj.—M.
   Sig.: Use as mouth-wash.   POTTER.

1142—℞ Potass. permanganat., . gr. ii–x.
      Aquæ, ... f℥j.—M.
   Sig.: Mouth-wash. (*To correct the fetor.*)
                          GARRETSON.

1143—℞ Atropiæ sulphat., . . gr. j.
      Aquæ, ... f℥j.—M.
   Sig.: Four minims three times a day.
                          BARTHOLOW.

1144—℞ Sodii borat., . . . ℥ij.
      Pulv. myrrhæ, . . . ℥j.
      Aquæ, ... f℥vj.—M.
   Sig.: Mouth-wash or gargle.   POTTER.

1145—℞ Tr. iodinii, . . . f℥ij.
      Aq. rosæ, ... f℥viij.—M.
   Sig.: Use as mouth-wash.

1146—℞ Potass. chlorat., . . . ℥ij.
      Infus. rhois glabri rad., . Oj—M.
   Sig.: Mouth-wash.   FAHNESTOCK.

1147—℞ Acid. tannic., . . . ℥j.
      Mellis rosæ, . . . ℥ij.
      Aquæ, . . . f℥vj.—M.
   Sig.: Mouth-wash.   BARTHOLOW.

PUERPERAL FEVER (See Fever).

PUERPERAL MANIA (See Mania).

PUERPERAL PERITONITIS (See Peritonitis).

PURPURA.

1148—℞ Ol. terebinth., . . . f℥iij.
       Ex. digitalis fl., . . f℥j.
       Mucil. acaciæ, . . . f℥ss.
       Aq. menthæ pip., . . f℥j.—M.
Ft. emuls.
Sig.: Teaspoonful every three hours. BARTHOLOW.

1149—℞ Strychniæ sulphat., . . gr. ss.
       Quiniæ sulphat., . . ℈j.
       Ferri sulphat. exsiccat., . ℈ij.
Et ft. pil. No. xx.
Sig.: One pill three times a day. NAPHEYS.

1150—℞ Liq. potass. arsenitis, . f℥ss.
Sig.: Five drops in water after meals three times
a day. (When due to iodism.) PHILLIPS.

1151—℞ Sodii sulphatis, . . . ℨij.
       Ferri sulphatis, . . . gr. iij.
       Acid. sulphuric. dil., . ♏xv.
       Tr. hyoscyami, . . . ♏xl.
       Infus. calumbæ, . . f℥ij.—M.
Sig.: To be taken in the morning. TANNER.

1152—℞ Ol. terebinthinæ, . . f℥ij.
       Ol. amygdalæ express., . f℥j.
       Tr. opii deod., . . . f℥ss.
       Mucil. acaciæ, . . . f℥j.
       Aq. lauro-cerasi, . ad f℥iij.—M.
Sig.: Teaspoonful every three or four hours.
                                   HUGHES.

1153—℞ Tr. rhois aromat.,
       Glycerinæ, . . . āā f℥iss.—M.
Sig.: Teaspoonful every four hours. MUNK.

PYÆMIA.

1154—℞ Acid. salicylici, . . . ℥ss.
       Sodii biborat., . . . ℨi.
       Glycerinæ, . . . f℥j.
       Aq. menthæ pip., . . f℥v.—M.
Sig.: Tablespoonful every two or three hours.
                                   BARTHOLOW.

143

PYÆMIA (Continued).

1155—℞ Syr. ferri hypophosphitis,
Liq. hydrogen. perox. (10
vol.)
Glycerinæ, . . āā f℥iss.
Aquæ, . . q. s. ad f℥vj.—M.
Sig.: Tablespoonful three times a day. GUITÉRAS.

1156—℞ Acid. gallici, . . . f℥ss.
Acid. sulphuric. dil.,
Tr. opii deod., . . āā f℥j.
Infus. rosæ comp., . . f℥iv.—M.
Sig.: Tablespoonful every four hours.
BARTHOLOW.

1157—℞ Acid. sulphurosi, . . f℥ss-j.
Aquæ, ... f℥ij.—M.
Sig.: Take every two to four hours. TANNER.

1158—℞ Potass. permanganat., . gr. xii-xxiv.
Aquæ, ... f℥iij.—M.
Sig.: Teaspoonful three times a day. BARTHOLOW.

1159—℞ Quiniæ sulphat., . gr. v-xx.
Sig.: Take at one dose.

PYROSIS (See also Acidity).

1160—℞ Acid. carbolic., . . . gr. ij.
Aquæ, ... f℥ij.—M.
Sig.: Twenty-five drops in water before each meal.
JONES.

1161—℞ Bismuth. subcarb., . . ℥ij.
Pulv. aromat., . . . gr. xxiv.—M.
Et ft. chart. No. xii.
Sig.: One powder one hour before meals.
HUGHES.

1162—℞ Carbonis animalis, . . gr. xxiv.
Bismuth. subnit., . . ℥j.
Pulv. aromat., . . . gr. xij —M.
Et ft. chart. No. xii.
Sig.: One at meal hour. RINGER.

1163—℞ Sodii bicarbonat., . ℥iss.
Ol. anisi, . . . gtt. j.
Syr. aurant. flor.,
Aquæ, . . . āā f℥j.—M.
Sig.: One dose. PIORRY.

144

PYROSIS *(Continued).*

1164—℞ Ex. nucis vomicæ. . gr. iss.
     Argent. nitrat., .   . gr. ij.
     Ex. lupuli,   .   . gr. xij.--M.
  Et ft. pil. No. vi.
  Sig.: One pill three times a day.   BARLOW.

1165—℞ Tr. nucis vomicæ, . . f3ii–iv.
     Acid. nitric. dil.,   . . f3vj.
     Syr. zingiber., .   . . f3iij.—M.
  Sig.: Teaspoonful in a wineglassful of water.
                              PHILLIPS.

1166—℞ Quiniæ sulphat.,   .   . gr. xij.
     Acid. sulphuric. dil.,
     Spt. chloroform.,   . āā f3ij.
     Syr. aurant. cort., . ad f3iss.—M.
  Sig.: Teaspoonful in water three times a day.

QUINSY.   MARTIN

1167—℞ Sodii bicarb.,   .   .   . 3j.
  Sig.: Apply locally to the tonsil in powder or in
  warm solution.   BAKER.

1168—℞ Salinaphthol.,   .   .   . gr. xx-xxv.
     Spt. vinii rectificat., . . f3j.—M.
  Sig.: One part to twenty of water, as an antiseptic
  gargle.   GEORGI.

1169—℞ Tr. guaiac. ammoniat.,
     Tr. cinchonæ comp., . āā f3iv.
     Potass. chlorat.,   .   . 3ij.
     Pulv. acaciæ,   .   .   . q. s.
     Aquæ,   .   . q. s. ad f3iv.—M.
  Sig.: Use as a gargle and take a teaspoonful every
  two hours.

1170—℞ Argenti nitrat., .   .   . gr. l.
     Aquæ, ... f3j.—M.
  Sig : Paint tonsil to abort impending attack.
                              POWELL.

1171—℞ Chloral hydrat., .   . gr. iv.
     Glycerinæ,   .   . . f3j.—M.
  Sig.: Use locally.   THE PACIFIC RECORD.

1172—℞ Tr. ferri chlor., . . . f3iss-iij.
     Glycerinæ,   .   . . f3j —M.
  Sig.: Use locally every two or three hours.
                              STARR.

145

QUINSY (*Continued*).

1173—℞ Jodi pur., ... gr. j.
    Potassii iodid., . . . gr. ij.
    Tr. opii, ... ℩xx.
    Glycerini, ... f℥iv.—M.

Sig.: Paint the tonsils morning and evening, and use as a gargle one-half a teaspoonful to a glass of warm water. (*For hypertrophy of the tonsils.*) MOURE.

1174—℞ Sodii salicylat., . . . gr. v-x.

Sig.: Take every three hours and use the following locally :—

1175—℞ Potass. chloratis, q. s. ad sat. sol.
    Tr. ferri chlor.,
    Glycerinæ,
    Aquæ, . āā f℥ss.—M.

Sig.: Use locally. PEPPER.

1176—℞ Tr. guaiaci ammoniat., . f℥ij.

Sig.: Teaspoonful in half a glassful of milk three or four times daily. (*Early stage.*) SAJOUS.

1177—℞ Sodii salicylat., . . . ℨiij.
    Syr. acaciæ, . . . f℥ss.
    Aq. cinnam., . . ad f℥iij.—M.

Sig.: Dessertspoonful every three hours. EASBY.

1178—℞ Tr. ferri chlor., . . . ℩xxiv-xlviij.
    Potass. chlorat., . . gr. xxiv.
    Syr. zingiberis, . . f℥j.
    Aquæ, . . q. s. ad f℥iij.—M.

Sig.: Teaspoonful every two hours for a child of two years. STARR.

1179—℞ Potass. chlorat., . . ℨij.
    Infus. rhus glabri baccar., ℥j.—M.

Sig.: Use as gargle. GERHARD.

1180—℞ Creolin., ... gr. xv.
    Aq. destillat., ... ℥j.
    Aq. menth. pip., . . . f℥iij.—M.

Sig.: Use as a gargle. (*For simple tonsillitis.*)

1181—℞ Acid. citric., . . . gr. xv.
    Potass. bicarbonat., . . Əj.
    Tr. guaiaci, . . . ℩x.
    Mucilag. acaciæ, . . f℥j.—M.

Sig.: One dose. To be taken while effervescing. (*For children.*) HAZARD.

1182—℞ Tr. belladonnæ, . . f℥ss.

Sig.: Five drops in water every one to three hours.
PHILLIPS.

1183—℞ Tr. verat. viridis (Norwood), gtt. xxx.
Morphiæ sulphat., . . gr. ⅓.
Aquæ, ... f℥vj.—M.

Sig.: Teaspoonful every hour for two hours, and
then every two or three hours, as needed. HUDSON.

1184—℞ Creosot., . . . gtt. viij.
Tr. myrrhæ,
Glycerini, . . . āā f℥ij.
Aquæ, . . . q. s. ad f℥viij.—M.

Sig.: To be used as a gargle every two hours. (*For
follicular tonsillitis.*)

1185—℞ Tr. aconiti rad., . . . f℥ss.
Tr. belladonnæ, . . . f℥j.
Tr. ferri chloridi, . . . f℥ij.
Tr. iodi comp., . . . f℥iiss.
Glycerini, . . q. s. ad f℥j.—M.

Sig.: Apply topically with a brush.

1186—℞ Tr. aconiti rad., . . f℥ss.

Sig.: From one-half to a drop every fifteen minutes
for two hours, and afterwards hourly. RINGER.

1187—℞ Acid. tannic., . . . gr. xv.
Tr. iodi, ... gtt. ij.
Acid. carbol., . . . f℥ss.
Glycerinæ, . . . f℥ss.
Aquæ, ... f℥iiss.—M.

Sig.: Apply locally. (*To abort abscess.*)
JOUR. RESPIRATORY ORGANS.

RACHITIS (RICKETS), SCROFULA, STRUMA.

1188—℞ Syr. ferri iodid., . . f℥iss.
Mist. ol. morrhuæ et lactophos. calcis, . q. s. ad f℥iij.—M.

Sig.: From one-half to a teaspoonful three times a
day. STARR.

1189—℞ Ol. morrhuæ, . . . f℥vj.
Syr. calcii lactophosphat.,
Liq. calcis, . . āā f℥iij —M.

Sig.: One-half to one teaspoonful three or four
times a day. SMITH.

1190—℞ Syr. ferri iodid., . . gtt. iii–xx.
     Aq. destillat., . q. s. ad f℥iij.—M.

Sig.: A teaspoonful every four or five hours during the day. (*Child six months or one year.*) SMITH.

1191—℞ Syr. calcii lactophos., . f℥iv.

Sig.: One teaspoonful three times a day after meals.
BARTHOLOW.

1192—℞ Phosphori, . . . gr. ⅙.
     Ol. amygdalæ, . . . f℥viiss.
     Pulv. acaciæ,
     Sacchar. alb., . ⸪ āā ℨiv.
     Aq. destillat., . . . f℥x.—M.
Ft. emuls.

Sig.: One teaspoonful three times a day after meals.

1193—℞ Phosphori, . . . gr. ⅓.
     Ol. morrhuæ, . . . f℥vj.—M.

Sig.: One teaspoonful three times a day after meals.
KASSOWITZ.

1194—℞ Calcii phosphatis,
     Ferri phosphatis, . āā gr. xxxvj.—M.
Ft. chart. No. xii.

Sig.: One powder morning and noon. NELIGAN.

1195—℞ Ol. morrhuæ, . . . f℥iv.
     Aq. calcis, ... f℥iij.
     Et ad—
     Syr. ferri iodidi, . . f℥iv.
     Ol. gaultheriæ, . . . f℥ss.
     Syr. simp., . q. s. ad f℥viij.—M.

Sig.: A tablespoonful three times a day.

1196—℞ Syr. ferri et manganesii
     iodid., ... f℥i–ij.
     Syr. simp., . q. s. ad f℥ij.—M.

Sig.: Teaspoonful three times a day. BARTHOLOW.

1197—℞ Creasoti, ... gtt. iv.
     Ol. morrhuæ, . . . f℥iss.
     Pulv. tragacanthæ comp., . ℨij.
     Aq. anisi, ... f℥ivss.—M.

Sig.: One-half to two tablespoonfuls three times a
day. THOMPSON.

RACHITIS (*Continued*).

1198—℞ Ferri bromid., . . gr. xij.
Div. in pil. No. xx.
Sig.: One pill three times a day. ROBERT DICK.

1199—℞ Ferri et quiniæ citrat., . gr. x.
Ol. morrhuæ,
Glycerinæ, . . āā f℥ij.—M.
Sig.: Tablespoonful three times a day.
HARTSHORNE.

1200—℞ Morrhuol, ... ℨj.
Div. in capsulæ No. xx.
Sig.: Three to four capsules daily. LAFARGUE.

1201—℞ Acid. tannic., . . . gr. vi–xij.
Div. in chart. No. xii.
Sig.: One powder two or three times a day.
ALISON.

1202—℞ Carbon. animalis,
Pulv. glycyrrhizæ, . āā ℨvj.—M.
Sig.: Half to a whole teaspoonful twice a day. (*In
children.*) RADIUS.

1203—℞ Ex. hæmatoxyli, . . gr. xx.
Vini ipecac., . . . ♏xx.
Vini opii, ... ♏x.
Mist. cretæ, . . . f℥ij.—M.
Sig.: Teaspoonful every four hours. (*In diarrhœa.*)
GOODHART and STARR.

1204—℞ Potass. iodidi, . . . ℨij.
Tr. stillingiæ comp.,
Syr. simp., . . āā f℥ij.—M.
Sig.: A teaspoonful four times a day. MENTZER.

1205—℞ Quiniæ sulphatis, . . gr. j.
Acid. sulphuric. dil., . ♏i–ij.
Vini ferri, ... f℥i–ij.—M.
Sig.: To be taken three times a day. JENNER.

1206—℞ Potass. iodid., . . gr. xxx.
Tr. iodinii, . . gtt. xv.
Acid. tannic., . . gr. xv.
Syr. quiniæ, . . f℥viiss.
Syr. acaciæ, . . f℥iv et f℥vss.—M.
Sig.: A fourth part to be taken every two hours
until four doses are taken. GUMOUT,

149

RACHITIS (Continued).

1207—℞ Iodol, ... gr. xxiij.
Ol. morrhuæ, . . . ℥viij.
Spt. menthæ pip., . . gtt. xx.—M.

Sig.: Tablespoonful after each meal. (*In enlarged glands.*) MONIN.

1208—℞ Acid. hydrocyanic. dil., . ℨj.
Glycerinæ, . . . ℥ij.
Acid. nitric. dil., . . ℨiij.
Infus. quassiæ, . . ad ℥xiiiss.—M.

Sig.: Tablespoonful three times a day. AITKEN.

1209—℞ Tr. nucis vomicæ, . . ℨj.
Ex. stillingiæ fl., . . ℨv.
Syr. sarsaparillæ comp., . ℨij.—M.

Sig.: Five to fifteen drops three times a day in water. BARTHOLOW.

1210—℞ Calcii chlorid., . . . ℨj.
Aquæ, ... ℥iiss.—M.

Sig.: Teaspoonful two or three times a day in milk. PHILLIPS.

1211—℞ Ammon. carbonat., . . gr. xxiv.
Potass. bicarb., . . . ℨij.
Ex. glycyrrhizæ fl., . . ℥ss.
Aquæ, . . q. s. ad ℥iij.—M.

Sig.: Teaspoonful every three or four hours. GOODHART.

RATTLESNAKE BITE.

1212—℞ Hydrarg. chlor. corros., . gr. ij.
Potass. iodid., . . . gr. iv.
Aquæ, ... ♏v.
Solve et ad—
Bromi, ... ℨv.—M.

Sig.: Take ten drops in a tablespoonful of wine or brandy every fifteen or twenty minutes. BIBRON.

1213—℞ Aq. ammoniæ, . . . ℨj.
Aquæ, ... ℨiij.—M.

Sig.: Inject thirty minims hypodermically into a superficial vein above seat of injury. HALFORD.

REMITTENT FEVER (See Fever).

RENAL CALCULI (See Calculi).

150

RENAL DROPSY *(See Dropsy).*

RENAL HEMORRHAGE *(See Hœmaturia).*

RHEUMATISM, ACUTE.

1214—℞ Sodii salicylat., . . . ℥ss.
　　　Tr. lavandulæ com., . . f℥iv.
　　　Glycerinæ, . . . f℥ss.
　　　Aquæ, . . q. s. ad f℥viij.—M.

Sig.: Tablespoonful every hour or two until pain and fever abate.　　MINOT (Mass. Gen. Hos.).

1215—℞ Ammonii salicylatis, . . ℈iij.
　　　Liq. pepsini, ... f℥iv.—M.

Sig.: Teaspoonful in water every two or three hours.

1216—℞ Liq. opii sed., . . . f℥j.
　　　Potass. bicarbonat., . . ℈iv.
　　　Glycerinæ, . . . f℥ij.
　　　Aq. bullientis, . . . f℥ix.—M.

Sig.: Soak a piece of flannel in the above hot solu-tion and wrap around painful joint.　　OSLER.

1217—℞ Sodii salicylat., . gr. xv.
　　　Ol. theobromæ, . q. s.—M.
　　　Ft. suppositoria.

Sig.: To be employed as a suppository five or six times in twenty-four hours.

1218—℞ Acid. salicylic., . . . ℈ij.
　　　Ferri pyrophosphat., . . ℈j.
　　　Sodii phosphat., . ℈j.
　　　Aquæ, . . q. s. ad ℥viij.—M.

Sig.: Tablespoonful every two hours.　　NICHOLS.

1219—℞ Salol., ... gr. xv.
　　　Chloroform., . . . ♏xv.
　　　Ol. amygdal. sterilisat., . . f℥ij.—M.

Sig.: Inject subcutaneously daily from two to four syringefuls.　　BOZZOLO.

1220—℞ Acid. salicylic., . . . ℈iij.
　　　Sodii borat., . . . gr. xv.
　　　Aq. menthæ pip., . ad f℥vj.—M.

Sig.: One-third to be taken during twenty-four hours. If there be no improvement in three or four days, discontinue and use—

151

1221—℞ Ammon. bromid., . . ℨiii–iv.
Div. in chart. No. xii.
Sig. A powder in water every four hours. When the acute symptoms abate add twelve to sixteen grains of quinine daily. DA COSTA.

1222—℞ Potass. iodid., . . . ℨj¼.
Sodii salicylat., . . . ℨv.
Syr. aurant. cort., . . f℥x.—M.
Sig.: One to two tablespoonfuls daily. For a chiid, teaspoonful t. i. d. AUDHOURI.

1223—℞ Potass. nitrat., . . . gr. xv.
Pulv. ipecac. comp., . . gr. iij.—M.
Et ft. chart. No. i.
Sig.: Take one powder every four hours. (*In sub-acute cases.*) DA COSTA.

1224—℞ Sodii salicylat., . . . ℨiss–ℨij.
Syr. aurantii amar. cort.,
Aq. destillat., . . . āā f℥ij.
Curacoa, ... f℥j.—M.
Sig.: To be taken in carbonated water in the course of twenty-four hours.

1225—℞ Ichthyol., . . . ℨj.
Div. in capsulæ No. xx.
Sig.: Three to six capsules during the twenty-four hours. SCHMIDT.

1226—℞ Sodii salicylatis,
Potass. iodidi,
Potass. acetatis, . āā ℨij.
Ex. cascaræ sagradæ fl.,
Glycerinæ,
Aq. cinnam., . . āā f℥ss.
Aq. menthæ pip., . . ℥iij.—M.
Ft. sol.
Sig.: Teaspoonful every four hours.
PROF. E. MARSHALL, Louisville.

1227—℞ Ol. gaultheriæ,
Ol. olivæ,
Lin. saponis,
Tr. aconiti,
Tr. opii, . . . ℨij.—M.
Ft. liniment.
Sig.: Apply freely and cover with cotton batting.
CANADA LANCET.

1228—℞ Lithii salicylat., . . ℈ii–iij.

Sig.: To be given in water during the twenty-four hours. ST. LUKE'S HOSPITAL, N. Y.

1229—℞ Lithii benzoat., . . . ʒss.
Sodii bromid.,
Potass. carbonat. pura, āā ʒij.
Potass. acetat., . . . ʒiss.
Sodii phosphat., . . ʒss.
Syr. zingiberis,
Aq. menthæ pip., . ad ʒvj.—M.

Sig.: Dessertspoonful to tablespoonful in half a glass of water every four or six hours, after food.
SATTERLEE.

1230—℞ Iodoform. deodorat., . . ʒiss.
Vaselini, ... ʒj.—M.
Sig.: Apply to the inflamed parts. BOTELER.

1231—℞ Ol. gaultheriæ,
Spt. chloroform, . āā fʒss.
Lin. saponis, . . . fʒiij.—M.
Sig.: Apply freely and wrap the joint in cotton batting. HATFIELD.

1232—℞ Acid. salicylic., . . . ʒss.
Ferri pyrophosphat., . . ʒj.
Sodii phosphatis, . . ʒx.
Aquæ, ... fʒvj.—M.
Sig.: Tablespoonful every two hours until relieved
PEABODY

1233—℞ Pimentæ, ... ʒvj, ʒij.
Aq. ammoniæ, . . . fʒiij, fʒj.
Ess. thymi,
Chloral hydrat., . āā ʒiiss.
Spt. vini rectif. (60), . . Oij.—M.
Sig.: Use pure or mixed with olive oil. (For friction about the joints.) POULET.

1234—℞ Acid. salicylici, . . . gr. x.
Sodii bicarb., . . . q. s.
Ex. glycyrrhizæ, . . gr. iij.
Glycerinæ, . . . fʒss.
Aquæ, . . q. s. ad fʒij.—M.
Sig.: Dose, dessertspoonful. VANDERBILT CLINIC.

RHEUMATISM, ACUTE (Continued).

1235—℞ Euonymin, .   .   . gr. ¼.
    Podophyllin,
    Aloin, .   .   . āā gr. ⅛.—M.

  Sig.: One tablet twice daily as required.

                                 SATTERLEE.

RHEUMATISM, CHRONIC.

1236—℞ Pulv. resinæ guaiaci,
    Potass. iodidi, .   . āā ℥j.
    Tr. colchici sem.,   .   . f℥iij.
    Aq. cinnam.,
    Syr. simp.,   q. s. ad ft. f℥vj.—M.

  Sig.: Dessertspoonful three times a day. PEPPER.

1237—℞ Liq. potass. arsenitis,   . f℥ij.
    Potass. iodid.,   .   .   . ℥ij.
    Syr. simp.,.   .   .   . f℥iij.—M.

  Sig.: Teaspoonful three times a day after meals.
                                  DA COSTA.

1238—℞ Tr. aconiti,
    Chloroform.,
    Aq. ammon.,   .   . āā f℥ij.
    Lini. saponis co.,   .   . f℥viij.—M.

  Sig.: Use locally. JEFFERSON HOSPITAL, PHILA.

1239—℞ Potass. et sodii tartratis,   . ℥ss.
    Potass. nitratis,   .   .   . ℥v.
    Vini colchici sem.,   .   . f℥ij.
    Aquæ,   .   . q. s. ad f℥ij.—M.

  Sig.: Teaspoonful three times a day.
                  BELLEVUE HOSPITAL, N. Y.

1240—℞ Tr. ferri chlor.,   .   .   . f℥ij.
    Sodii salicylat.,   .   .   . ℥ij.
    Acid. citric.,   .   .   . gr. x.
    Glycerinæ,   .   .   . ℥j.
    Liq. ammoniæ citratis (B. P.),
              q. s. ad ℥iv.
    Ol. gaultheriæ,   .   .   . gr. xv.—M.

  Sig.: Dose, one or two teaspoonfuls every two
hours until ringing of the ears is produced, and
then increase the intervals to four or six hours.
(*In anæmic cases.*) PHILADELPHIA HOSPITAL.

1241—℞ Acid. salicylic.,
    Ol. terebinthinæ,
    Lanolin.,   .   . āā ℥iss.
    Adipis, ... ℥iij.—M.
  Ft. ung.
  Sig.: Apply topically.

1242—℞ Chloroformi, ... fʒv.
     Tr. opii, ... f℥iv.
     Acid. salicylic., . . . ℨiv.
     Alcohol., ... f℥iv.
     Ol. olivæ, . . . ad fʒxij.—M.
  Sig.: Rub into the parts thoroughly.

1243—℞ Phenazoni, ... ℨij.
     Sodii salicylat., . . . ℨiij.
     Ammonii bromid., . . . ℨiv.
     Aq. cinnamomi, . . . f℥iij.—M.
  Sig.: A teaspoonful every three or four hours.
                                  ESHNER.

1244—℞ Potass. et sodii tartrat., . ℥ss.
     Vini colchici sem., . . fʒij.
     Aquæ, . . q. s. ad fʒij.—M.
  Sig.: Teaspoonful three times a day.
                CHARITY HOSPITAL, N. Y.

1245—℞ Sodii salicylat.,
     Sodii acetat.,
     Potass. bicarb., . . āā fʒiss.
     Tr. digitalis, . . . fʒiij.
     Aquæ, . . q. s. ad f℥ij.—M.
  Sig.: Teaspoonful four times a day. MAYS.

1246—℞ Potass. iodid.,
     Salicin, . . . āā ʒij.
     Ex. manacæ fl., . . . fʒij.
     Tr. cimicifugæ, . . . f℥j.
     Hydrangeæ lithiat., q. s. ad f℥vj.—M.
  Sig.: Teaspoonful, diluted, every three or four hours.

1247—℞ Potassii bromid., . . . ʒj.
     Ext. rhus toxicodendron fl., . fʒv.
     Syr. sarsap. comp., . . . f℥iss.
     Aquæ, ... f℥iv.—M.
  Sig.: A teaspoonful after each meal. BENEDICT.

1248—℞ Ol. gaultheriæ,
     Ol. olivæ,
     Liniment. saponis,
     Tr. aconiti,
     Tr. opii, . . . āā ʒij.—M.
  Ft. liniment.
  Sig.: Apply to part.

1249—℞ Liniment. aconiti (B. P.),
    Liniment. belladonnæ, āā f℥ij.
    Glycerinæ, . . ad f℥ij.—M.
  Sig.: Apply over the seat of pain.   FOTHERGILL.

1250—℞ Potass. iodid., . . ℨiij.
    Vini colchici sem.,
    Tr. opii camph., . āā f℥ij.
    Tr. stramonii, . . . f℥vj.
    Tr. cimicifugæ, . . . f℥iij.
  Sig.: Teaspoonful three times a day.
                   ST. LUKE'S HOSPITAL, N. Y.

1251—℞ Chloroform.,
    Tr. aconiti rad.,
    Ol. terebinthinæ, . āā f℥ss.
    Ol. sassafras, . . . ℳv.
    Lini. saponis camphorat., . f℥iiss.—M.
  Sig.: Apply locally.   GERHARD.

1252—℞ Ol. cajuputi,
    Tr. opii, . . . āā f℥ij.
    Ol. terebinthinæ, . . f℥iv.
    Liniment. ammoniæ, . . f℥j.—M.
  Sig.: Use locally.   FULLER.

1253—℞ Tr. iodinii,
    Spt. vini rect., . . āā f℥j.—M.
  Sig.: Apply with a camel's-hair brush night and
morning.   DA COSTA.

RHINITIS (See Catarrh).

RICKETS (See Rachitis).

RINGWORM (See Skin Diseases).

RUBEOLA (See Fever).

RUPIA (See Skin Diseases).

SALIVATION (See Ptyalism).

SARCINÆ AND TORULÆ.

1254—℞ Sodii hyposulphitis, . . ℨij.
    Infus. quassiæ, . . . f℥vj.—M.
  Sig.: Tablespoonful three times a day.   NEALE.

SARCINÆ AND TORULÆ (Continued).

1255—℞ Sodii sulphitis, . . gr. xxx-xl.
Infus. quassiæ, . . f℥iss.—M.

Sig.: To be taken three times a day. JENNER.

1256—℞ Acid. sulphurosi, . . f℈i-iss.
Infus. calumbæ, . . f℥xij.—M.

Sig.: Wineglassful ten minutes before meals.
LAWSON.

1257—℞ Acid. sulphurosi, . . f℈ss-j.
Aquæ, ... f℥ij.—M.

Sig.: To be taken three times a day. TANNER.

SATYRIASIS (See Nymphomania).

SCABIES (See Lice).

SCARLATINA (See also Fever and Diphtheria).

1258—℞ Tr. ferri chlor., . . . f℈j.
Potass. chlorat., . . gr. xlviij.
Glycerinæ, . . . f℥j.
Aquæ, . . q. s. ad f℥iij.—M.

Sig.: Teaspoonful every two hours for a child of
four years. MORRIS.

1259—℞ Acid. boracic., . . . ℈ss.
Potass. chlor., . . . ℈ij.
Tr. ferri chlor., . . . f℈ij.
Glycerinæ,
Syr. simp., . . āā f℥j.
Aquæ, ... f℥ij.—M.

Sig.: Teaspoonful every two hours for a child of
five years. J. LEWIS SMITH.

1260—℞ Infus. digitalis, . . . f℥iv.

Sig.: One-half to one teaspoonful every two or
three hours. BARTHOLOW.

1261—℞ Acid. carbol., . . . ♏xx.
Vaseline, ... ℥j.—M.

Sig.: Apply to body night and morning. STARR.

1262—℞ Acid. salicylic., . . . gr. xlviij.
Aquæ, ... f℥ij.
Syr. aurantii, . q. s. ad f℥iij.—M.

Sig.: Teaspoonful every hour during the day and
every two or three hours at night. HARE.

1263—℞ Ol. menthæ pip.,   .   .   ♏xv.
       Ol. olivæ, ...   f℥iij.—M.
    Sig.: Apply to body night and morning.   STARR.

1264—℞ Tr. digitalis,   .   .   .   fℨss.
       Liq. ammon. acetat., .   .   f℥iss.
       Spt. æth. nit.,   .   .   .   fℨij.
       Syr. tolu, ...   f℥ss.
       Aq. cari,   .   .   q. s. ad   f℥iij.—M.
    Sig.: Teaspoonful every two hours for a child of six or eight years.   GOODHART and STARR.

1265—℞ Chloralis, ...   gr. xxx.
       Syr. lactucarii (Aubergier),
       Aquæ,   .   .   .   āā   f℥ss.—M.
    Sig.: Teaspoonful in cold water every two, three, or four hours.   J. C. WILSON.

1266—℞ Hydrarg. biniodid.,   .   .   gr. i-vj.
       Ex. glycyrrhizæ,   .   .   gr. xij.—M.
    Et ft. pil. No. xxiv.
    Sig.: One pill every four hours.   DUKES.

1267—℞ Resorcin, ...   ℨij.
       Lanolini, ...   ℥iss.
       Ol. sesami,   .   .   .   ℥ss.—M
    Sig.: Rub well into the skin. (*To hasten desquamation.*)   JAMIESON.

1268—℞ Pulv. digitalis fol.,   .   .   ℨj.
       Aq. bullientis,   .   .   .   f℥vj.—M.
    Ft. infusio.
    Sig.: Give one teaspoonful every hour until you get the physiological effect.   ATKINSON.

1269—℞ Ex. jaborandi fl.,   .   .   f℥ss.
       Liq. potass. citrat., q. s. ad   f℥iij.—M.
    Sig.: Teaspoonful every four hours at the age of six years. (*Scarlatinal anasarca.*)   STARR.

1270—℞ Antifebrin,   .   .   .   gr. xv.
       Sacch. alb.,   .   .   .   gr. xxx.—M.
    Et ft. chart. No. x.
    Sig.: A powder as required to relieve fever, for a child of three or four years.   WIDOWITZ.

1271—℞ Acid. carbol., . . . gr. xx.
    Thymol, ... gr. x.
    Vaseline, vel ung. simp., . ℥j.—M.
  Sig.: Rub in well.   STARR.

SCIATICA (See also Neuralgia).

1272—℞ Saloli,
    Sacch. lact., . . āā ℨiij.—M.
  Div. in pulv. No. xii.
  Sig.: One powder every four to six hours.
                  ASCHENBACH.

1273—℞ Antipyrin, . . . ℨij.
    Syr. aurant. cort., . . f℥ss.
    Aq. aurant. flor., . . f℥ij.—M.
  Sig.: A dessertspoonful every hour to four hours,
until three to six doses are taken.   GERMAIN SÉE.

1274—℞ Pulv. sulphuris sub., . ℥iv.
  Sig.: Dust thickly on the limb and envelop it in
soft flannel.   RINGER.

1275—℞ Veratriæ, ... ℈i-ij.
    Adipis, ... ℥j.—M.
  Sig.: Rub well into painful part.   TURNBULL.

1276—℞ Morphiæ sulph., . . gr. ss-$\frac{2}{3}$.
    Atropiæ sulph., . . . gr. $\frac{1}{25}$.
    Aq. destillat., . . . ♏xx.—M.
  Sig.: Inject deeply into the muscle over the course
of the nerve.   BROWN SÉQUARD.

1277—℞ Quininæ sulphat., . . gr. ij.
    Morphinæ sulphat., . . gr. $\frac{1}{20}$.
    Strychninæ sulphat., . gr. $\frac{1}{30}$.
    Acid. arseniosi, . . . gr. $\frac{1}{20}$.
    Ex. aconiti, . . . gr. $\frac{1}{4}$.—M.
  Et ft. pil. No. i.
  Sig.: Take one pill every one, two, or three hours.
                 GROSS.

1278—℞ Spt. glonoin., . . . f℥ss.
    Tr. capsici, . . . f℥iss.
    Aq. menth. piper., . . f℥iij.—M.
  Sig.: Five drops three times daily for three days,
then ten drops three times a day.

1279—Methyl chlorid. sprayed along the course of the
    nerve.   HUGHES.

1280—℞ Sodii salicylat.,   .   .   . ʒss.
        Ol. cajuputi, ... fʒss.
        Ol. eucalypti, ... ♏xv.
        Liniment. saponis, .   .   . fʒss.
        Spt. rectif.,   .   . q. s. ad fʒviij.—M.
    Sig.: Apply with friction topically.

1281—℞ Potass. iodid.,   .   .   . ℈j.
        Decoct. sarsap. co., .   . fʒij.—M.
    Sig.: To be taken three times a day. (*Chronic
cases.*)   WARING.

1282—℞ Tr. aconiti rad.,
        Tr. colchici sem.,
        Tr. belladonnæ,
        Tr. cimicifugæ,   . āā fʒj.—M.
    Sig.: Twelve drops every four to eight hours.
                  J. T. METCALF.

1283—℞ Chloroformi,   .   .   . fʒij.
    Sig.: Five to fifteen minims hypodermically near
the seat of pain.   BARTHOLOW.

1284—℞ Tr. colchici sem.,   .   . gtt. xv.
        Potass. iodid.,   .   .   . gr. x.
        Tr. zingiber.,   .   .   . gtt. x.
        Syr. simp.,
        Aquæ,   . āā q. s. ad fʒij.—M.
    Sig.: Apply a strip of blistering plaster over the
course of the nerve, and give the above in water
three times a day.   DA COSTA.

1285—℞ Pulv. opii,
        Pulv. ipecacuanhæ, .   . āā gr. xv.
        Sodii salicylat.,   .   .   . ʒiss.
        Ex. cascaræ sagrad.,   .   . q. s. ad.—M.
    Ft. pil. No. xx.
    Sig.: From one to three pills daily. RICHARDSON.

1286—℞ Saloli,   .   •   •   • ʒss.
        Ol. vaselini,   .   .   . ʒv.—M.
    Sig.: Inject twenty or thirty minims over course of
the nerve.   MEUNIER.

SCIRRHUS (See Cancer).

SCLEROSIS, POSTERIOR SPINAL *(See also Locomotor Ataxia).*

1287—℞ Ex. belladonnæ, . . gr. iv.
    Ol. terebinthinæ, . . f3ij.
    Ol. theobromæ, . . . q. s.—M.
 Et ft. capsulæ No. xii.
 Sig.: One three times a day. A. McL. HAMILTON.

1288—℞ Antipyrin, . . . 3ij.
    Syr. sarsaparillæ comp., . f3ij.
    Aq. cinnamomi, . . ad f3vj.—M.
 Sig.: Tablespoonful every hour or two until relieved.   SUCKLING.

1289—℞ Tr. ferri chlor.,
    Tr. nucis vomicæ,
    Acid. phosphoric. dil.,
    Syr. simplicis, . . āā f3j.—M.
 Sig.: Teaspoonful in water an hour before meals.
             SWERINGEN.

1290—℞ Argenti nitratis,
    Ex. belladonnæ, . āā gr. i–viij.
    Ex. gentian., . . . q. s.—M.
 Et ft. pil. No. xxiv.
 Sig.: One after each meal. A. McL. HAMILTON.

1291—℞ Potass. iodid., . . . 3vi–viij.
    Ferri et ammon. citrat., . 3ij.
    Tr. aurant. cort.,
    Syr. simp., . . āā f3iij.
    Aq. menthæ pip., . ad f3iv.—M.
 Sig.: Teaspoonful in water an hour after meals.
             SWERINGEN.

SCROFULA *(See Rachitis).*

SCURVY *(See also Purpura).*

1292—℞ Potass. bitartratis, . . 3j.
    Ol. limonis, . . . ♏xv.
    Sacch. alb., . . . 3ij.
    Aq. bullientis, . . . Oij.—M.
 Ft. haustus.
 Sig.: Use when cold as a drink. TANNER.

1293—℞ Acid. muriat., . . . f3j.
    Mellis,
    Aq. rosæ, . . . āā f3j.—M.
 Sig.: Apply three or four times daily to the gums.
             BRANDA.

SCURVY (Continued).

1294—℞ Succi limonis, . . . f℥viij.—M.
    Sig.: Two tablespoonfuls daily.   PARKES.

SEA-SICKNESS.

1295—℞ Cerii oxalat., . . . gr. ij.
    Tr. valerian. co., . . f℥j.
    Aquæ, ... f℥j.—M.
    Sig.: Take every thirty minutes until relieved.
         WALSH.

1296—℞ Chloroform., . . . f℥ss.
    Sig.: Two to five minims on sugar every half hour
until relieved.   BARTHOLOW.

1297—℞ Chloral hydrat., . . ℥ss.
    Syr. aurant. cort., . . f℥j.
    Aq. aurant. flor., . ad f℥ij.—M.
    Sig.: One or two teaspoonfuls every four hours.
         RINGER.

1298—℞ Amyl nitritis, . . . ℨij.
    Sig.: Inhale three to five drops on a handkerchief,
with care.   BARTHOLOW.

1299—℞ Cocaini hydrochlor., . . gr. xxx.
    Aquæ, ... fℨivss.—M.
    Sig.: Four or five drops on a small piece of ice
three times a day.   OTTO.

1300—℞ Hyoscyami,
    Strychniæ, . . āā gr. ss.
    Ex. gentian., . . . Əj.—M.
    Et ft. pil. No. xxxiii.
    Sig.: One every ten minutes.   EMBLETON.

SEPTICÆMIA (See Pyæmia).

SHINGLES (See also Skin Diseases and Herpes Zoster).

1301—℞ Veratriæ, ... Əi–ij.
    Vaselini, ... ℥j.—M.
    Sig.: Apply locally.   RINGER.

1302—℞ Hydrarg. chlor. mit., . gr. v.
    Sacch. alb., . . ℥ss.—M.
    Et ft. chart. No. x.
    Sig.: One powder every two hours, to be followed
by a saline aperient.   GERHARD.

SHINGLES (Continued).

1303—℞ Zinci phosphidi,
  Ex. nucis vomicæ, . ãã gr. x.—M.
Et ft. pil. No. xxx.
Sig. One pill every two to four hours. BULKLEY.

1304—℞ Magnesii carbonat., . . gr. xx.
  Vini colchici rad.,
  Tr. opii, . . . ãã f3ss.
  Aq. camphoræ, . . . f3j.—M.
Sig.: For one dose. (*To relieve the deep-seated pain
in the chest.*)   THOMPSON.

1305—℞ Sulphuris sublimat., . Ɖj.
  Hydrarg. ammoniat., . 3ss.
  Ungt. simplicis, . . 3j.—M.
Sig.: Apply two or three times a day. CORFE.

1306—℞ Collodii flex., . . . f3j.
Sig.: Apply with a brush to the affected area constantly, to exclude the air.   AUSTIE.

1307—℞ Pulv. amyli, . . . 3iv.
Sig.: Apply as a dusting powder. BULKLEY.

SICK-HEADACHE (See Headache).

SINGULTUS (See Hiccough).

SKIN, DISEASES.

1308—℞ Liq. potassæ, . . . f3j.
  Aquæ, ... f3j.—M.
Sig.: Apply to the acne spots only, then use :—

1309—℞ Plumbi nitrat., . . . gr. xv.
  Ungt. petrolei, . . . 3j.—M.
Sig.: Apply twice daily. (*In acne indurata.*)
   BARTHOLOW.

1310—℞ Sulphuris præcip., . . 3j.
  Glycerinæ, . . . f3ss.
  Adipis benzoat., . . 3j.
  Ol. rosæ, . . . gtt. iij.—M.
Sig.: To be thoroughly rubbed into the skin at
night.   DUHRING.

1311—℞ Hydrarg. chlor. corros., . gr. ij.
  Ungt. petrolei, . . . 3j.—M.
Sig.: Apply thoroughly. (*In acne rosacea.*)
   HUGHES.

SKIN DISEASES *(Continued).*

1312—℞ Sulphuris præcip., . . ℨiv.
    Pulv. camphoræ, . . gr. x.
    Pulv. tragacanthæ, . . ℈j.
    Aq. calcis, . . . f℥ij.
    Aq. rosæ, ... f℥ij.—M.

Sig.: Shake the bottle before using, and apply
every few hours. (*In acne rosacea.*)
"KUMMERFELD'S LOTION."

1313—℞ Ichthyol.,
    Resorcin., . . . āā gr. xv-lxxv.
    Lanolin., ... ℨvj.
    Aq. destillat., . . q. s. ad f℥iss.—M.

Sig.: Apply topically. (*Acne rosacea.*)

1314—℞ Sulphur. præcip.,
    Cretæ præcip.,
    Aq. laurocerasi,
    Spt. vini rect.,
    Glycerinæ, . . āā ℨij.—M.

Sig.: Bathe the face with hot water and dry it
with friction, then apply the lotion. (*In acne of the
face.*) LEROY.

1315—℞ Magnesii sulphat., . . ℥j.
    Ferri sulphat., . . . gr. iv.
    Sodii chloridi, . . . ℨss.
    Acid. sulphuric. dil., . f℥ij.
    Infus. quassiæ, . . ad f℥iv.—M.

Sig.: Tablespoonful in a tumbler of cold water
before breakfast. (*In acne.*) STARTIN.

1316—℞ Liq. potass. arsenitis, . f℥ij.
    Vini ferri, . . ad f℥iv.—M.

Sig.: Teaspoonful in water after meals. (*In acne
with anæmia.*) VAN HARLINGEN.

1317—℞ Chrysarobini, . . . ℨss.
    Collodii, ... f℥j.—M.

Sig.: Put a brush through the cork and paint
lesion every night. G. H. FOX.

1318—℞ Potass. acetat., . . . ℨiv.
    Tr. nucis vomicæ, . . f℥ij.
    Ex. rumicis fl., . . ad f℥iv.—M.

Sig.: Teaspoonful, well diluted, after meals, three
times a day. (*In acne vulgaris.*) BULKLEY.

1319—℞ Zinci oleat.,
Pulv. talc, . . āā ʒj.—M.
Sig.: Dust on every morning. (*In acne.*)
JAMIESON.

1320—℞ Potass. acetat., . . . ʒj.
Sodii et potass. tart., . ʒij.
Syr. zingiberis, . . fʒij.
Aquæ, . . q. s. ad fʒviij.—M.
Sig.: Tablespoonful in a wineglassful of water,
after meals. (*In acne.*) TAYLOR.

1321—℞ Chloral. hydrat., . . ʒj.
Acid. carbolic.,
Tr. iodi, ... āā ſʒss.—M.
Sig.: Apply with a brush. (*Chloasma.*)

1322—℞ Ol. theobromæ,
Ol. ricini, . . āā ʒiiss.
Zinci oxidi, . . . gr. ivss.
Hydrarg. ammon., . . gr. ij.
Ol. rosæ, ... q. s.—M.
Sig.: Apply morning and evening. (*In chloasma.*)
MOREIER.

1323—℞ Hydrarg. pur., . . . gr. c.
Ungt. hydrarg.,
Sevi benzoinati, . āā gr. c.
Adipis benzoinati, . ad fʒiv.—M.
Sig.: Spread on muslin and bind in patches at
night, or rub in thoroughly with the finger. (*In
chloasma.*) VAN HARLINGEN.

1324—℞ Zinci oxidi, . . . gr. iij.
Hydrarg. ammoniat., . gr. iss.
Ol. theobromæ,
Ol. ricini, . . āā ʒiiss.
Essent. rosæ, . . . gtt. x.—M.
Sig.: Apply to the face night and morning. (*In
chloasma of pregnancy.*) MONIN.

1325—℞ Quiniæ sulphat., . . ʒss.
Acid. sulphuric. aromat., fʒss.
Tr. cardamomi comp., . fʒiss.
Aquæ, . . q. s. ad fʒiv.—M.
Sig.: Dessertspoonful three times a day. (*In
ecthyma.*) RINGER.

1326—℞ Sodii biborat., . . . ʒii–iij.
Aq. rosæ, ... f̄ʒvj.—M.
Sig.: Apply two or three times a day. (*In ecthyma.*)
COPLAND.

1327—℞ Ex. opii, ... gr. x–xx.
Acid. tannic., . . . Ꭰj.
Unguent., . . . ʒj.—M.
Sig.: Apply after the inflammatory condition has
been subdued with lead lotion. (*In idiopathic ecthyma.*)
TILBURY FOX.

1328—℞ Hydrarg. iodid. rub., . gr. xij.
Cerati simp., . . . ʒviiss.—M.
Sig.: Apply locally. (*In ecthyma syphilitica.*)
DIDAY.

1329—℞ Pulv. camphoræ, . ʒss.
Zinci oxidi,
Bismuthi subnit., . . āā ʒj.
Talci, ... ʒiss.—M.
Sig.: Use as dusting-powder. (*Eczema.*) BROCQ.

1330—℞ Formalin., . gr. iiss.
Zinci oxidi,
Pulv. talc., . . . āā ʒss.
Vaselin., ... ʒj.—M.
Sig.: Apply topically. (*Eczema.*) ROTTER.

1331—℞ Picis liquidæ, . . . fʒj.
Sulphur, ... Ꭰj.
Ungt. simplicis, . . fʒj.—M.
Sig.: To be rubbed in morning and evening. (*In
eczema squamosum.*) STELWAGON.

1332—℞ Hydrarg. ammoniat.,
Acid. boric., . .
Zinci oxidi, . . āā ʒj.
Plumbi acetat., . . gr. v.
Vaselini, ... ʒj.—M.
Sig.: Apply night and morning. (*In eczema of the
nares.*) MEDICAL PRESS.

1333—℞ Glyceriti amyli, . . ʒviiss.
Acid. tannic.,
Hydrarg. chlor. mit., āā gr. xv.—M.
Sig.. Apply morning and evening. (*In dry eczema
with itching.*) VIDAL.

SKIN DISEASES (Continued).

1334—℞ Pulv. rhei,
    Sodii bicarb.,   .   . āā ʒi–iij.
    Aq. menthæ pip.,   . . f℥iv.—M.
  Sig.: Teaspoonful after meals.   VAN HARLINGEN

1335—℞ Ungt. zinci oxidi,
    Ungt. plumbi subacetat., āā ℥ss.
    Chloral hydrat.,
    Pulv. camphoræ,   . āā gr. xv.—M.
  Sig.: Use two or three times daily, after bathing
with warm water. (In general eczema.)

1336—℞ Bismuth. subnitrat., .   . ℥iij.
    Zinci oxidi,   . . . gr. xxx.
    Glycerinæ,   . . . f℥iss.
    Acid. carbolic. liquid., . ℳxx.
    Vaselin. alb., . . . ℥vj.—M.
  Sig.: Use night and morning. (In eczema.)
                           MACKINTOSH.

1337— ℞ Lin. calcis,   .   .   . f℥iv.
    Ext. belladonnæ,   .   . gr. xij.
    Zinci oxidi,   .   .   . ʒij.
    Glycerini,   .   .   . f℥ij.
    Aq. calcis,   .   .   . f℥iv.—M.
  Sig.: To be applied at night after bathing the parts
in hot water. (Eczema of genitals.)   FINNY.

1338—℞ Lin. calcis,   .   .   . f℥iv.
    Ac. hydrocyan. dil.,   . . f℥j.
    Liq. plumbi subacetat., . . f℥ij.
    Glycerini,   .   .   . f℥ij.
    Aq. rosæ,   . . q. s. ad f℥viij.—M.
  Sig.: Apply on strips of old linen. (Eczema of
genitals.)   FINNY.

1339—℞ Acid. salicylic., .   . . gr. xlv.
    Zinci oxidi,   .   . ʒiij.
    Pulv. amyli,   .   . ℥v.—M.
  Sig. Dust the surface and cover with wadding.
                           ELLIOTT.

1340—℞ Ammon. sulpho-ichthyol., . ʒij.
    Aq. rosæ,
    Glycerinæ,   . . āā f℥ss.—M.
  Sig.: Use locally. (In nervous eczema.)   RAVOGHI.

1341—℞ Ex. grindeliæ robust. fl., . f℥ij.
    Aquæ,   .   .   . Oj.—M.
  Sig.: Apply on cloths. (In eczema covering a large
surface.)   VAN HARLINGEN.

1342—℞ Pulv. camphoræ, . . ℨss.
　　　 Pulv. zinci ox., . . . ℥iij.
　　　 Glycerinæ, . . . ♏xl.
　　　 Ungt. benzoatis, . . ℥j.—M.
　　Sig.: Apply locally. (*In vesiculous eczema.*)
　　　　　　　　　　　　　　　　　　DUURING.

1343—℞ Hydrarg. chlor. mit., . . gr. xx.
　　　 Acid. carbol., . . . gtt. xx.
　　　 Ungt. zinci ox.,
　　　 Vaselini, . . . āā ℥ss.—M.
　　Sig.: Apply night and morning. (*In infantile eczema.*)
　　zema.)　　　　　　　　　　　　　POWELL.

1344—℞ Acid. salicylic., . . . gr. xxv.
　　　 Pulv. amyli,
　　　 Pulv. zinci ox., . . āā ℥ij.
　　　 Petrolati, ... ℥ss.—M.
　　Sig.: Use twice a day. (*In eczema of the hand.*)
　　　　　　　　　　　　　　　　　STELWAGON.

1345—℞ Bismuth. oxidi, . . . ℨj.
　　　 Acid. oleic. pur., . . ℥j.
　　　 Ceræ albæ, . . . ℥iij.
　　　 Vaselini, ... ℥ix.
　　　 Ol. rosæ, ... ♏ij.—M.
　　Sig.: Apply twice a day.　　ANDERSON.

1346—℞ Zinci oxidi, ... ℨj.
　　　 Talci, ... ℨj.
　　　 Ol. olivæ, ... f℥ss.
　　　 Aq. calcis, ... f℥ss.
　　　 Lanolin., ... ℥ijss.
　　　 Tr. benzoin., ... ♏x.—M.
　　Sig.: Apply topically. (*Eczema.*)

1347—℞ Ol. cadini, . . . f℥ss.
　　　 Glycerinæ, . . . f℥j.
　　　 Ungt. diachyli, . . f℥iiss.—M.
　　Sig.: Apply locally. (*In squamous eczema with
thickened skin.*)　　　　　TILBURY FOX.

1348—℞ Resorcin, ... gr. xl.
　　　 Glycerinæ, . . . ♏xv.
　　　 Alcohol., ... ℨj.
　　　 Aquæ, ... ℥iv.—M.
　　Sig.: To be used in conjunction with an ointment.
　　(*For eczema of the hands.*)　　STELWAGON.

1349—℞ Hydrarg. chlor. mit., . . gr. lxxx.
    Mucil. tragacanthæ, . . f℥j.
    Liq. calcis, . . ad f℥viij.—M.
   Sig.: Apply locally and then use the following :—

1350—℞ Pulv. zinci oxidi, . gr. lxxx.
    Ungt. aq. rosæ,
    Ungt. petrolei, . . āā ℨiv.—M.
   Sig.: Apply after the above wash. (*In eczema.*)
                           Van Harlingen.

1351—℞ Pulv. bismuth. subnit., . ℨss.
    Ungt. aq. rosæ, . . . ℥j.—M.
   Sig.: Apply night and morning. (*In eczema of the scalp.*)
                           Van Harlingen.

1352—℞ Liq. carb. detergen., . gtt. xxx.
    Hydrarg. ammoniat., . gr. xx.
    Ung. zinci oxidi,
    Vaselin., ... āā ℥ss.—M.
   Sig.: Apply topically. (*Chronic eczema.*)

1353—℞ Liq. plumbi subacetat., . f℥j.
    Glycerinæ,
    Aquæ, . . . āā f℥iv.—M.
   Sig.: To be applied two or three times a day with a camel's-hair brush. (*In infantile eczema.*)
                           J. Lewis Smith.

1354—℞ Acid. boric., . . . gr. lxxx.
    Balsam. Peru., . . . gr. viij.
    Vaselini, ... ℥j.—M.
   Sig.: Apply twice a day. (*In eczema of children.*)

1355—℞ Menthol., ... gr. xxx.
    Resorcin., ... gr. xv.
    Sulph. præcip., . . . ℥iiss.
    Zinci oxidi, . . . ℥iiiss.
    Vaselini, ... ℥j.—M.
   Sig.: Apply topically. (*Dry eczema with pruritus.*)
                           Thibierge.

1356—℞ Hydrarg. ammon., . . gr. x.
    Acid. carbol. cryst., . . gr. viiss.
    Ungt. petrolei,
    Ungt. zinci oxidi, . āā ℥ss.
    Ol. olivæ, . . . ℨss.—M.
   Sig.: Apply two or three times daily. (*In infantile eczema.*)
                           Stelwagon.

1357—℞ Resorcin,
Zinci oxidi, . . āā ℥j.
Ungt. aq. rosæ, . . . ℥x.—M.
Sig.: Apply locally. (*In indurated eczema of infant.*)
FLIESBURG.

1358—℞ Ungt. hydrarg. ox. rub.,
· Ungt. sulphuris, . āā ℥ij.
Acid. carbol., . . . gr. iij.
Ungt. simp., . . . ℥ss.—M.
Sig.: Apply to the affected parts. (*In chronic eczema.*)
DA COSTA.

1359—℞ Pulv. camphoræ, . . ℥ss-j.
Zinci oxidi, . . . ℥iv.
Pulv. amyli, . . . ℥j.—M.
Sig.: Use as a dusting powder. (*In erythema.*)
BULKLEY.

1360—℞ Pulv. zinci carbonat. præcip.,
Pulv. zinci oxidi,
Pulv. amyli,
Glycerinæ, . . āā ℥iv.
Aquæ, ... Oss.—M.
Sig.: Apply twice a day. (*Erythema.*)
VAN HARLINGEN.

1361—℞ Zinci acetat., . . . gr. ij.
Aq. rosæ, ... f℥j.
Ungt. aq. rosæ, . . . ℥j.—M.
Sig.: Apply locally. (*In erythema.*)
TILLBURY FOX.

1362—℞ Calcis præcip., . . . gr. iss.
Bismuth. subnit., . . gr. ij.
Sacch. alb., . . . gr. iij.—M.
Et ft. chart. No. i.
Sig.: One three times a day. (*Erythema intertrigo.*)
VAN HARLINGEN.

1363—℞ Bismuth. subnit., . . ℥ss.
Sig.: Dust the affected parts. (*In erythema about the genitals.*)
BARTHOLOW.

1364—℞ Hydrarg. chlor. mit., . . gr. xx.
Lycopodii, ... ℥ij.—M.
Sig.: Use as a dusting powder. (*In erythema inter-trigo.*)
POWELL.

1365—℞ Quiniæ sulphat., . . ℨss.
Acid. sulphuric. aromat., . f̃ℨss.
Ex. taraxaci fl., . . f̃ℨvj.
Aquæ, . . q. s. ad f̃ℨiv.—M.
Sig.: A dessertspoonful three times a day. (*In erythema nodosum.*) BARTHOLOW.

1366—℞ Plumbi acetat., . . . gr. xv.
Acid. hydrocyanic. dil., . . ℳxx.
Alcoholis, ... f̃ℨss.
Aquæ, . . . q. s. ad f̃ℨvj.—M.
Sig.: Apply with a sponge. (*Freckles and sunburn.*) TILBURY FOX.

1367—℞ Potass. carbonat., . . ℨiij.
Sodii chlor., . . . ℨij.
Aq. aurant. flor., . . f̃ℨij.
Aq. rosæ, . . . ad f̃ℨviij.—M.
Sig.: Use night and morning. (*For freckles.*) BARTHOLOW.

1368—℞ Hydrarg. ammoniat.,
Bismuth. subnit., . āā ℨj.
Glycerit. amyli, . . ℨiv.—M.
Sig.: Apply every second day. (*For freckles.*) PHARMACEUTICAL RECORD.

1369—℞ Hydrarg. chlor. cor., . gr. viiss.
Zinci sulph.,
Plumbi acet., . . . āā ℨss.
Aquæ, ... f̃ℨiv.—M.
Sig.: Use as a lotion. (*Freckles.*)

1370—℞ Morphiæ sulphat., . . gr. viij.
Collodii, ... f̃ℨj.—M.
Sig.: Paint affected surfaces. (*In herpes zoster.*) VAN HARLINGEN.

1371—℞ Potass. iodid., . . . gr. xii–xv.
Ungt. hydrarg. nitrat., . ℨss.—M.
Sig.: Apply twice daily. (*In herpes exedens.*) BLASIUS.

1372—℞ Cocainæ hydrochlorat.,
Morphinæ, . . āā gr. ij.
Sodii borat., . . . ℨiss.
Mellis, ... ℨj.—M.
Sig.: A portion the size of a pea to be applied on cotton several times a day. (*For herpes of the mouth and lips.*) HUGENSCHMIDT.

SKIN DISEASES *(Continued)*.

1373—℞ Pulv. morphiæ sulphat., . gr. ij.
      Pulv. zinci oxidi,
      Pulv. amyli, . . āā ʒss.—M.
   Sig.: Use as a dusting powder. *(In herpes zoster.)*
                              VAN HARLINGEN.

1374—℞ Aluminis, ... ʒj.
      Aquæ, ... fʒj—M.
   Sig.: Saturate a piece of lint and apply to the
glans penis. *(In herpes preputialis.)* WARING.

1375—℞ Camphoræ, ... gr. v.
      Pulv. marantæ, . . . gr. xxx.
      Bismuth. subnitrat., . . gr. xxx.
      Aq. rosæ, ... fʒiv.—M.
   Sig.: Apply topically. *(Herpes of lips.)*

1376—℞ Hydrarg. chlor. mit., . gr. x.
      Adipis benzoat., . . ʒj.—M.
   Sig.: Apply three times a day. *(In chronic herpes
labialis.)*   NELIGAN.

1377—℞ Potass. chlorat., . . ƺij.
      Acid. muriat. dil.,
      Spt. chloroform.,
      Liq. cinchonæ, . . āā fʒj.
      Aq. destillat., . q. s. ad fʒvj.—M.
   Sig.: Two tablespoonfuls three times a day. *(In
herpes zoster.)*   STURGES.

1378—℞ Zinci oxidi, . . . ʒij.
      Glycerinæ, . . . fʒij.
      Liq. plumbi subacetat. dil., fʒiss.
      Liq. calcis, . . . fʒvi–viij.—M.
   Sig.: Apply locally. *(In herpes.)* TILBURY FOX.

1379—℞ Pulv. camphoræ,
      Chloral hydrat., . āā ʒiv.—M.
   Sig.: Apply locally with a camel's-hair brush.
(In herpes labialis and preputialis.) JAMIESON.

1380—℞ Acid. tannici, . . . ʒj.
      Alcoholis, ... fʒviij.—M.
   Sig.: Use as a lotion. *(In hyperidrosis.)*
                              VAN HARLINGEN.

1381—℞ Ungt. picis (U. S. P.),
      Ungt. sulphuris (U. S. P.), āā ʒss.—M.
   Sig.: Use twice a day. *(In hyperidrosis.)*
                              VAN HARLINGEN.

1382—℞ Pulv. camphoræ, . . gr. x.
Ungt. zinci oxidi, . . ℥j.—M.
Sig.: Apply night and morning. (*In ichthyosis.*)
ERASMUS WILSON.

1383—℞ Adipis benzoat, . . ℥ij.
Ungt. petrolei, . . . ℥ss.
Glycerinæ, . . . ℈ij.—M.
Sig.: Apply night and morning. (*In icuthyosis.*)
VAN HARLINGEN.

1384—℞ Zinci sulphat., . . . ℨj.
Adipis, ... ℥j.—M.
Sig.: Use locally. (*In ichthyosis.*)
ERASMUS WILSON.

1385—℞ Resorcin, ... gr. xv.
Adipis, ... ℨj.—M.
Sig.: Rub in twice a day. (*In ichthyosis.*)
ANDEER.

1386—℞ Cupri sulphat., . . gr. xx.
Ungt. sambuci, . . ℨj.—M.
Sig.: Apply night and morning. (*In ichthyosis.*)
ERASMUS WILSON.

1387—℞ Sodii bicarbonat., . . gr. xx–℥ss.
Adipis benzoat., . . ℨj.—M.
Sig.: Use twice a day. (*In ichthyosis.*) DEVERGIE.

1388—℞ Sulphuris, . . . gr. xxv-l.
Ungt. simp., . . . ℥j.—M.
Sig.: Rub in at night. (*In ichthyosis.*) UNNA.

1389—℞ Ulmi corticis, . . . ℥iss.
Aq. bullientis, . . . Oj.—M.
Sig.: Wineglassful two or three times a day. (*In
ichthyosis.*) LETTSOM.

1390—℞ Potass. iodid., . . . ℈j.
Ol. pedis bubuli,
Adipis, . . . āā ℥ss.
Glycerinæ, . . . f℥j.—M.
Sig.: Apply twice a day. (*In ichthyosis.*)
VAN HARLINGEN.

1391—℞ Bismuth. subnit., . . ℥ss–j.
Ungt. aquæ rosæ, . . ℥j.—M.
Sig.: Apply night and morning. (*In impetigo.*)
VAN HARLINGEN.

1392—℞ Acid. salicylici, . . ℥ss.
    Ex. cannabis ind., . . gr. x.
    Collodii, ... f℥j.—M.
Sig.: Paint the surface twice daily. (*In ichthyosis hystrix.*)   VAN HARLINGEN.

1393—℞ Acid. carbol., . . . gr. x.
    Glycerinæ,
    Aq. rosæ, . . . āā f℥j.—M.
Sig.: Apply locally. (*Impetigo.*)   HEADLAND.

1394—℞ Tr. ferri chlor., . . . f℥ss.
    Magnesii sulphat., . . ℥ij.
    Tr. calumbæ, . . . f℥iss.
    Infus. quassiæ, . . . f℥xviij.—M.
Sig.: Wineglassful every morning. (*In impetigo of old people.*)   NELIGAN.

1395—℞ Acid. salicylic., . . gr. xxx.
    Petrolati, . . . ℥j.
    Zinci oxidi,
    Amyli, ... āā ℥ss.—M.
Sig.: Apply after removal of crusts and cleansing. (*Contagious impetigo.*)   LASSAR.

1396—℞ Acid. hydrocyanic. dil., . f℥iij.
    Spt. rectificat., . . . f℥ss.
    Aq. destillat., . . . f℥vij.—M.
Sig.: Apply with lint and cover with oiled-silk. (*Impetigo.*)   PLUMBE.

1397—℞ Hydrarg. chlor. corros., . gr. iss.
    Ol. theobromæ,
    Vaselini, . . . āā gr. ccxxv.—M.
Sig.: Use twice a day. (*In impetigo of the scalp.*)   JORISSENNE.

1398—℞ Creasoti, ... ℥ss.
    Aq. destillat., . . . Oj.—M.
Sig.: Use as a wash. (*In impetigo sparsa.*)   DUNGLISON.

1399—℞ Glyceriti acid. tannic., . f℥ij.
Sig.: Apply with a camel's-hair brush during the day and poultice at night. (*Impetigo.*)   RINGER.

1400—℞ Hydrarg. chlor. mit., . gr. xx.
    Lycopodii, . . . ℥j.—M.
Sig.: Use as a dusting powder. (*Impetigo.*)   POWELL.

1401—℞ Hydrarg. ammon., . . gr. v.
       Adipis, ... ℥j.—M.
Sig.: Apply to the surface beneath the scabs after poulticing. (*Impetigo contagiosa.*)   Tilbury Fox.

1402—℞ Ungt. zinci oxidi, . . ℥j.
Sig.: Apply locally. (*Impetigo.*)   Ringer.

1403—℞ Lini aq. calcis, . . . f℥vj.
Sig.: Use locally. (*Intertrigo.*)   Tilbury Fox.

1404—℞ Acid. tannic., . . . ℥ss.
       Glycerinæ,   . . . f℥ij.—M.
Sig.: Use locally. (*Intertrigo.*)   Bartholow.

1405—℞ Acid. boracic., . . . ℨiss.
       Vaselini, ... ℥j.—M.
Sig.: Apply locally. (*Intertrigo.*)   Waring.

1406—℞ Hydrarg. chlor. mit., . . gr. xv.
       Vaselini, ... ℥j.—M.
Sig.: Use night and morning. (*Intertrigo.*)
                      Starr.

1407—℞ Pulv. camphoræ, . ℨiss.
       Pulv. zinci ox.,
       Pulv. amyli, . . āā ℥j.—M.
Sig.: Use as a dusting powder. (*Intertrigo.*)
                 Van Harlingen.

1409—℞ Pulv. amyli,
       Pulv. lycopodii, . . āā   parts v.
       Cretæ præparatæ,
       Bismuth. subnit., . . āā   parts x.—M.
Sig.: Gently bathe the affected parts once daily with a watery solution of picric acid (1 : 120). When the irritation has subsided and the epidermis has re-formed, keep approximated surfaces separated by thin layers of absorbent cotton upon which the foregoing powder is spread. (*Intertrigo.*)

1410—℞ Ol. gurjon., . . . f℥j.
       Liq. calcis, . . f℥iij.—M.
Sig.: Apply to ulcers. (*Lepra.*) Van Harlingen.

1411—℞ Acid. carbol. cryst., . . ℨj.
       Ol. amygdalæ dulc., . . f℥ij.—M.
Sig.: **Apply** to the tubercules. (*In tuberculous lepra.*)   Fleming.

1412—℞ Chyrsarobin, . . . gr. x-xx-ℨj.
Ætheris et alcoholis, . ad q. s.
Collodii, ... fℨj.—M.

Sig.: Rub the chrysarobin with a little alcohol
and ether and add the collodion.
Paint the affected patch with a camel's-hair brush.
(In chronic lepra.) G. H. Fox.

1413—℞ Acid. arseniosi, . . . gr. x-xxx.
Adipis, ... ℨj.—M.

Sig.: Apply over a small patch of skin once a day
for two weeks ; then treat a fresh portion. *(Lepra.)*
Tilbury Fox.

1414—℞ Sodii carbonat., . . ℨss-j.
Aquæ, ... fℨvj.—M.

Sig.: Dessertspoonful twice a day. *(In lepra where
mercurials are contraindicated.)* Beauperthuy.

1415—℞ Sodii arseniat., . . . gr. iss.
Aq. destillat., . . . fℨxxv.—M.

Sig.: Teaspooful every morning at meal-time.
Double the dose in the course of a week. *(In
lichen.)* Vidal.

1416—℞ Potassæ caustic, . . gr. xv.
Picis liquidæ, . . . gr. xxx.
Aquæ, ... fℨiv.—M.

Sig.: Use locally. *(In lichen ruber.)*
Van Harlingen.

1417—℞ Liq. potassæ, . . . fℨij.
Acid. hydrocyanic. dil., . fℨj.
Mist. amygdalæ, . . fℨviij.—M.

Sig.: Use as a wash. *(In lichen.)* Burgess.

1418—℞ Ol. rusci crudi, . . . fℨj.
Ungt. aq. rosæ, . . . fℨj.
Ol. rosæ, ... ℳxx.—M.

Sig.: Apply twice a day. *(In lichen ruber.)*
Van Harlingen.

1419—℞ Hydrarg. chlor. corros., . gr. vij.
Cretæ prep., . . . ℨiss.
Acid. carbol.,
Ol. olivæ, . . . aa fℨv.
Ungt. zinci oxidi, . . ℨxv.—M.

Sig.: Rub in thoroughly. *(In lichen planus.)*
Unna.

SKIN DISEASES *(Continued).*

1420—℞ Liq. plumbi subacetat., . f℥i–iij.
      Infusi althææ, . . . Oj.—M.
    Sig.: Apply locally. *(In lichen agrius.)* BURGESS.

1421—℞ Ol. cadini, . . . f℥ij.
      Glyceriti amyli, . . . f℥iss.—M.
    Sig.: Apply locally. *(In chronic lichen of the genitals.)* VIDAL.

1422—℞ Chloroformi, . . . ♏xv.
      Ol. olivæ, ... f℥j.—M.
    Sig.: After a tepid bath, and well dried. *(In lichen.)* NELIGAN.

1423—℞ Sodii carbonatis, . . ℈j.
      Aq. rosæ, ... f℥vj.
      Glycerinæ, . . . f℥ij.—M.
    Sig.: Use locally. *(In infantile lichen.)* TILBURY FOX.

1424—℞ Hydrarg. bichlor., . . gr. ij.
      Acid. carbol., . . . gr. x.
      Ungt. zinci oxidi, . . ℥j.—M.
    Sig.: Apply twice a day. *(In lichen ruber.)* VAN HARLINGEN.

1425—℞ Acid. nitric. vel muriatic., ℥j.
      Aq. ferventis, . . cong. xxx.—M.
    Sig.: Acid bath. *(In chronic lichen and prurigo.)* TILBURY FOX.

1426—℞ Ungt. hydrarg. nitrat., . ℥ij.
      Ungt. simplicis, . . ℥vj.—M.
    Sig.: Use twice daily and take the following internally :—

1427—℞ Potass. iodid., . . . ℥j.
      Aquæ, ... f℥iij.—M.
    Sig.: Teaspoonful with cod-liver oil three times a day. *(In syphilitic and strumous cases of pemphigus.)* WARING.

1428—℞ Liq. potass. arsenitis, . f℥ij.
      Aq. menthæ pip., q. s. ad f℥iij.—M.
    Sig.: Teaspoonful three times a day, after meals. *(In pemphigus.)* WARING·

1429—℞ Argenti nitrat., . . . gr. ij.
Aq. destillat., . . . f℥j.—M.
Sig.: Use locally. *(In pemphigus after the bullæ have burst.)* E. WILSON.

1430—℞ Lini. calcis, . . . f℥j.
Sig.: Apply after the bullæ have been punctured. *(In pemphigus.)* CHAMBARD.

1431—℞ Hydrarg. chlorid. corrosiv., . gr. iv.
Ol. lavandulæ, . . . ℥xvj.
Tr. lavandulæ, . . . f℥j.
Sapo viridis, ... ℥v.—M.
Sig.: Apply, let dry, and wash off in three days.

1432—℞ Saponis viridis, . . . ℥ij.
Alcoholis, ... f℥j.—M.
Sig.: Dissolve by the aid of heat and filter. Add a teaspoonful to an equal quantity of water and rub into the scalp, and wash after with warm water. *(In pityriasis capitis.)* VAN HARLINGEN.

1433—℞ Acid. carbolic., . . . Əj.
Alcoholis, ... f℥iss.
Glycerinæ, . . . f℥iss.
Ol. limonis, . . . ℥iss.—M.
Sig.: Drop a few drops here and there over the surface and then rub well into the scalp. *(In pityriasis capitis.)* VAN HARLINGEN.

1434—℞ Sodii sulphuret.,
Sodii carbonatis, . ãã ℥ij.
Ungt. simplicis, . . ℥iiss.—M.
Sig.: Apply twice a day. *(In pityriasis.)* BAREGES.

1435—℞ Acid. salicylic., . . . ℥j.
Sulphuris præcip., . . ℥v.
Vaselini, ... ℥iij.—M.
Sig.: Apply after soaking the affected part in hot water. *(In pityriasis.)* L'UNION MÉDICALE.

1436—℞ Hydrarg. sulphat. flavæ, . gr. xlv.
Vaselini, ... ℥xv.
Ess. limonis, . . . gtt. xx.—M.
Sig.: Keep in a porcelain jar. Apply at night and wash off the following morning. *(In pityriasis capitis.)* VIGIER.

SKIN DISEASES (Continued).

1437—℞ Potass. sulphuret., . . ℨj.
Aq. destillat., . . . f℥iij.—M.
Sig.: Apply once a day. (In pityriasis capitis.)
WINZAR.

1438—℞ Acid. tannic., . . ℨj.
Ungt. aquæ rosæ,
Ungt. petrolii, . . ãã ℨiv.—M.
Sig.: Apply. (In pityriasis capitis.)
VAN HARLINGEN.

1439—℞ Liq. iodinii comp.,
Liq. potass. arsenitis, ãã f℥ij.—M.
Sig.: Ten drops, well diluted, three times a day.
(In pityriasis.)
ELLIS.

1440—℞ Sulphur præcip., . . ℨi–ij.
Ungt. petrolii, . . . ℥j.—M.
Sig.: Apply. (In pityriasis capitis.)
VAN HARLINGEN.

1441—℞ Hydrarg. ammoniat., . ℈j.
Ungt. petrolii, . . . ℥j.—M.
Sig.: Apply. (In pityriasis capitis.)
VAN HARLINGEN.

1442—℞ Acid. hydrocyanic. dil., . f℥iss.
Aq. rosæ, ... f℥viiss.—M.
Sig.: Use locally. (In prickly heat.)
A. T. THOMPSON.

1443—℞ Sodii bicarb., . . . ℨj.
Aquæ, ... Oij.—M.
Sig.: Bathe parts night and morning. (In prickly
heat.)
STARR.

1444—℞ Liq. potass. citrat., . . ℥vj.
Sig.: Tablespoonful in ice-water every two or three
hours. (In prickly heat.)

1445—℞ Hydrarg. chlor. mit., . gr. xx.
Lycopodii, . . . ℨij.—M.
Sig.: Use as a dusting powder. (In prickly heat.).
POWELL.

1446—℞ Zinci carbonat. præcip., . ℨiv.
Zinci oxidi, . . . ℨij.
Glycerinæ, . . . f℥ij.
Aq. rosæ, ... f℥viij.—M.
Sig.: Apply locally. (In prickly heat.)
TILBURY FOX.

1447—℞ Spt. æther. nitro., . . f℥j.
    Magnesii sulphat., . . ℥j.
    Ol. cajuputi, . . . ℳj.
    Syr. tolu., . . . f℥ij.
    Liq. magnesii carb., . . f℥ij.—M.

Sig.: Teaspoonful two or three times a day. (*In prickly heat.*)   GOODHART and STARR.

1448—℞ Sodii bicarb., . . . ℥j.
    Tr. nucis vomicæ, . . ℳvj.
    Tr. cardamom. comp., . f℥ij.
    Syr. simp., . . . f℥ij.
    Aq. chloroform., . . f℥ss.
    Aquæ, . . q. s. ad f℥ij.—M.

Sig.: Teaspoonful every six hours. (*In prickly heat.*)   EUSTACE SMITH.

1449—℞ Ungt. hydrarg. nitrat., . ℥i-ij.
    Zinci oxidi, . . . ℥ij.
    Liq. plumbi subacetat., . f℥ss.
    Acid. carbol., . . . gtt. ij.
    Ol. olivæ, ... f℥i-iss.—M.

Sig.: Apply after removing the scabs. (*In psoriasis.*)   TILBURY FOX.

1450—℞ Acid. chrysophanic., . gr. x.
    Adipis benzoat., . . ℥j.—M.

Sig.: Use night and morning. (*In psoriasis.*)

1451—℞ Tr. cantharidis,
    Liq. potass. arsenit., . āā f℥ss.—M.

Sig.: Take ten minims, well diluted, twice a day. (*In psoriasis.*)   BENNETT.

1452—℞ Ol. cadinii,
    Ungt. hydrarg., . āā ℥ij.
    Vaselini, ... f℥j.—M.

Sig.: Apply locally. (*In psoriasis syphilitica.*)
     MAURIAC.

1453—℞ Hydrarg. chlorid. mit.,
    Lanolin.,
    Adipis, . . . āā ℥iv.—M.

Sig.: To be rubbed in at night and washed off in the morning. (*Palmar psoriasis.*)

1454—℞ Ungt. picis liquidæ,
    Ungt. sulphuris, . āā ℥j.—M.

Sig.: Apply at night. (*In psoriasis.*)
     GUY'S HOSPITAL.

1455—℞   Acid. chrysophanic.,   .   gr. x.
   Liq. carbonis detergent.,   ℥x.
   Hydrarg. am. chlorid.,   .   gr. x.
   Adipis benzoat.,   .   .   ℥j.—M.
 Ft. unguentum.

Sig.: At night the patient should wash the diseased surfaces free from all scales ; then, standing before a fire, rub on the ointment, devoting, if possible, half an hour to the operation.   (*In psoriasis.*)
       JONATHAN HUTCHINSON.

1456—℞   Acid. salicylic.,   .   .   ℥j.
   Alcoholis, ...   f℥iv.—M.

Sig.: Apply twice a day when the patches are few and scaly.   (*In psoriasis.*)   VAN HARLINGEN.

1457—℞   Ichthyol.,
   Acid. salicylic.,
   Acid. pyrogallic.,   .   .   āā   ℥iss.
   Ol. olivæ, ...   f℥j.
   Lanolin., ...   ℥j.—M.

Sig.: Apply topically.   (*Psoriasis.*)   RICHTER.

1458—℞   Chrysarobin.,
   Ichthyol.,   .   .   āā   gr. xx.
   Acid. salicylici,   .   .   .   gr. viij.
   Ung. zinci oxidi,   .   .   .   ℥iiiss.
   Vaselin.,   .   .   q. s. ad   ℥j.—M.

Sig.: Apply topically.   (*Psoriasis.*)   UNNA.

1459—℞   Hydrarg. iodid. rub.,   .   gr. i–ij.
   Ex. gentian.,   .   .   .   Đij.—M.
 Et ft. pil. No. xii.

Sig.: One pill three times a day.   (*In rupia.*)
       TILBURY FOX.

1460—℞   Hydrarg. chlor. corros.,   .   Đj.
   Potass. iodid.,   .   .   .   ℥vj.
   Tr. iodinii comp.,   .   .   f℥ij.
   Aquæ,   .   .   ad ft.   f℥xvj.—M.

Sig.: One-half to one teaspoonful three times a day.   (*In rupia.*)   STARTIN.

1461—℞   Hydrarg. iodid. rub.,   .   gr. iij.
   Potass. iodid.,   .   .   .   ℥i–ij.
   Alcoholis, ...   f℥ij.
   Syr. zingiberis, .   .   .   f℥iv.
   Aquæ,   .   .   .   ad   f℥iss.—M.

Sig.: Thirty drops three times a day.   (*In rupia*)
       PUCHE.

1462—℞ Hydrarg. oxidi rub.,
    Hydrarg. ammoniat.,   āā   gr. vj.
    Adipis, ...   ℨj.—M.

Sig.: Apply locally. (*In rupia.*)   STARTIN.

1463—℞ Hydrarg. cyanidi, . . gr. vj.
    Cerat. simplicis, . . ℨj.—M.

Sig.: Use locally. (*In rupia when the crusts become loosened.*)   TILBURY FOX.

1464—℞ Tr. ferri chlor.,
    Acid. phosphoric. dil., . fℨj.
    Syr. limonis, . . fℨij.—M.

Sig.: One-half to one teaspoonful in water three times a day. (*In seborrhœa.*)   VAN HARLINGEN.

1465—℞ Sulphuris loti, . . . gr. ccxxv.
    Ol. ricini, ... fℨxiiss.
    Ol. theobromæ, . . . ℨiij.
    Balsami Peruviani, . . ℨss.—M.

Sig.: Apply twice a day. (*In dry seborrhœa of scalp.*)
   VIDAL.

1466—℞ Sulphuris præcipitat., . ℨss.
    Ungt. petrolii, . . . ℨiv.—M.

Sig.: Rub a small quantity in once a day. (*In seborrhœa of the scalp.*)   VAN HARLINGEN.

1467—℞ Sulphuris loti, . . . ℨij.
    Balsami Peruviani, . . ℨss.
    Vaselini, ... ℨx.—M.

Sig.: After bathing the part apply the ointment. (*In seborrhœa.*)   G. H. FOX.

1468—℞ Zinci sulphat.,
    Potass. sulphureti, . āā gr. xxx.
    Alcoholis, ... ℳc.
    Aq. rosæ, . . q. s. ad fℨij.—M.

Sig.: Wet a rag with ether and rub the nose at night, and then apply the lotion. (*In seborrhœa of the nose.*)   G. H. FOX.

1469—℞ Acidi carbol., . . . Ƌi-fℨj.
    Ol. amygdalæ, . . . fℨiv.
    Ol. limonis, . . . fℨj.
    Aq. destillat., . . ad fℨij.—M.

Sig.: Apply after washing. (*In seborrhœa of the scalp.*)   VAN HARLINGEN.

1470—℞ Potass. carbonat.,   .   . ʒiij.
        Sodii chloridi,   .   .   . ʒij.
        Aq. aurant. flor.,   .   . fʒij.
        Aq. rosæ, ... fʒviij.—M.
  Sig.: Face-wash. (*In tan and freckles*.)
                                    BARTHOLOW.

1471—℞ Lactis recentis, .   .   . ʒxiiss.
        Glycerinæ,   .   .   . fʒviiss.
        Acid. muriat.,   .   .   . ℳlxxv.
        Ammon. muriat.,   .   . ʒj.—M.
  Sig.: Apply morning and evening with camel's-
hair brush. (*In tan and freckles*.)   MONIN.

1472—℞ Plumbi acetat., .   .   . gr. xv.
        Acid. hydrocyanic. dil.,   . ℳxx.
        Alcoholis, ... fʒss.
        Aquæ,   .   . q. s. ad fʒvj.—M.
  Sig.: Apply with a sponge. (*In freckles and sunburn.*)   TILBURY FOX.

1473—℞ Acid. chrysophan.,   .   . ʒj.
        Hydrarg. ammon. chlor.,   . gr. xx.
        Lanolin, ... ʒj.
        Adipis benzoat.,   .   . ʒvj.
        Liq. carb. deterg.,   .   . ℳx.—M.
  Sig.: Use locally. (*Tinea circinata.*)
                                    J. HUTCHINSON.

1474—℞ Cupri oleat.,   .   .   . ʒss.
        Adipis benzoat.,   .   . ʒj.—M.
  Sig.: Use locally. (*Tinea circinata.*) SHOEMAKER.

1475—℞ Creasoti, ... ℳxx.
        Ol. cadini, ... fʒiij.
        Sulphuris,   .   .   . ʒiij.
        Potass. bicarb., .   .   . ʒj.
        Adipis, ... ʒj.—M.
  Sig.: Use locally. (*Tinea circinata.*)
                                    VAN HARLINGEN.

1476—℞ Sodii hyposulphit.,   .   . ʒij.
        Aquæ, ... fʒij.—M.
  Sig.: Apply locally. (*Tinea circinata.*) DUHRING.

1477—℞ Aceti cantharidis,   .   . ʒss.
  Sig.: Apply lightly with camel's-hair brush; then
use the following :—
                    183

1478—℞ Hydrarg. chlor. corros., . gr. ij.
Adipis, ... ℥j.—M.

Sig.: Rub in well for ten days ; then use cantharidal ointment. (*Tinea decalvans.*) TILBURY FOX.

1479—℞ Sodii hyposulphitis, . . ℥j.
Aquæ, ... f℥xiij.—M.

Sig.: Use locally. (*Tinea favosa.*) TILBURY FOX.

1480—℞ Potassii carbonat., . . . ℨij.
Flor. sulphur., . . . ℥j.
Tr. iodi,
Picis liquid., . . . āā f℥iij.
Adipis, ... ℥viij.—M.

Sig.: Apply daily in thin layer on lint. (*Tinea favosa.*) PIROGOFF.

1481—℞ Sulphuris loti, . . . ℥j.
Ol. cadini,
Hydrarg. chlor. corros., āā gr. v.—M.

Sig.: Apply four times a day. (*Tinea favosa.*) BAZIN.

1482—℞ Acid. sulphurosi, . . f℥ij.
Aquæ, ... f℥viij.—M.

Sig.: Apply constantly. (*In tinea favosa.*) SIR W. JENNER.

1483—℞ Sulphuris iodid., . . ℥j.
Ungt. simplicis, . . ℥iss.—M.

Sig.: Apply. (*Tinea favosa.*) DONOVAN.

1484—℞ Acid. salicylici,
Acid. chrysophanic., . āā ℨij.
Cretæ præp., . . . ℨij.
Vaselini, ... ℨxviiss.—M.

Sig.: Remove the crusts and rub the ointment in for fifteen minutes at night. (*Tinea favosa.*) MONROE.

1485—℞ Hydrarg. chlor. corros., . gr. x.
Aquæ, ... f℥j.—M.

Sig.: Apply with camel's-hair brush, after epilation. (*Tinea sycosis.*) HARLEY.

1486—℞ Sodii hyposulphitis, . ₀ ℥j.
Aquæ, ... f℥j.—M.

Sig.: Sponge the part freely, then apply ungt. sulphur. (*Tinea sycosis.*) HUGHES.

1487—℞ Hydrarg. oleat. (5–10 per cent.)
Sig.: Paint over the affected part. (*Tinea sycosis.*)
CANE.

1488—℞ Naphthol, . . . ℨi–iiss.
Saponis viridis,
Cretæ præp.,
Sulphuris loti,
Lanolini, . . āā ℨvi, gr. xv.—M.
Sig.: Apply locally. (*Tinea sycosis.*) LIEBREICH.

1489—℞ Sulphuris, . . . ℨi–ij.
Ol. rosæ, ... gtt. v.
Vaselini, ... ℨj.—M.
Sig.: Use locally. (*Tinea sycosis.*)

1490—℞ Acid. carbolic. cryst.,
Ungt. hydrarg. nitrat.,
Ungt. sulphuris, . āā ℨss.—M.
Sig.: Apply twice a day. (*Tinea tonsurans.*)
VAN HARLINGEN.

1491—℞ Hydrarg. ammoniat.,
Hydrarg. oxidi rub., . āā gr. vj.
Adipis, ... ℨj.—M.
Sig.: Use after epilation and washing. (*Tinea tonsurans.*) STARTIN.

1492—℞ Sodii biborat., . . . ℨj.
Aceti destillat., . . fℨij.—M.
Sig.: Use locally. (*Tinea tonsurans.*)
ABERCROMBIE.

1493—℞ Hydrarg. chlorid. corrosiv., . gr. x.
Balsami Peruvian., . . . ℨiij.
Ol. lavandulæ, . . . fℨj.
Alcoholis, . . . ad fℨj.—M.
Sig.: Apply topically.

1494—℞ Acid. carbol., . . . ℨj.
Glycerinæ, . . . fℨss–j.—M.
Sig.: Rub in well night and morning. (*Tinea tonsurans.*) TILBURY FOX.

1495—℞ Cupri oleat., . . . ℨss.
Sig.: Apply twice a day. (*Tinea tonsurans.*)
WEIR.

1496—℞ Ol. cadini, ... f℥iss.
      Sulphuris, . . . ℨiss.
      Tr. iodinii, . . . f℥iss.
      Acid. carbolic., . . . ℳxx–xl.
      Adipis benzoat., . . ℨiv.—M.
Sig.: Use night and morning. (*Tinea tonsurans.*)
                          Van Harlingen.

1497—℞ Hydrarg. chlor. corros., . ℈j.
      Saponis viridis, . . . ℥ij.
      Alcoholis, ... f℥iv.
      Ol. lavandulæ, . . . f℥j.—M.
Sig.: To be rubbed in well night and morning.
(*Tinea versicolor.*)   Van Harlingen.

1498—℞ Hydrarg. chlor. corros., . gr. iv.
      Alcoholis, ... f℥vj.
      Ammon. muriat., . . ℨss.
      Aq. rosæ, . . . ad f℥vj.—M.
Sig.: Apply frequently. (*Tinea versicolor.*)
                          Tilbury Fox.

1499—℞ Acid. salicylici, . . gr. xxx.
      Sulphuris loti, . . . ℨiss.
      Lanolini, ... ℨxxv.—M.
Sig.: Apply with friction. (*Tinea versicolor.*)
                          Liebreich.

1500—℞ Sodii sulphitis, . . ℨiij.
      Glycerinæ, . . . f℥ij.
      Aquæ, . . . ad f℥iv.—M.
Sig.: Apply frequently. (*Tinea versicolor.*)
                          Tilbury Fox.

1501—℞ Resorcin, ... ℨi–iiss.
      Ol. ricini, ... f℥xiss.
      Alcoholis, ... f℥xxxviiiss.
      Balsami Peruviani, . . gr. viiss.—M.
Sig.: Apply locally. (*Tinea versicolor.*)   Ihle.

1502—℞ Sodii bicarbonat., . . ℥ii–x.
      Aq. ferventis (90°–95° F.),
                  cong. xx–xxx.—M.
Sig.: Alkaline bath. (*In skin diseases where there
is much local irritation.*)   Tilbury Fox.

1503—℞ Potass. carbonat., . . ℥ii–vj.
       Sodii borat., . . . ℥ij.
       Aq. ferventis (90°–95° F.),
                      cong. xx–xxx.—M.
   Sig.: Alkaline bath.   TILBURY FOX.

SLEEPLESSNESS (See Insomnia).

SMALLPOX.

1504—℞ Tr. aconiti rad., . . gtt. i–ij.
       Spt. æth. nitro., . . f℥ss.
       Liq. ammon. acetat., . f℥ij.
       Aquæ, . . . f℥iss.—M.
   Sig.: Take every hour or two. (*For the initial
fever.*)   HUGHES.

1505—℞ Atropinæ sulphat., . . gr. j.
       Aquæ, ... f℥ss.—M.
   Sig.: Three to five minims every three or four
hours.   HITCHMAN.

1506—℞ Pulv. iodoform., . . ℥ss.
       Pulv. camphoræ, . . ℥j.
       Vaselini, ... ℥j.—M.
   Sig.: Apply to the affected parts of the skin. (*To
prevent pitting.*)   WITHERSTINE.

1507—℞ Tr. aconiti rad., . . gtt. iv–viij.
       Liq. potass. citrat., . . f℥j.—M.
   Sig.: Teaspoonful every twenty minutes until four
doses are taken for a child from three to eight years.
(*In the initial fever.*)   STARR.

1508—℞ Ungt. hydrarg.,
       Ungt. aq. rosæ, . . āā ℥ij.—M.
   Sig.: Apply on mask night and morning. STARR.

1509—℞ Acid. salicylic., . gr. xx.
       Sodii bicarbonat.,
       Ammon. carbonat.,   āā gr. iv.—M.
   Et ft. chart. No. i.
   Sig.: Take in water every two to four hours.
                    PRIDEAUX.

1510—℞ Argent. nitrat., . . ℈ij.
       Aquæ, ... f℥ij.—M.
   Sig.: Paint the skin that is exposed to the light.
(*To prevent pitting.*)   RINGER.

SMALLPOX *(Continued)*.

1511—℞ Hydrarg. chlor. corros., . gr. ii–iv.
　　　Aquæ, ... f℥vj.—M.
　Sig.: Wet compresses and apply to the eruption.
　　　　　　　　　　　　　　　　SKODA.

1512—℞ Acid. boric., . . . ℥iss.
　　　Glycerinæ, . . . f℥j.
　　　Listerini, ... f℥ij.
　　　Aquæ, . . q. s. ad f℥vj.—M.
　Sig.: Use as mouth-wash. POWELL.

1513—℞ Chloral, ... gr. xv–xx.
　　　Mucil. acaciæ, . . . f℥ij.
　　　Aquæ, ... f℥ij.—M.
　Sig.: Give by the rectum. *(In cerebral excitement.)*
　　　　　　　　　　　　　　　　HUGHES.

1514—℞ Collodii flexilis, . . f℥j.
　Sig.: Apply every day or two with a camel's-hair
brush to the eruption. *(To prevent pitting.)*
　　　　　　　　　　　　　　　　RINGER.

1515—℞ Sodii salicylat., . . ℥ij.
　　　Glycerinæ, . . . f℥j.
　　　Aq. menthæ pip., . ad f℥iij.—M.
　Sig.: One or two teaspoonfuls three or four times
a day. *(To abort the pustules.)* REIMER.

1516—℞ Liq. ammon. acetat., . f℥iiiss.
　　　Spt. æth. nitro., . . f℥ss.—M.
　Sig.: Tablespoonful in a wineglassful of water
every two or three hours. HARTSHORNE.

SPERMATORRHŒA.

1517—℞ Tr. cimicifugæ, . . f℥iij.
　Sig.: Teaspoonful three times a day. MORSE.

1518—℞ Potass. brom., . . . ℥j.
　　　Aquæ, . . q. s. ad f℥ij.—M.
　Sig.: Teaspoonful, well diluted, three times a day.
(In the strong and plethoric.) BARTHOLOW.

1519—℞ Antipyrin, . . . ℥ij.
　　　Syr. acaciæ, . . . f℥ss.
　　　Aq. cinnam., . . ad f℥iv.—M.
　Sig.: One or two dessertspoonfuls at night. THOR.

1520—℞ Tr. gelsemii, . . . f3j.
      Tr. belladonnæ, . . f3ij.—M.
Sig.: Fifteen drops at bedtime.   BARTHOLOW.

1521—℞ Digitalinæ, . . . gr. j.
      Pulv. acaciæ, . . . ℈ij.
      Syr. simp., . . . q. s.—M.
Et ft. pil. No. xxxv.
Sig.: One pill three times a day.   CORVISART.

1522—℞ Tr. cantharidis, . . f3ij.
      Tr. ferri chlor., . . f3vj.—M.
Sig.: Twenty drops in water three times a day.
                    H. C. WOOD.

1523—℞ Potass. brom., . . . 3j.
      Sodii bicarb., . . . gr. xv.
      Infus. digitalis, . . f3ss.
      Atropinæ sulphat., . . gr. $\frac{1}{60}$.
Sig.: To be taken at bedtime.   GROSS.

1524—℞ Infus. digitalis, . . . f3iv.
Sig.: One or two teaspoonfuls two or three times a
day.   RINGER.

1525—℞ Lupulinæ, . . . gr. x.
      Pulv. camphoræ, . . gr. vj.
      Ex. belladonnæ, . . gr. ij.—M.
Et ft. pil. No. xii.
Sig.: One pill three times a day.   BARTHOLOW.

1526—℞ Pulv. opii, . . . gr. v.
      Pulv. camphoræ, . . ℈iv.
      Pulv. acaciæ,
      Syr. simplicis, āā q. s. ut ft. mass.—M.
Et ft. pil. No. xl.
Sig.: Two pills three times a day.   WARING.

1527—℞ Acid. tannici, . . . 3j.
      Glycerinæ, . . . q. s.—M.
Sig.: Apply to the deep urethra with a cupped
sound.   VAN BUREN and KEYES.

1528—℞ Pulv. digitalis, . . gr. ij.
      Lupulinæ, . . . gr. xv.—M.
Et ft. chart. No. i.
Sig.: Take powder at bedtime.   PESCHECK.

SPLEEN, ENLARGEMENT OF (See Fever, Intermittent Fever, and Leucocythæmia).

STRANGURY.

1529—℞ Decoct. uvæ ursi, . f℥viij.
  Liq. potassæ, . . gtt. cxxx.
  Tr. belladonnæ, . gtt. xlviij.—M.
  Sig.: Tablespoonful every four hours. AGNEW.

1530—℞ Balsam. copaibæ, . . ℥ss.
  Acid. benzoici., . . . ℨj.
  Vitelli unius ovi,
  Aq. camphoræ, . . . f℥vij.—M.
  Sig.: Take two tablespoonfuls twice a day.
  SODEN.

1531—℞ Aceti scillæ,
  Spt. æth. nitrosi, . āā fℨij.
  Aq. anisi, . q. s. ad Oj.—M.
  Sig.: A wineglassful every hour or oftener.
  WARING.

1532—℞ Ex. belladonnæ, . gr. ii–iv.
  Ft. suppos. No. ii.
  Sig.: Introduce one into the rectum, and repeat in four hours if necessary. HARTSHORNE.

1533—℞ Ex. opii, . . . gr. iv.
  Ex. hyoscyami, . gr. ij.—M.
  Et ft. suppos. No. iv.
  Sig.: Introduce one into the rectum.

1534—℞ Tr. cannabis indicæ, . f℥ij.
  Sig.: Thirty drops every few hours. RINGER.

STRUMA (See Rachitis).

STYE.

1534a—℞ Acid. boric., . • . ℈iv.
  Aq. destillat., . . . ℥v.—M.
  Sig.: Apply to the eyelids several times a day.
  ABADIE.

SUPPURATION (See Abscess).

SWEATING (See Phthisis and Fetor).

SYCOSIS (See Tinea in Skin Diseases).

SYNOVITIS.

1535—℞ Acid. carbolic., . . . gr. viij.
      Aq. destillat., . . . f℥j.—M.
Sig.: Use ether spray, and inject ten minims into
joint and repeat every three days. (*In chronic form.*)
MARTIN.

1536—Paint joint with tr. iodini and apply—
      ℞ Ungt. hydrarg.,
        Ungt. belladonnæ, . ℥j.—M.
Sig.: Apply on lint. ASHHURST.

1537—℞ Ungt. hydrarg., . . ℥ij.
        Pulv. ammon. chlorid., . ℥j.—M.
Sig.: For inunction. DUPUYTREN.

1538—℞ Morphiæ sulphat., . . gr. viij.
        Hydrarg. oleat. (5 to 10 per
          cent.), ... ℥j.—M.
Sig.: Apply twice daily with a soft brush. (*In
acute form.*) MARSHALL.

1539—℞ Iodi, ... ℥iv.
        Potass. iodid., . . . ℥j.
        Aquæ, ... f℥vj.—M.
Sig.: Apply externally with a brush. MARTIN.

1540—℞ Chloral., ... ℥j.
        Acid. carbolic., . . . ℥j.
        Aquæ, ... Oij.—M.
Sig.: Apply hot hourly upon layers of lint and
cover with oil-silk.

SYPHILIS.

1542—℞ Hydrarg. prot., . . . gr. v.
        Pulv. ipecac. et opii, . . gr. xl.
        Ex. gentian., . . . q. s.—M.
Et ft. pil. No. xx.
Sig.: One pill three times a day. SIMES.

1543—℞ Ungt. hydrarg., . . ℥j.
Ft. chart. No. viii.
Put in waxed papers.
Sig.: Rub, after bathing, for fifteen minutes the
contents of one paper into body in following order:
First night, axilla and side of chest; next night,
same on opposite side ; next night, groin and inner
part of thigh ; next, same on opposite side ; next,
chest and abdomen, and repeat. Wear same shirt
next to skin under other clothing.

1544—℞ Hydrarg. salicylat., . . gr. vij.
Confec. rosæ, . . . ℥ss.—M.
Et ft. pil. No. lx.

Sig.: One three times a day, after meals. CHAVES.

1545—℞ Hydrarg. prot., . . gr. vj.
Ft. pil. No. xxiv.

Sig.: One pill three times a day; every second
day increase by one pill until first symptoms of
ptyalism appear ; then cut down dose one-half and
continue for eighteen months this tonic dose ; after
that give—

1546—℞ Potass. iodid., . . . ℥iss–iv.
Hydrarg. chlor. corros., . gr. i–iss.
Syr. aurant. cort., . . f℥j.
Aquæ, . . q. s. ad f℥ij.—M.

Sig.: Teaspoonful three times a day for from six to
twelve months. MARTIN.

1547—℞ Mass. hydrarg., . . gr. xxiv.
Pulv. ferri sesquichlor., . gr. xij.—M.
Ft. pil. No. xii.

Sig.: One pill three times a day ; increase one pill
every two days up to physiological limit ; then cut
down dose one-half and continue for eighteen months.

1548—Mucous patches in mouth are healed by application of solid stick of silver or sulphate of
copper. If elsewhere, wash with 1–2000
bichloride solution and dust with—

℞ Hydrarg. chlor. mit.,
Bismuth. subnit., . aa ℥ij.—M.

Sig.: Dusting powder.

1549—℞ Hydrarg. chlor. corros., . . gr. iss.
Tr. ferri chlor., . . . f℥v.
Glycerini, ... f℥ij.
Aquæ, . . . q. s. ad f℥iv.—M.

Sig.: Teaspoonful in water every three hours.

1550—℞ Potass. iodid., . . . ℥iiss.
Syr. aq. hydriodic, . . ℥j.
Aq. destillat., . . . ℥iij.—M.

Sig.: Dessertspoonful thrice daily in a wineglassful of rice-water. (*To detect free iodine.*) GERHARD.

SYPHILIS (Continued).

1551—℞ Hydrarg. iodid. rub., . . gr. j.
 Potass. iodid., . . . ℨiv.
 Syr. sarsaparillæ co.,
 Aquæ, . . . āā f℥ij.—M.
Sig.: Teaspoonful three times a day after meals.
         R. W. TAYLOR.

1552—℞ Hydrarg. chlor. mit., . . ℨss.
Sig.: Vaporize by means of heat, beneath a blanket
covering, the naked body.

1553—℞ Hydrarg. chlor. corros., . gr. vj.
 Sodii chlorid., . . . gr. xxxvj.
 Aq. destillat., . . . f℥x.—M.
Sig.: Inject daily five to eight drops hypodermic-
ally.   HEBRA.

1554—℞ Pil. hydrargyri, . . gr. xx.
 Ferri sulph. exsiccat., . gr. x.
 Ex. opii, ... gr. v.—M.
Ft. pil. No. xx.
Sig.: One pill three times a day.   OTIS.

1555—℞ Tr. myrrh, . . . f℥ss.
 Potass. chlorat., . . ℨiij.
 Aquæ, . . q. s. ad f℥vj.—M.
Sig.: Wash mouth every two or three hours. (For
mucous patches.)

1556—℞ Hydrarg. chlor. mit.,
 Lycopodii, . . āā ℨij.—M.
Sig.: Use as snuff three times daily, in syphilitic
lesions of nose.   GROSS.

1557—℞ Hydrarg. chlorid. mitis, . . gr. xxiv.
 Ol. olivæ sterilisat., . . f℥j.—M.
Sig.: Inject ♏xv once a week. FOURNIER.

1558—℞ Hydrarg. iodid. rubri, . . gr. iv.
 Ol. olivæ sterilisat., . . f℥j.—M.
Sig.: Inject from ♏xv to ♏xxx t. d.
       DE LAVARENNE.

1559—℞ Hydrarg. cyanat., . . . gr. x.
 Aq. sterilisat., . . . f℥ij.—M.
Sig.: For intravenous injection 15 minims; for sub-
cutaneous injection 25 minims. ABADIE.

SYPHILIS (Continued).

1560—℞ Hydrarg. chlor. corros., . gr. j.
      Potass. iodidi, . . . ℥ij.
      Tr. gentian. comp., . . f℥iij.—M.
  Sig.: A teaspoonful three times a day.
CHARITY HOSPITAL, N. Y.

1561—℞ Hydrarg. prot.,
      Lactucarii, . . āā gr. xv.
      Ex. opii, ... gr. ii¼.
      Ex. guaiaci, . . . ℥ss.—M.
  Et ft. pil. No. xx.
  Sig.: One pill at breakfast and after supper, followed by a large draught of water. DIDAY.

1562—℞ Acid. nitro-muriat. dil., . f℥iiss.
      Syr. stilliugiæ co., . . f℥xiiiss.
      Aquæ, ... f℥ij.—M.
  Sig.: One or two teaspoonfuls three times a day.
(In cases saturated with approved remedies, but still presenting mucous patches.) BARTHOLOW.

TABES MESENTERICA (See Marasmus).

TAPE WORM (See Worms).

TETANUS.

1563—Control the spasm by inhalations of ether, chloroform, or nitrite of amyl. Give ℥ij to ℥iv of bromide of potash in divided doses during the day, and chloral, gr. xxx to xl, at bedtime.
  Also give opium, if necessary. Support with food and stimulants. WOOD.

1564—℞ Potass. bromid., . . ℥iss.
  Div. in pulv. No. xii.
  Sig.: One powder in a half tumblerful of water every three or four hours. H. C. WOOD.

1565—℞ Chloral hydrat., . . ℥ss.
      Syr. aurant. cort., . . f℥iss.
      Aquæ, . . . ad f℥iij.—M.
  Sig.: Dessertspoonful as required. BARTHOLOW.

1566—℞ Pulv. opii, . . . ℥j.
      Pulv. camphoræ, . . gr. xv.
      Adipis præp., . . . ℥ss.—M.
  Sig.: Rub the parts affected with the spasm.
THOMAS.

1567—℞ Cocain. muriat.,
      Morphiæ muriat.,   . āā gr. xij.
      Aq. destillat.,   .   .   . f℥j.—M.

Sig.: Twenty to sixty minims hypodermically, as required.   LOPEZ.

1568—℞ Strychniæ sulphat., .   . gr. j.
      Aq. bullientis,   .   . . f℥j.—M.

Sig.: Eight to sixteen minims hypodermically, as required.   BARTHOLOW.

1569—℞ Liq. potass. arsenitis,   . f℥j.

Sig.: Five to eight drops, well diluted, every three hours.   DALTON.

1570—℞ Ex. belladonnæ,   . gr. ss–j.
    Ft. pil. No. i.

Sig.: One pill every two hours, to be increased *pro re nata;* also apply belladonna locally.
        HUTCHINSON.

1571—℞ Tr. cannabis indicæ,   . f℥ss.
      Syr. acaciæ,   .   . . f℥ij.
      Aq. cinnam.,   .   . . f℥ss.
    Ft. haustus.

Sig.: Take at once, and repeat in two hours, or sooner if necessary.   NELIGAN.

1572—℞ Ex. physostigmatis, .   . gr. iss.
      Pulv. zingiberis,   . . gr. iij.—M.
    Et ft. pil. No. iii.

Sig.: One pill every hour.   E. WATSON.

TETANY.

1572*a*—℞ Bismuthi salicyl.,   .   . ℥j.
      Benzonaphthol.,   .   . ℥ss.
      Sacchari,   .   .   . q. s.—M.
    Div. in chart. No. xii.

Sig.: One powder four times daily.

In conjunction with the foregoing administer the following:

1572*b*—℞ Potass. bromid.,   .   . . gr. xlv.
      Chloral. hydrat.,   .   . . gr. xv.
      Syr. aurant. cort.,   .   . f℥iss.
      Aq. destillat., .   .   . f℥iij.—M.

Sig.: One teaspoonful three times daily for a child two or three years of age.

THREAD-WORMS (See Worms).

THRUSH (See Aphthœ).

TIC DOULOUREUX (See Neuralgia).

TINEA (See Skin Diseases).

TINNITUS AURIUM.
1573—℞ Tr. cimicifugæ, . . ℳclx.
Aquæ, ... f℥ij.—M.
Sig.: Teaspoonful three times a day. PATTON.

TONSILLITIS (See Quinsy).

TOOTHACHE.
1574—℞ Collodii flexilis,
Acid. carbolic. cryst., āā f℈ij.—M.
Sig.: Apply to the tooth-cavity by means of a probe wrapped on the end with cotton. GUILD.

1575—℞ Morphiæ sulphat., . . gr. iv.
Atropiæ sulphat., . . gr. j.
Aq. destillat., . . . f℥j.—M.
Sig.: A few drops on cotton placed in the cavity.
BARTHOLOW.

1576—℞ Creasoti, ... f℈ij.
Sig.: Moisten a very small pledget of cotton and lay it in the carious cavity; then pack a larger piece of plain cotton over it to retain it. HENSON.

1577—℞ Acid. tannic., . . . ℈j.
Mastichis, ... gr. x.
Ætheris, ... f℈iv.—M.
Sig.: A few drops on cotton placed in the cavity.
DRUITT.

1578—℞ Chloroform., . . . gtt. v.
Tr. opii (Sydenham's), . gtt. ij.
Tr. benzoini, . . . gtt. x.
Sig.: Apply on cotton. LE BULLETIN MÉD.

1579—℞ Ol. caryophylli, . . f℈ij.
Sig.: Moisten a small piece of cotton and place in the cavity. HARTSHORNE.

TOOTHACHE (Continued).

1580—℞ Acid. arseniosi,   .   .
     Cocaini muriat.,   .   āā   gr. xv.
     Menthol cryst.,   .   .   gr. iiiss.
     Glycerinæ,   .   .   .   f℥iij.—M.

Sig.: A pledget of cotton moistened with this, and placed in the cavity of the tooth, will quickly check the pain.   L'UNION MÉDICALE.

1581—℞ Lini. aconiti (B. P.),
     Chloroformi,   .   .   āā   f℥iij.
     Tr. capsici,   .   .   .   f℥j.
     Tr. pyrethri,
     Ol. caryophylli,
     Pulv. camphoræ,   .   āā   ℨss.—M.

Sig.: A few drops on cotton placed in the cavity.   MASON.

1582—℞ Camphor. vas.,   .   .
     Chloral hydrat.,   .   āā   gr. lxxv.
     Cocaini hydrochlor.,   .   gr. xv.—M.

Sig.: To be introduced into the tooth-cavity.

1583—℞ Tr. iodinii,   .   .   .   f℥iv.
     Tr. aconiti,   .   .   .   f℥j.—M.

Sig.: Paint the gums twice daily around the painful tooth.   RODIER.

1584—℞ Cocaini hydrochlor.,   .   .   gr. xv.
     Opii,   .   .   .   gr. lx.
     Menthol,   .   .   .   gr. xv.
     Althææ pulv.,   .   .   gr. xlv.—M.

Et div. in pellets weighing one-half grain each.

Sig.: Place pellet in cavity of the aching tooth.

1585—℞ Cocaini hydrochlor.,
     Morphiæ sulphat.,
     Chloral hydrat.,
     Acid. carbolic.,   .   .   āā   gr. x.
     Aq. rosæ,   .   .   .   f℥x.—M.

Sig.: Inject with a hypodermic syringe into the gums. (For painless tooth extraction.)

TRICHINOSIS.

1586—℞ Sodii sulpho-carbolat.,   .   gr. ii–x.
     Aquæ,   .   .   .   f℥ij.—M.

Ft. haustus.

Sig.: To be taken three or four times daily.   FUREY.

TRICHINOSIS (Continued).

1587—Dr. Ferrer has cured a case with alcohol. He began with six and increased to nine ounces daily, in sweetened water. The cure was complete in eighteen days.

NAPHEYS' MED. THERAPEUTICS.

1588—Ergot or ergotini is suggested by—

RHODE, OF BERLIN.

TRISMUS NEONATORUM (See also Tetanus).

1589—℞ Ex. gelsemii fl., . . ℳviii–xvj.
Syr. simplicis, . . . f℥j.
Aquæ, . . q. s. ad f℥iv.—M.

Sig.: Half teaspoonful every two to four hours.

BARTHOLOW.

1590—℞ Tr. opii, ... gtt. v.
Tr. assafœtidæ, . . . f℥iss.
Syr. simplicis, . . . f℥v.
Aquæ, . . . ad f℥xv.—M.

Sig.: Half teaspoonful every hour. EBERLE.

1591—℞ Tr. opii, ... ℳj.
Ol. ricini, ... f℥j.—M.

Sig.: A teaspoonful every four hours, with a warm bath. DRUITT.

1592—℞ Chloral hydrat., . . gr. i–iv.
Syr. simplicis, . . . f℥j.—M.

Sig.: One dose. BARTHOLOW.

TUBERCULOSIS (See Rachitis and Phthisis).

TYMPANITES.

1593—℞ Naphthol,
Magnesii carbonat.,
Carbo. lig., . . āā gr. lxxv.
Ol. menthæ pip., . . gtt. x.—M.

Et ft. chart. No. xv.

Sig. One powder when required. MEDICAL NEWS.

1594—℞ Ol. terebinthinæ, . . f℥j.
Pulv. acaciæ, . . . q. s.—M.

Et adde—
Decocti hordei, . . f℥xix.—M.

Et ft. enema.

Sig.: Inject into the bowel. HOOPER.

1595—℞ Ol. terebinthinæ, . . f℥j.
　　　Ol. amygdalæ express., . f℥ss.
　　　Tr. opii, ... f℥ij.
　　　Mucil. acaciæ, . . . f℥v.
　　　Aq. lauro-cerasi, . . f℥ss.—M.

Sig.: Teaspoonful every three to six hours.

BARTHOLOW.

1596—℞ Ol. terebinthinæ,
　　　Ol. ricini, . . . āā f℥iij.
　　　Ol. cajuputi, . . . ℳvj.
　　　Magnesii calcinatæ, . . ℈j.
　　　Aq. menthæ pip., . . f℥iss.—M.

Et ft. haustus.

Sig.: Take at one dose. JOY.

1597—℞ Pulv. capsici, . . . gr. vi-xxiv.
　　　Sacch. lact., . . . ℈iss.—M.

Et ft. chart. No. xii.

Sig.: One powder every four hours. PHILLIPS.

TYPHOID AND TYPHUS FEVERS (*See Fever*).
ULCER.

1598—℞ Zinci oxidi,
　　　Gelatin puris, . . āā f℥j.
　　　Glycerinæ,
　　　Aq. destillat., . . āā f℥iv.—M.

Sig.: Wash the leg thoroughly with soap and water, and apply the paste in a thick layer to the parts, excepting the site of the ulcer. The ulcer is then sprinkled with iodoform, and covered with a layer of cotton and sublimate or iodoform gauze. Over this is applied tightly a double-headed wet mull-bandage, the ends crossing in front of the leg. The bandage should extend at least from the middle of the foot to the calf, and is supplemented by a second one similarly applied. The dressings are changed in from two to four or even eight days, according to the amount of discharge. (*Leg ulcer.*)

UNNA.

1599—℞ Argenti nitrat. fusæ, . q. s.

Sig.: Apply to the surface and edges, and strap with adhesive plaster. (*Leg ulcer.*) MARKOE.

1600—℞ Calcii phosphatis, . . f℥j.
　　　Aquæ, ... f℥x.—M.

Sig.: Saturate compresses and apply, renewing three or four times daily. (*Leg ulcers.*) GROSSICH.

ULCER (*Continued*).

1601—℞ Bismuth. subnit., . . ℥ij.
   Pulv. opii, . . . gr. iij.—M.
Et ft. chart. No. xii.
Sig.: One powder three times a day, followed by—

1602—℞ Acid. nitrici, . . . ℳxij.
   Aquæ, ... f℥xvj.—M.
Sig.: Use locally. (*Indolent ulcers.*)   HOWE.

1603—℞ Cupri sulphat., . . gr. vj.
   Aquæ, ... f℥viij.—M.
Sig.: Use locally. (*Sloughing ulcer.*)   COOPER.

1604—℞ Argenti nitratis, . . gr. v.
   Tr. opii, ... f℥iss.
   Aq. anisi, . . . ad f℥iiss.—M.
Sig.: Teaspoonful three times a day. (*Gastric
ulcer.*)   THOMPSON.

1605—℞ Argenti oxidi,
      Ex. hyoscyami, . . āā gr. v.—M.
Et ft. pil. No. x.
Sig.: One pill three times a day. (*Gastric ulcer.*)
   BARTHOLOW.

1606—℞ Codeini phosph.,
      Ext. belladonnæ, . . āā gr. v.
      Bismuthi subcarb., . . . gr. l.
      Lactos., ... ℥j.—M.
Ft. chart. No. xv.
Sig.: Take two or three powders daily. (*Gastric
ulcer.*)   LEUBE.

1607—℞ Argenti nitrat., . gr. iv.
      Ext. hyoscyami, . gr. x-xx.—M.
Ft. pil. No. xx.
Sig.: One twenty minutes before each meal. (*Gastric
ulcer.*)   HARE.

1608—℞ Iodol., . . ℥ss.
      Vaselin.,
      Lanolin., . . . āā ℥iiss.—M.
Sig.: Spread in a thin layer on aseptic lint and
apply topically.

ULCER (*Continued*).

1609—℞ Creasoti, ... ♏iv.
   Tr. galbani, . . . f℥ij.
   Aquæ, ... f℥ij.—M.
 Sig.: Use locally. (*In indolent ulcers with excessive discharge.*)   NELIGAN.

1610—℞ Chloral hydrat., . . ℨss–ij.
   Aquæ, ... f℥vj.—M.
 Sig.: Use as a wash. (*In sluggish ulcers.*) KEYES.

1611—℞ Hydrarg. chlor. corros., . gr. xv.
   Acid. carbol., . . . ♏xxx.
   Aquæ, . . q. s. ad f℥iv.—M.
 Sig.: Apply on cotton daily. (*Syphilitic ulcers.*)
             FOX.

1612—℞ Emplast. plumbi, . . ℥ij.
   Ungt. hydrarg., . . ℥ss.
   Ol. cadini, . . . ℥ij.—M.
 Sig.: Spread on linen and apply. (*Inflamed syphilitic ulcers.*)   BUMSTEAD and TAYLOR.

1613—℞ Pulv. camphoræ,
   Carbonis animal., . āā ℥j.—M.
 Sig.: Use as a dusting powder. (*In deep chronic ulcers.*)   BARBACCI.

1614—℞ Aluminis, . . . ℥ij.
   Aquæ, ... f℥viij.—M.
 Sig.: (*Foul ulcers.*)   PENNYPACKER.

1615—℞ Acid. tannic., . . . gr. lxxv.
   Hydrarg. nitrat. acid., . gtt. xij.
   Adipis, ... ℥viiss.—M.
 Sig.: Apply as a dressing. (*For chronic syphilitic ulcers.*)   VENOT.

1616—℞ Sodii chlorid. pulv., . . ℥j.
   Menthol., ... gr. vj.—M.
 Sig.: Apply to cleansed and washed surface. (*Varicose ulcers.*)   SIMONELLI.

URÆMIA (*See also Albuminuria*).

1617—℞ Acid. benzoic., . . . ℈v.
   Div. in chart. No. v.
 Sig.: One powder in a half-tumblerful of water every three hours.   DA COSTA.

1618—℞ Pulv. scillæ,
  Pulv. scammonii,
  Pulv. digitalis, . . āā gr. xv.—M.
Et ft. pil. No. xx.
Sig.: Take from four to six pills daily, for six days.
          LANCEREAUX.

1619—℞ Ext. pilocarpi alc.,
  Ext. scillæ,
  Res. jalapæ,
  Res. scammonii, . āā gr. xv.—M.
Ft. pil. No. xx.
Sig.: Four or five pills daily during as many days.

1620—℞ Ex. colocynth. comp., . gr. xiv.
  Hydrarg. chlor. mit., . gr. vj.—M.
Et ft. pil. No. iv.
Sig.: Take at one dose, and follow in four hours
with a purge.   JOHNSON.

1621—℞ Tr. scillæ, ... f℥ij.
  Liq. ammon. acetat., . . f℥ij.
  Decoct. scoparii, q. s. ad f℥vj.—M.
Sig.: Two tablespoonfuls three times a day.
          CHARTERIS.

1622—℞ Acid. benzoic., . . . gr. xx.
  Syr. tolu., ... f℥j.—M.
Sig.: Take every three hours, well diluted.
         DA COSTA.

1623—℞ Pilocarpinæ muriat., . . gr. ij.
  Aquæ, ... f℥ij.—M.
Sig.: Inject hypodermically ten minims; half the
quantity for a child.   E. R. STONE.

1624—℞ Ol. tiglii, ... gtt. viij.
  Elaterii, ... gr. ss–j.
  Micæ panis, . . . q. s.—M.
Et ft. pil. No. viii.
Sig.: One or two pills as a purge.   BARTHOLOW.

URIC ACID DIATHESIS (See also Gout).
1625—℞ Sodii bicarbonat., . . ℥j.
  Tr. calumbæ, . . . f℥j.
  Infus. quassiæ, . . f℥iij.—M.
Sig.: Tablespoonful four times a day. HAZARD.

1626—℞ Liq. potass. arsenitis,   . ♏︎ v.
     Potass. bicarbonat.,
     Ferri et potass. tart.,   āā gr. v.
     Infus. quassiæ, .   .   . f℥j.—M.

Sig.: Take three times daily, two hours after meals.   FOTHERGILL.

1627—℞ Lithii carbonat.,
     Potass. iodid.,   .   . āā ℨiiss.
     Pulv. acaciæ,   .   .   . gr. xxiij.
     Ex. gentianæ,   .   . ℈iiss.—M.
Et ft. pil. No. c.
Sig.: One pill after each meal.   VIGIER.

1628—℞ Acid. muriat. dil.,   .   . f℥j.
     Acid. lactici,   .   .   . f℥iij.
     Syr. simp.,   .   .   . f℥ss.
     Aquæ, ... f℥ij.—M.

Sig.: Dessertspoonful after each meal. (*When excess of acid is due to indigestion.*)   BARTHOLOW.

1629—℞ Sodii boratis,   .   . ℨiij.
     Sodii bicarbonat.,
     Potass. nitratis,   . āā ℨiss.—M.
Et ft. chart. No. xii.
Sig.: One powder in a tumblerful of water.   DRUITT.

1630—℞ Lithii benzoat., .   .   . ℨiiss.
     Ex. gentianæ,   .   .   . gr. cv.—M.
Et ft. pil. No. c.
Sig.: One pill morning and evening.   VIGIER.

URINE, INCONTINENCE OF.

1630*a*—℞ Tr. belladonnæ,
     Ext. ergotæ fld., .   . āā f℥iv.—M.

Sig.: Gtt. ij–x t. d.

1630*b*—℞ Ferri carbonat., .   . gr. x–xxx.
     Ext. belladonnæ,
     Ext. nucis vomicæ,   . āā gr. iij–xv.—M.
Ft. pil. No. xx.

Sig.: Begin with one pill daily, and increase gradually until the physiologic effects of the belladonna appear.

URTICARIA (See also Pruritus).

1631—℞ Magnesii sulphat., . . ℨj.
     Ferri sulphat., . . . gr. iv.
     Sodii chloridi, . . . ℨss.
     Acid. sulphuric. dil., . f℥ij.
     Infus. quassiæ, . . ad f℥iv.—M.
Sig.: Tablespoonful in tumblerful of water before
breakfast.   VAN HARLINGEN.

1632—℞ Acid. carbolic., . . . f℥iss.
     Glycerinæ, . . . f℥ij.
     Alcoholis, ... f℥viij.
     Aq. amygdal. amar., . . f℥viij.—M.
Sig.: Use locally two or three times a day.
                  DUHRING.

1633—℞ Chloroformi, . . . f℥j.
     Ungt. zinci ox., . . ℥ij.—M.
Sig.: Apply with hand.   HUGHES.

1634—℞ Sodii bicarbonat., . . ℨj.
     Glycerinæ, . . . f℥iss.
     Aq. sambuci, . . . f℥viss.—M.
Sig.: Apply to allay the itching.   TILBURY FOX.

1635—℞ Ammon. carbonat., . . ℨj.
     Plumbi acetat., . . . ℨij.
     Aq. rosæ, ... f℥viij.—M.
Sig.: Use locally.   AITKEN.

1636—℞ Pulv. pilocarpii,
     Ex. guaiaci, . . āā gr. iss.
     Lithii benzoat., . . . gr. iij.—M.
Et ft. pil. No. i.
Sig.: Take from two to four each twenty-four hours.
                HUGHES.

1637—℞ Sodii borat., . . . ℨij.
     Aq. lauro-cerasi, . . f℥j.
     Aq. sambuci, . . . f℥xj.—M.
Sig.: Use locally. (*To allay itching.*)   NELIGAN.

1638—℞ Chloralis,
     Camphoræ, . . āā ℨj.
     Pulv. amyli, . . . ℥i-ij.—M.
Sig.: Keep tightly corked in a wide-mouthed bottle.
Rub in with hand.   BULKLEY.

1639—℞ Plumbi acetat.,
   Ammon. carbonat., . āā ℨj.
   Tr. opii, ... fℨss.
   Aq. rosæ, ... fℨviij.—M.
  Sig.: Use locally.   HAZARD.

1640—℞ Chloroformi, . . . fℨj.
   Glycerinæ, . . . fℨiv.—M.
  Sig.: Apply with a brush.   DUPARC.

1641—℞ Potass. cyanidi, . . gr. vj.
   Pulv. cocci, . . . gr. j.
   Ungt. aq. rosæ, . . . ℨj.—M.
  Sig.: Apply locally.   ANDERSON.

1642—℞ Potass. brom., . . . ℨss.
   Aq. menthæ pip., . . fℨiij.—M.
  Sig.: Dessertspoonful four times a day.
          ANDERSON.

1642*a*—℞ Menthol., . . gr. xx.
   Chloroform.,
   Æther.,
   Spt. camphoræ, . . āā fℨj.—M.
  Sig.: After using as a spray or lotion, dust the part with powdered starch or zinc oxid.   GAUCHER.

1642*b*—℞ Acid. carbolic., . . . gr. xv.
   Ess. menthæ pip., . . . ℳxv.
   Zinci oxidi, ... ℨiij.
   Lanolin., ... ℨss.
   Vaselin., ... ℨij.—M.
  Sig.: The application of the ointment can be preceded by antipruriginous lotions of chloral in eau-de-cologne.   BROCQ.

1642*c*—℞ Plumbi acet., ... gr. xv.
   Acid. hydrocyanic. dil., . . fℨiv.
   Alcohol., ... fℨviiss.
   Aq. destillat., . . q. s. ad fℨij.—M.
  Sig.: To be applied on cotton wool.
     MED. TIMES AND HOSP. GAZ.

UVULA, RELAXATION OF.

1643—℞ Acid. tannic., . . . ℨss.
   Glycerinæ, . . . fℨij.—M.
  Sig.: Apply with camel's hair brush.   HILLIER.

1644—℞ Liq. ferri perchlor., . . f3ij.
   Aquæ, ... f℥ij.- M.
 Sig.: Apply with a camel's-hair brush.
          MACKENZIE.

1645—℞ Aluminis, .   . 3j.
   Infus. gallæ,   . f℥vj.—M.
 Sig.: Use as gargle.   WARING.

1646—℞ Trochisci acid. tannic.,   . No. xx.
 Sig.: Take one every two or three hours. AITKEN

1647—℞ Zinci chloridi, . . . 3j.
   Aquæ, ... f℥ij.—M.
 Sig.: Apply with a camel's-hair brush.
          MACKENZIE.

VAGINITIS.

1648—℞ Acid. tannic., . . . 3j.
   Morphiæ sulphat., . . gr. iij.
   Ol. theobromæ, . . . ℥v.—M.
 Et ft. suppos. No. x.
 Sig.: After freely syringing the vagina night and
morning insert suppository.   T. GAILLARD THOMAS.

1649—℞ Argent. nitrat., . . . Ðij.
   Aq. destillat., . . . f℥j.—M.
 Sig.: Apply on a cotton pledget within the cervical
canal and over the vaginal mucous membrane.
          EMMET.

1650—℞ Glyceriti acid. tannic., . f℥j.
 Sig.: Apply locally.   RINGER.

1651—℞ Ex. hydrastis fl., . . f℥iv.
 Sig.: Apply to the cervix and vagina, and place a
tampon smeared with vaseline between the vulvæ
and in the vagina.   MUNDÉ.

1652—℞ Acid. boracic., . . . ℥iss.
   Glycerinæ, . . . f℥xxx.—M.
 Sig.: Three or four dessertspoonfuls in a quart of
water as a vaginal injection.   CHÉRON.

1652a—℞ Acetanilid., ... gr. lxxv.
   Ac. tannici, ... gr. viij.
   Ext. hyoscyami, . . . gr. iv.
   Sacchari lactis, . . . gr. cl.—M.
 Sig.: Use such a suppository two or three times a day.

VAGINITIS (*Continued*).

1652*b*—℞ Pulv. aluminis,
  Zinci sulphatis,
  Sodii biboratis,
  Acid. carbolici, . . āā ʒj.
  Aquœ, ... f ʒvj.—M.

Sig.: A tablespoonful to a quart of lukewarm water as a vaginal injection twice daily.

VANDERBILT CLINIC.

VALVULAR DISEASE (See Heart Disease).

VARICOSE VEINS.

1653—℞ Ex. hamamelis fl., . . fʒij.

Sig.: Teaspoonful three or four times a day, with compresses applied externally. J. V. SHOEMAKER.

1654—℞ Ergotini (aq. ext.),
  Glycerinæ, . . āā fʒj.
  Aq. destillat., . . . fʒvij.—M.

Sig.: Fifteen minims hypodermically alongside of the veins, care being taken not to puncture a vein.

BARTHOLOW.

VARIOLA (See Smallpox).

VENEREAL DISEASE (See Syphilis).

VERTIGO (See also Biliousness, Indigestion, etc.).

1655—℞ Pulv. rhei, . . . ʒj.
  Sodii bicarb.,
  Pulv. gentian., . āā ʒij.
  Aq. menthæ pip.,
  Aq. destillat., . . āā fʒiij.—M.

Sig.: Tablespoonful before each meal. MANN.

1656—℞ Potass. bitartrat., . . ʒvj.
  Pulv. jalapæ, . . . ʒij.—M.

Sig.: Teaspoonful in milk every two or three hours. (*In plethoric cases.*) SWERINGEN.

1657—℞ Tr. gelsemii, . . . fʒj.

Sig.: Ten minims three times a day. (*In aural vertigo.*) RINGER.

VERTIGO *(Continued).*

1658—℞ Pil. hydrarg.,
　　　Pil. rhei co.,
　　　Ex. hyoscyami, . . āā ℈j.—M.
Et ft. pil. No. xii.

Sig.: Two pills occasionally at bedtime. *(In plethoric cases.)* Tanner.

1659—℞ Pulv. jalapæ, . . . gr. xij.
　　　Hydrarg. chlor. mit., . . gr. iij.
　　　Potass. sulphat., . . gr. vij.—M.
Et ft. chart. No. i.

Sig.: Take at bedtime. *(In bilious vertigo.)*
A. T. Thompson.

VOMITING *(See also Morning Sickness and Sea-sickness).*

1660—℞ Liq. calcis,
　　　Aq. cinnam., . . āā f℥iij.—M.

Sig.: Tablespoonful in ice-water, to be repeated
until relieved. Starr.

1661—℞ Acid. carbol., . . . gr. iv.
　　　Bismuth. subnitrat., . ℥ij.
　　　Mucil. acaciæ, . . ℥j.
　　　Aq. menth. pip., . . f℥iij.—M.

Sig.: Tablespoonful every two to four hours.
Bartholow.

1662—℞ Vini ipecac., . . . f℥ss.

Sig.: One minim every half hour. Ringer.

1663—℞ Creasoti, ... ♏iv.
　　　Aquæ, ... f℥vj.—M.

Sig.: Tablespoonful repeated as necessary.
Niemeyer.

1664—℞ Aloini, ... gr. v.
　　　Strychniæ sulphat., . . gr. j.
　　　Ex. colocynth. comp., . gr. v.
　　　Ex. hyoscyami, . . ℥j.—M.
Et ft. pil. No. lx.

Sig.: One pill after each meal. *(In obstinate vomiting due to chronic constipation.)* Da Costa.

1665—℞ Tr. benzoin. comp.,
　　　Acid. sulphuric. dil., āā f℥ss.—M.

Sig.: Give thirty drops with sugar.
E. G. Clark.

1666—℞ Bismuth. subnit,,   .   . ℥ij.
      Acid. hydrochlor. dil.,   . f℥ss.
      Mucil. acaciæ,
      Aq. menthæ pip.,   . āā f℥ij.—M.

Sig.: Tablespoonful three times a day. (*With gastric ulcer.*)   Da Costa.

1667—℞ Liq. calcis,
      Lactis recentis, .   . āā f℥iij.—M.

Sig.: Tablespoonful every half hour or hour.
                              Wood.

1668—℞ Liq. potass. arsenitis,   . f℥ss.

Sig.: Half drop every half hour for six or eight doses. (*Vomiting of drunkards and pregnancy.*)
                            A. A. Smith.

1669—℞ Chloroformi,   .   .   . f℥ss.

Sig.: Two to five minims on sugar. (*In non-inflammatory vomiting.*)   Ringer.

1670—℞ Ex. belladonnæ,
      Ex. physostigmat.,
      Ex. nucis vomicæ,
      Aloini,   .   .   . āā gr. xv.
      Ferri sulphat. exsiccat.,   . ℥j.—M.
Et ft. pil. No. lx.

Sig.: Pill at bedtime. One grain of permanganate of potash in water is also taken three times a day. (*In hysterical vomiting.*)   Bartholow.

1671—℞ Sodii bicarb.,   .   .   . gr. xv.
      Acid. hydrocyauic. dil.,   . ℳiss.
      Aq. camphoræ,   .   .   . f℥x.—M.

Sig.: To be taken three times a day after meals (*When due to acidity.*)   Chambers.

1672—℞ Ex. nucis vomicæ,   .   . gr. j.
      Ex. conii, ... gr. xij.—M.
Et ft. pill No. vi.

Sig.: One pill three times a day. (*When due to malignant disease of the stomach.*)   Barlow.

1673—℞ Cerii oxalat.,   .   .   . gr. j.
      Ipecacuanhæ,   .   .   . gr. j.
      Creasoti, ... gtt. ij.—M.

Sig.: This is to be taken every hour until nausea is controlled. (*In pregnancy.*)   Goodell.

VOMITING (Continued).

1674—Take the fourth part of a Seidlitz powder every
fifteen minutes.   WOODBURY.

1675—℞ Ceri oxalat, . . . gr. j.
       Pulv. ipecac., . . . gr. j.
       Creasoti, ... gtt. j.—M.
  Sig.: Take every hour.

1676—℞ Cocain. muriat., . . gr. ¼.
       Ex. nucis vomicæ, . . gr. ⅛.
       Pulv. assafœtidæ, . . gr. ij.—M.
  Et ft. capsulas No. i.
  Sig.: Take one capsule three times a day, half
hour before eating.   M. W. EVERSON.

1676a—℞ Spt. vini rectif., . . . f℥iiss.
       Menthol., ... ℨj.
       Tr. nucis vom., . . . f℥ss.—M.
  Sig.: Ten drops every hour in a teaspoonful of chlo-
roform-water.   PRACTITIONER.

1676b—℞ Menthol., ... gr. ij.
       Cocain. hydrochlor., . . gr. iv.
       Spt. vini rectif., . . f℥ij.
       Syrup., ... f℥j.—M.
  Sig.: Teaspoonful every half hour for several doses.

VULVITIS (See Vaginitis).

WAKEFULNESS (See Insomnia).

WARTS (See Condylomata).

WHITLOW (See Onychia).

WHOOPING-COUGH,

1677—℞ Ex. belladonnæ, . . gr. ss.
       Pulv. aluminis, . . gr. xxiv.
       Syr. zingiber.,
       Aquæ, . . . āā f℥iss.—M.
  Sig.: Teaspoonful every two hours for a child of
one year. ·   GOODHART and STARR.

1678—℞ Tr. opii camph.,
       Syr. ipecac., . . āā f℥j.
       Syr. scillæ, . . . f℥iij.
       Syr. tolu., . . . f℥ss.
       Liq. potass. citrat., q. s. ad f℥iij.—M.
  Sig.: Teaspoonful every two hours for catarrhal
stage.   PENROSE.

1679—℞ Ex. belladonnæ,   . . gr. j.
       Syr. tolutan., . . . f℥iv.

Sig.: Three to four coffeespoonfuls for a child one year old.   L'UNION MÉDICALE.

1680—℞ Antipyrin,
       Quiniæ sulphat.,   . āā ℈ss.
       Elix. glycyrrhizæ, . . f℥iv.—M.

Sig.: Teaspoonful every two to four hours.
                        WAUGH.

1681—℞ Pulv. belladonnæ rad.,   . gr. ⅕.
       Pulv. Dover., . . . gr. ss.
       Sulphuris sub., . . . gr. iv.
       Sacch. alb.,   . . . gr. x.—M.
   Et ft. chart. No. i.

Sig.: One powder from two to ten times a day, according to age.   GERMAIN SÉE.

1682—℞ Thymolis, .   .   . gr. xx.
       Acid. carbolici,
       Ol. sassafras,
       Ol. eucalypti,
       Picis liquidæ,
       Ol. terebinthinæ,   . āā f℈ij.
       Ætheris, .   .   . f℈iv.
       Alcoholis, . . q. s. ad f℥iij.—M.

Sig.: Put about thirty drops upon a pad of such a size as to be conveniently hung around the child's neck, renewing the application every two or three hours.

In severe cases the inhalation treatment is supplemented by the internal administration of—

1683—℞ Acid. carbolici, .   .   . gr. iij.
       Sodii bromidi, .   .   . gr. j.
       Tr. belladonnæ,   . . gtt. xx.
       Glycerinæ,   .   .   . f℈iij.
       Aquæ,   . . q. s. ad f℥ij.—M.

Sig.: Teaspoonful for a child three or four years of age occasionally.   BEALL

1684—℞ Ammon. brom.,
       Potass. brom.,   . . āā ℈j.
       Tr. belladonnæ,   . . f℈j.
       Glycerinæ,   .   . f℈j.
       Aq. rosæ, .   .   . f℥iv.—M.

Sig.: Use as spray from four to six times daily.
                        KEATING.

1685—℞ Quiniæ sulphat.,   . . gr. xij.
      Ol. theobrom., .   . . q. s.—M.
Et ft. suppos. No. xii.

Sig.: Use one or two three times a day for a child of two years.

1686—℞ Terpine,
      Antipyrin,   . . āā gr. xv.
      Syr. aurant.,   .   . . fℨi–ʒvj.
      Mucilaginis,   . . fℨij.—M.

Sig.: One or two teaspoonfuls several times a day for a child under four years.   SALAMON.

1687—℞ Acid. carbolic.,
      Alcohol.,   .   . . āā gtt. xv.
      Tr. iodin., ... gtt. x.
      Tr. belladonnæ,   . . gr. xxx.
      Aq. menth. pip.,   . . fℨiss.
      Syr. opiat.,   .   . . fℨij.—M.

Sig.: A teaspoonful every hour to a child of one year.   ROTHE.

1688—℞ Chloroformi,   .   . . fℨj.
      Æther. sulphuri.,   . . ℨij.
      Ess. terebinthinæ rect.,   . fℨiiss.—M.

Sig.: Pour a teaspoonful upon a compress and hold close to the child's mouth. (*During paroxysm.*)
    WILDE.

1689—℞ Pulv. acid. boric.,   . gr. xxxvj.
Div. in chart. No. xii.

Sig.: Blow one powder into nose with insnfflator every three hours.   MONTI.

1690—℞ Codeinæ sulphat.,   . . gr. j.
      Acid. carbolic., .   . . ℳviij.
      Syr. simplicis,   .   . . fℨss.
      Glycerinæ,   .   . . fℨj.
      Syr. limonis,   .   . . fℨss.—M.

Sig.: Teaspoonful every two or three hours.
    HUGHES.

1691—℞ Ex. castaneæ fl.,   . . fℨiij.
Sig.: Dose for a child five years old, teaspoonful every two hours for three days (during the night after each paroxysm); afterwards three or four times a day.   GERHARD.

1692—℞ Antipyrin, . . gr. ij.
 Sacch. alb., . . Ɔj.—M.
 Et ft. chart. No. xiv.

Sig.: One powder three times a day and once at night for very young children. SONNENBERGER.

1693—℞ Sol. cocaini muriat. (5 per
 cent.), ... f℥ss.

Sig.: Paint the throat and fauces several times a day. LABRIC.

1694—℞ Tr. lobeliæ,
 Syr. scillæ, . . āā f℥j.
 Ex. belladonnæ, . . gr. iv.—M.

Sig.: Thirty drops three times a day. HAZARD.

1695—℞ Acid. carbolic., . . . f℥ss.
 Potass. chlorat., . . ℥ij.
 Glycerinæ, . . . f℥iv.
 Aquæ, . . q. s. ad f℥vj.—M.

Sig.: Use with a steam atomizer three times a day.
 J. LEWIS SMITH.

1696—℞ Acid. carbolic. puri, . . gtt. xv–xx.

Sig.: Drop on cotton or in an inhaler, and inhale for several hours daily. PECK.

1696*a*—℞ Tr. belladonnæ, . . . f℥ij.
 Tr. valerianæ,
 Tr. digitalis, . : . āā f℥j.—M.

Or

1696*b*—℞ Tr. belladonnæ, . . . f℥ij.
 Tr. digitalis,
 Tr. moschi, . . . āā f℥j.—M.

Sig.: For children under two years 5 drops daily, increased to 30 drops; between two and five years, 10 drops daily, increased to 60; for adults, from 15 drops increased to 90.

1696*c*—℞ Phenocoll. hydrochlor.,
 Antipyrin., . . . āā gr. x.
 Potassii bromid., . . . gr. viij.
 Syr. aurantii cort. amaræ,
 Aq. aurantii floris, . . āā f℥j.—M.

Sig.: A child, eight years old, may take the whole amount in four doses in the course of twenty-four hours.

1696*d*—℞ Bromoformi, ... f℥iij.
 Tr. gelsemii, ... f℥iij.
 Syr. lactucarii, . . . f℥ij.—M.
 Sig.: Teaspoonful three or four times a day.

1696*e*—℞ Tr. belladonnæ, . . . ℈iss.
 Phenacetin., ... gr. xl.
 Spt. vini rectif., . . . f℥ij.
 Ex. castaneæ fluid., . . f℥j.—M.
 Sig.: Ten drops at intervals of from two to six hours for children under a year old; up to a teaspoonful for children ten years old. LANCASTER.

1696*f*—℞ Potassii bromid., . . . ℈j.
 Chloral. hydrat., . . . gr. xl.
 Tr. belladonnæ, . . . ℈ss.
 Syr. aurantii, ... f℥j.
 Aq. cinnamomi, . . ad f℥iij.—M.
 Sig.: Teaspoonful at bedtime for a child one year old, and increase according to age.

1696*g*—℞ Syr. ipecac. comp., . . . f℥ijss.
 Syr. belladonnæ, . . . f℥j.
 Ammonii bromidi, . . . gr. xvss.
 Creosoti, ... gtt. x.—M.
 Sig.: One teaspoonful every three hours.

1696*h*—℞ Bromoformi, ... ♏xl.
 Mucilag. gummi Arabic.,
 Syr. tolutani, . . . āā f℥vij.—M.
 Sig.: Teaspoonful from three to five times a day.

1696*i*—℞ Pulv. benzoini,
 Bismuthi salicylat., . āā ℈ijss.
 Quininæ sulphat., . . . ℈ss.—M.
 Sig.: Insufflate into nares five times a day.
 MOIZARD.

1696*k*—℞ Bromoform., ... ♏xl.
 Spt. vini rectif., . . . f℥iv.
 Aq. destillat., ... f℥j.
 Syr. of tolu, . . q. s. ad f℥iij.—M.
 Sig.: Teaspoonful, in water, every three hours.
 PHILA. POLYCLINIC.

1696*l*—℞ Tr. belladonnæ, . . . ♏xxxij.
 Acid. carbol., C. P., . . gtt. viij.
 Ammon. bromid., . . . ℈ij.
 Potassii bromid., . . . ℈vj.
 Aq. menth. pip., . q. s. ad f℥iv.—M.
 Sig.: Spray the child's throat every two hours.

1697—℞ Chloroformi,
   Ex. aspidi fl.,   .   .   āā   fℨj.
   Emul. ol. ricini (B. Ph.),   f℥iij.—M.

Sig.: To be taken in the early morning; no food until after thorough action of the bowels. (*Tapeworm.*)   Hughes.

1698—℞ Peponis decort.,   .   .   ℥v-x.
   Sacch. alb.,   .   .   .   ℥vj–gr. xv.
   Lactis recentis, .   .   .   ℥xv.—M.

Sig.: Take before breakfast. Follow in two hours by a dose of castor-oil. (*Tapeworm.*)   Dupont.

1699—℞ Thymoli, ...   ℥ij.
   Div. in chart. No. xii.

Sig.: First take a dose of castor-oil, then one powder every fifteen minutes, and follow with a second dose of oil. (*Tapeworm.*)   Campi.

1700—℞ Granati corticis,   .   .   ℥ij.
   Ft. infusum.

Sig.: To be taken before 11 A. M., and followed after two hours by—

1701—℞ Ol. ricini, ...   f℥iij.
   Ol. terebinth.,   .   .   fℨj.
   Ex. filicis maris æther.,   .   fℨj.—M.
   Ft. haustus.

Sig.: Fasting unnecessary. (*Tapeworm.*)   Wilde.

1702—℞ Pulv. kamalæ,   .   .   .   gr. v–x.
   Syr. aurantii,   .   .   .   fℨss.
   Mucil. tragacan.,   .   .   ℨj.
   Aquæ, ...   f℥j.—M.

Sig.: Take early in the morning, and follow by a purge in four hours. For a child from two to five years. (*Tapeworm.*)   T. H. Tanner.

1703—℞ Ol. terebinthinæ,
   Oleoresin. filicis maris,   āā   ℨj.
   Mucil. acaciæ,   .   .   f℥ij.—M.

Sig.: Give day before treatment liquid diet and one drachm of compound jalap powder. Give the above the following morning, fasting. Half-hour later a dose of castor-oil. (*Tapeworm.*)   F. A. A. Smith

1704—℞ Chloroformi, . . . f℥j.
      Syr. simp., . . . f℥j, ℳxl.—M.

Sig.: Take in three equal doses at 7 A. M., 9 A. M., and 11 A. M. At midday give two tablespoonfuls of castor-oil. (*Tapeworm.*)   Le Courier Médical.

1705—℞ Ol. filicis maris æther., . ℨii–iij.
      Emuls. amygdal. dulc., ad ℥vj.—M.

Sig.: In the evening a light meal is eaten. At bedtime, about twenty minutes apart from each other, this medicine is taken in two doses. The next morning early, about five o'clock, two tablespoonfuls of castor-oil are administered, and these followed about an hour later by another tablespoonful. (*Tapeworm.*)   Hugo Engel.

1706—℞ Ol. filicis maris, . . f℥iij.
      Ol. chenopodii, . . . f℥j.
      Ol. terebinth., . . . f℥ij.
      Emul. ol. ricini (50 per cent.)
                q. s. ad f℥ij.—M.

Sig. Teaspoonful twice a day for a child of six years. (*Tapeworm.*)   L. Starr.

1707—℞ Tauret's pelletierini, . 1 bottle.

Sig.: In the evening use a large laxative injection and take only milk. The next morning mix the contents of a bottle with a glass of water, and take at one dose; one hour after, take one ounce of compound tincture of jalap mixed with a half glass of water. (*Tapeworm.*)   L. Starr.

1708—℞ Tr. kamalæ, . . . f℥ss.
      Syr. zingiber., . . . f℥j.
      Syr. acaciæ, . . . f℥ss.—M.

Sig.: Take at one dose at bedtime, followed by a purge in the morning. (*Tapeworm.*)   L. Starr.

1709—℞ Flor. koosso, . . . ℨiiss–iv.
      Ex. filic. mar. æth., . . f℥iss–ij.
      Aq. destillat., . . . f℥iij.—M.

Sig.: Take in three portions half hourly. (*Tapeworm.*)   Kinder-Arzt

1710—After a light diet the evening before, give the
          following on an empty stomach :—
    ℞ Ol. tiglii, ... gtt. j.
      Chloroform, purif., . . f℥j.
      Glycerinæ, . . . f℥j, f℥ij.—M.

Sig.: Take in two doses, half an hour apart. (*Tapeworm.*)   Pharmaz. Zeit.

1711—℞ Pelletierine sulphat., . gr. vi–viiss.
   Pulv. acid. tannic., . . gr. viiss.
   Syr. simp., . . . f℥ij.—M.

Sig.: Take only milk the night before, and at bedtime an injection. Take the above the following morning before breakfast. Fifteen minutes after take two tablespoonfuls of castor-oil. (*Tapeworm.*)
              LABBÉ.

1712—℞ Sodii chloridii, . . . ℥x.
   Aquæ, ... f℥vj.—M.

Sig.: Inject into the rectum. (*Seatworms.*)
             EILLARD.

1713—℞ Tr. rhei, ... gtt. xxx.
   Magnesii carbonat., . . gr. iij.
   Tr. zingiber., . . . gtt. j.
   Aquæ, . . q. s. ad f℥iv.—M.

Sig.: Warm and use as an injection three times a day. (*Seatworms.*)   ANNALS OF GYNECOLOGY.

1714—℞ Ferri sulphat., . . . ℥j.
   Infus. quassiæ, . . Oj.—M.

Sig.: After cleansing the lower bowel with an enema of warm soap-suds, inject the third part of the above on alternate mornings. (*Seatworms.*)
             L. STARR.

1715—℞ Santonini, . . . gr. i–ij.
   Hydrarg. chlor. mit., . . gr. i–iij.
   Pulv. aromat., . . . gr. iv.—M.
Et ft. chart. No. iv.

Sig.: One at bedtime, to be followed by a dose of castor oil in the morning. GOODHART and STARR.

1716—℞ Santonini, . . gr. xij.
   Ol. theobromæ, . . ℥j.—M.
Et ft. suppos. No. iv.

Sig.: Insert one at night. (*Seatworms.*)
            HARTSHORNE.

1717—℞ Ol. chenopodii, . . . gtt. lx–℥j.
   Mucil. acaciæ, . . . f℥ij.
   Syr. simplicis, . . . f℥j.
   Aq. cinnam., . . . f℥ij.—M.

Sig.: Dessertspoonful three times a day for three days, and repeat after three days. For a child of two years.   MEIGS and PEPPER.

WORMS (*Continued*).

1718—℞ Trochisci santonini (U. S.
P.), ... No. xxiv.

Sig.: One to six at bedtime, followed by a dose of castor oil in the morning. (*For lumbrici.*)

BARTHOLOW.

1719—℞ Hydrarg. chlor. mit., . . gr. j.
Resinæ jalapæ, . . . gr. ij.
Pulv. scammonii, . . gr. v.—M.
Et ft. chart. No. i.

Sig.: To be taken at bedtime for a child of six years. (*Seatworm.*) GOODHART and STARR.

1720—℞ Tr. ferri chlor., . . f℥ss.
Aquæ, ... Oj.—M.

Sig.: Inject one-fourth to one-third. (*Seatworms.*)

RINGER.

1721—℞ Tr. kamalæ, . . . f℥iss.
Syr. aurant. cort., . . f℥ss.
Aquæ, . . q. s. ad f℥iv.—M.

Sig.: Take in broken doses and at frequent intervals until all is taken. If the worm is not expelled within two hours after the last dose, give castor' oil. (*For lumbrici.*) DU JARRDIN BEAUMETZ.

1722—℞ Ex. spigeliæ et sennæ fl., . f℥j.
Santonini, . . . gr. viij.—M.

Sig.: Teaspoonful for a child of five years. (*For lumbrici.*) J. LEWIS SMITH.

1722a—℞ Oleores. aspidii, . . . ℥j.
Tr. quillaiæ, ... f℥ss.
Tr. aurantii dulcis, . . f℥j.
Syr. aurantii, . . q. s. ad f℥vij.—M.

Sig.: For a child five years old. (*Tapeworm.*)
The teniacide should be given after fasting, and be followed in an hour by a cathartic to carry off the worm. The best teniacides are pomegranate or its alkaloid, pelletierine; filix mas; kousso; pumpkin-seed; turpentine; and cocoanut.

TOWNSEND.

1722b—℞ Benzonaphthol.,
Santonicæ, . āā gr. xxx.
Sacchari alb., . . gr. lxxx.—M.
Div. in chart. No. xx.

Sig.: From two to five powders daily.

218

1723—℞ Iodoform., ... gr. c.
Thymoli, : . . . gr. cc.
Sacch. lact., . . . gr. j.—M.
Et ft. pulv.
Sig.: Apply as a powder three times a day.
WITHERSTINE.

1724—℞ Iodoform., ... ℥ij.
Sig.: Use as a dusting powder with dry dressings.
BARTHOLOW.

1725—℞ Acid. carbolic.,
Ol. rjcini, . . . āā f℥ss.
Collodii, ... f℥j.—M.
Sig.: "Carbolized collodion."

1726—℞ Hydrarg. chloridi corros., . gr. viiss.
Aq. ferventis. . . . Oij.—M.
Sig.: Solution (1 to 2000).

1727—℞ Acid. boracic., . . . ℥iss.
Ess. eucalypti, . . . f℥iss.
Vaselini, . . . ℥xxv.—M.
Sig.: Use as a dressing. BRONDEL.

1728—℞ Tr. eucalypti, . . f℥ij.
Aq. destillat., . . f℥iv.—M.
Sig.: GIMBERT.

1729—℞ Phénol sodique, . . f℥vj.
Sig.: Use pure or diluted with water.
J. W. WHITE.

1730—℞ Iodol,
Glycerinæ, . āā ℥j.
Vaselini, . . . ℥vij.—M. •
Sig.: Use locally. WOLFENDEN.

1731—℞ Pulv. acid. salicylic., . . ℥j.
Sig.: Use as a dusting powder. THIERSCH.

1732—℞ Iodoform., ... ℥j.
Collodii flex., . . . ℥vij.—M.
Sig.: Stitch the edges of the wound together and apply with a brush. BRUNS.

WORMS *(Continued).*

1733—℞ Pulv. naphthol.,   .   . ℥j.
    Sig.: Use as a dusting powder.   BOUCHARD.

1734—℞ Acid. carbol.,   .   . f℥j.
    Glycerinæ,   .   . f℥ij.—M.
    Sig.: Use locally.   HAZARD.

1734*a*—℞ Iodoformi,
    Salol.,
    Bismuthi subnitrat.,
    Carbo. lignis,
    Cinchonæ,
    Benzoini,   .   . āā ℥ij.—M.
    Sig.: Dusting-powder.

XERODERMA *(See Ichthyosis in Skin Diseases).*

YELLOW FEVER *(See Fever).*

DOSE TABLE.

THE doses given below are for adults. For children, Dr. Young's rule will be found most convenient. Add 12 to the age, and divide by the age to get the denominator of the fraction, the numerator of which is 1. Thus, for a child two years old, $\dfrac{2+12}{2} = 7$, and the dose is one-seventh of that for an adult. Of powerful narcotics scarcely more than one-half of this proportion should be used. Of mild cathartics two or even three times the proportion may be emploved.

For Hypodermic Injection the dose should be one-half of that used by the mouth ; by rectum, four-fifths of the same.

REMEDIES.	DOSE.	GRAMMES.
Abstract. aconiti, . . .	¼ to ½ grain.	0.015 to 0.03
aspidospermæ, . . .	5 to 20 grains.	0.35 to 1.3
belladonnæ, . . .	½ to 1½ grains.	0.03 to 0.1
cannab. ind., . . .	1 to 3 grains.	0.06 to 0.2
conii, ...	1 to 2 grains.	0.06 to 0.1
digitalis, ...	1 to 3 grains.	0.06 to 0.2
gelsemii, ...	1 to 3 grains.	0.06 to 0.2
hyoscyami, . . .	2 to 5 grains.	0.1 to 0.3
ignatiæ, ...	1 to 3 grains.	0.06 to 0.2
ipecac., ...	3 to 30 grains.	0.2 to 2.
jalapæ, ...	6 to 10 grains. -	0.4 to 0.65
nuc. vom., . . .	¼ to ½ grain.	0.015 to 0.03
phytolaccæ. . . .	5 to 15 grains.	0.3 to 1.
pilocarpi, . . .	6 to 30 grains.	0.4 to 2.
podophylli, . . .	4 to 10 grains.	0.25 to 0.65
senegæ, ...	4 to 10 grains.	0.25 to 0.65
valerianæ, . . .	10 to 15 grains.	0.65 to 1.
veratr. vir., . . .	1 to 3 grains.	0.06 to 0.2
Acetanilid, . . .	8 grains.	0.5
Acetphenetidine, . . .	1 to 2 grains.	0.06 to 0.1
Acet. lobeliæ, . . .	15 to 30 minims.	1. to 2.
opii, ...	5 to 16 minims.	0.3 to 1.
sanguinar., . . .	15 to 30 minims.	1. to 2.
scillæ, ...	10 to 30 minims.	0.65 to 2.
Acid. acet. dil., . . .	60 to 90 minims.	4. to 6.
arsenios., ...	⅟₆₄ to ⅟₆ grain.	0.001 to 0.003
benzoic., ...	5 to 15 grains.	0.3 to 1.
boric., ...	5 to 10 grains.	0.3 to 0.65
camphoric. (*to check night sweats*)	15 to 30 grains.	1. to 2.
carbolic., ...	1 to 3 grains.	0.06 to 0.2
gallic., ...	3 to 15 grains.	0.2 to 1.
gallic., in albuminuria, .	10 to 60 grains.	0.65 to 4.
hydriodic dilut., . . .	10 to 60 minims.	0.65 to 4.
hydrobrom. (34 per cent.),	10 to 15 grains.	0.65 to 1.
hydrobrom. dil., . .	40 m. to 2 fl. drms.	2. to 8.

REMEDIES.	DOSE.	GRAMMES.
Acid. hydrochlor., . . .	3 to 10 minims.	0.2 to 0.65
hydrochlor. dil., . .	10 to 30 minims.	0.65 to 2.
hydrocyan. dil., . .	2 to 6 minims.	0.1 to 0.35
lactic., ...	15 to 60 grains.	1. to 4.
nitr., ...	3 to 10 minims.	0.2 to 0.65
nitr. dil., . . .	10 to 30 minims.	0.65 to 2.
nitro-hydrochlor., . .	3 to 10 minims.	0.2 to 0.65
nitro-hydrochlor. dil., .	5 to 20 minims.	0.3 to 1.3
phosphoric (50 per cent.),	3 to 15 grains.	0.2 to 1.
phosphoric. dil., . .	10 to 30 minims.	0.65 to 2.
salicylic., . . .	5 to 20 grains.	0.35 to 1.3
sulphuric., . . .	5 to 10 minims.	0.35 to 0.65
sulphuric. dil., . .	5 to 30 minims.	0.35 to 2.
sulphuric. arom., . .	5 to 10 minims.	0.35 to 0.65
sulphuros., . . .	30 to 60 minims.	2. to 4.
tannic., ...	2 to 10 grains.	0.1 to 0.65
Aconitina (white crystals) .	$\frac{1}{100}$ to $\frac{1}{30}$ grain.	0.0001 to 0.0003
Adoninin, ...	$\frac{1}{3}$ grain.	0.02
Agarcin, . . .	$\frac{1}{8}$ to $\frac{1}{4}$ grain.	0.008 to 0.015
Aloe, ...	2 to 5 grains.	0.1 to 0.35
Aloinum, ...	1 to 3 grains.	0.06 to 0.2
Alumen, ...	10 to 15 grains.	0.65 to 1.
Ammonii benzoas, . .	10 to 20 grains.	0.65 to 1.3
bromid., . . .	5 to 30 grains.	0.3 to 2.
carb., ...	3 to 10 grains.	0.2 to 0.65
chlorid., . . .	10 to 30 grains.	0.65 to 2.
iodid., ...	3 to 15 grains.	0.2 to 1.
phosp., ...	5 to 20 grains.	0.35 to 1 3
picras., ...	$\frac{1}{4}$ to $\frac{1}{2}$ grain.	0.015 to 0.03
sulph., ...	3 to 15 grains.	0.2 to 1.
valer., . . .	3 to 15 grains.	0.2 to 1.
Amylene hydrate, . . .	10 to 60 grains.	0.65 to 4.
Amyl nitris, ...	2 to 5 minims.	0.1 to 0.35
Amylum iodatum, . . .	3 to 30 grains.	0.2 to 2.
Analgen (analgesic, antipyr.),	8 to 30 grains.	0.5 to 2.
Antifebrin, ...	8 grains.	0.5
Antimonii et pot. tartr.(diaph.)	$\frac{1}{20}$ to $\frac{1}{12}$ grain.	0.003 to 0.005
et pot. tartr. (emetic), .	1 to 2 grains.	0.06 to 0.1
oxid., ...	1½ to 2 grains.	0.1 to 0.1
oxysulphuret, . .	½ to 2 grains.	0.03 to 0.1
sulphid., . . .	½ to 2 grains.	0.03 to 0.1
sulphuret., . . .	½ to 2 grains.	0.03 to 0.1
Antipyrin, ...	5 to 30 grains.	0.35 to 2.
Aplol, ...	3 to 5 grains.	0.2 to 0.35
Apomorph. hydrochlor., .	$\frac{1}{30}$ to $\frac{1}{5}$ grain.	0.003 to 0.006
Aqua ammoniæ, . .	6 to 30 minims.	0.4 to 2.
amygd. amar., . .	2 to 4 fl. drms.	8. to 16.
camphoræ, . .	½ to 2 fl. ounces.	16. to 64.
chlori, . . .	1 to 4 fl. drms.	4. to 32.
creasoti, . . .	1 to 4 fl. drms.	4. to 32.
laurocerasi, . .	6 to 30 minims.	0.4 to 2.
Arbutin, ...	5 to 15 grains.	0.35 to 1.
Argenti iodidum, . .	½ to 2 grains.	0.03 to 0.1
nitras, . . .	$\frac{1}{6}$ to $\frac{1}{3}$ grain.	0.01 to 0.065
oxid., ...	½ to 2 grains.	0.03 to 0.1
Arsenii bromid. . .	$\frac{1}{64}$ to $\frac{1}{16}$ grain.	0.001 to 0.004
iodidum, . .	$\frac{1}{64}$ to $\frac{1}{10}$ grain.	0.001 to 0.006
sodium . .	$\frac{1}{30}$ to $\frac{1}{10}$ grain.	0.003 to 0.006
Asaprol (locally, 2 per cent.),		
(internally), . .	5 to 20 grains.	0.3 to 1.3
Aspidosperminæ hydrochlor.,	$\frac{1}{60}$ to $\frac{1}{20}$ grain.	0.001 to 0.003
Assafœtida, ...	5 to 20 grains.	0.35 to 1.3
Atropina, ...	$\frac{1}{120}$ to $\frac{1}{30}$ grain.	0.0005 to 0.002
Atropinæ sulph., . .	$\frac{1}{120}$ to $\frac{1}{30}$ grain.	0.0005 to 0.002
Auri et sodii chlorid., .	$\frac{1}{32}$ to $\frac{1}{16}$ grain.	0.002 to 0.004
Balsamum gurjunæ, . .	20 to 30 minims.	1.3 to 2.
Barii chloridi . . .	½ to 5 grains.	0.032 to 0.3
Belladonnæ fol., . .	1 to 10 grains.	0.06 to 0.65

REMEDIES.	DOSE.	GRAMMES.
Belladonnæ rad.,	1 to 5 grains.	0.06 to 0.35
Benzacetin (antineuralgic),	10 to 20 grains.	0.65 to 1.3
Benzanilide,	1 to 6 grains.	0.06 to 0.35
Benzonaphthol.	2 to 10 grains.	0.13 to 0.65
Berberina and its salts,	3 to 15 grains.	0.2 to 1.
Berberinæ sulph.,	3 to 10 grains.	0.2 to 0.65
Betanaphthol,	2 to 5 grains.	0.13 to 0.35
Bismuthi citras,	3 to 15 grains.	0.2 to 1.
et ammon. citr.,	1 to 15 grains.	0.06 to 1.
salicylat.,	2 to 10 grains.	0.1 to 0.65
subcarb.,	6 to 30 grains.	0.4 to 2.
subgallas,	5 to 20 grains.	0.3 to 1.3
subnitr.,	30 to 60 grains.	2. to 4.
tannas,	6 to 30 grains.	0.4 to 2.
valer.,	1 to 3 grains.	0.06 to 0.2
Brayera,	2 to 6 drachms.	8. to 24.
Bromoformum (in pertussis),	5 to 10 grains.	0.35 to 0.65
Brucina	$\frac{1}{64}$ to $\frac{1}{16}$ grain.	0.001 to 0.004
Butyl-chloral hydrate	5 to 10 grains.	0.3 to 0.65
Caffeina,	1 to 5 grains.	0.06 to 0.35
Caffeinæ citras,	1 to 5 grains.	0.06 to 0.35
Calcii bromidum,	5 to 30 grains.	0.35 to 2.
carb.,	15 to 60 grains.	1. to 4.
chlorid. hydrat.,	5 to 20 grains.	0.3 to 1.3
hypophosphis,	3 to 15 grains.	0.2 to 1.
iodidum.	1 to 3 grains.	0.06 to 0.2
lactophosphas	5 to 10 grains.	0.3 to 0.65
phosphas,	15 to 30 grains.	1. to 2.
Calx sulphurata,	$\frac{1}{3}$ to 1 grain.	0.02 to 0.06
Camphora,	3 to 10 grains.	0.2 to 0.65
Camph. monobrom.,	2 to 5 grains.	0.1 to 0.35
Cantharis,	$\frac{1}{2}$ to 2 grains.	0.03 to 0.1
Capsicum,	1 to 3 grains.	0.06 to 0.2
Castoreum,	6 to 15 grains.	0.4 to 1.
Catechu,	15 to 30 grains.	1. to 2.
Cerii nitras,	1 to 3 grains.	0.06 to 0.2
oxalas,	1 to 3 grains.	0.06 to 0.2
Chinoidinum,	3 to 30 grains.	0.2 to 2.
Chloral,	3 to 20 grains.	0.2 to 1.3
Chloralamid (hypnotic),	15 to 60 grains.	1. to 4.
Chloralose (hypnotic),	3 to 15 grains.	0.2 to 1.
Chloroformum,	1 to 5 minims.	0.06 to 0.35
Chrysarobinum,	3 to 15 grains.	0.2 to 1.
Cinchona,	15 to 60 grains.	1. to 4.
Cinchonidina and its salts,	1 to 30 grains.	0.06 to 2.
Cinchonina and its salts,	1 to 30 grains.	0.06 to 2.
Cinnamomum,	6 to 30 grains.	0.4 to 2.
Cocaine,	1 to 4 per ct. sol.	
Codcina,	$\frac{1}{2}$ to 2 grains.	0.03 to 0.1
Colchicin,	$\frac{1}{100}$ to $\frac{1}{50}$ grain.	0.0006 to 0.0013
Colocynthin,	$\frac{1}{6}$ to 2 grains.	0.01 to 0.1
Confectio sennæ,	1 to 2 grains.	0.06 to 0.1
Coniina and its salts,	$\frac{1}{64}$ to $\frac{1}{32}$ grain.	0.001 to 0.002
Copaiba,	15 to 60 minims.	1. to 4.
Cota,	1 to 2 grains.	0.06 to 0.1
Cotoina,	$\frac{1}{6}$ to $\frac{1}{2}$ grain.	0.01 to 0.03
Creolin,	$\frac{1}{2}$ to 5 grains.	0.03 to 0.35
Creosote valerianas	3 to 30 grains.	0.19 to 2.
Creosotum,	1 to 3 minims.	0.06 to 0.2
Creta præpar.,	15 to 75 grains.	1. to 5.
Croton chloral,	1 to 6 grains.	0.06 to 0.35
Cubeba,	15 to 60 grains.	1. to 4.
Cupri acetas	$\frac{1}{2}$ grain.	0.03.
arsenis,	$\frac{1}{100}$ grain.	0.0006.
sulphas,	$\frac{1}{4}$ to $\frac{1}{2}$ grain.	0.015 to 0.03
am.,	$\frac{1}{6}$ to 1 grain.	0.01 to 0.06
Curare,	$\frac{1}{32}$ to $\frac{1}{6}$ grain.	0.002 to 0.01
Curarina,	$\frac{1}{64}$ to $\frac{1}{20}$ grain.	0.001 to 0.003

REMEDIES.	DOSE.	GRAMMES.
Daturine, ...	$\frac{1}{160}$ to $\frac{1}{80}$ grain.	0.0006 to 0.0013
Decoct. aloes comp., . .	$\frac{1}{2}$ to 2 fl. ounces. 16.	to 64.
sarsap. comp., . .	2 to 6 fl. ounces. 64.	to 192.
Digitalinum, . . .	$\frac{1}{64}$ to $\frac{1}{32}$ grain.	0.001 to 0.002
Digitalis, ...	$\frac{1}{2}$ to 2 grains.	0.03 to 0.1
Digitoxin	$\frac{1}{240}$ to $\frac{1}{48}$ grain.	0.00026 to 0.0013
Diuretin, . . .	5 to 20 grains.	0.35 to 1.3
Duboisina and its salts, .	$\frac{1}{120}$ to $\frac{1}{40}$ grain.	0.0005 to 0.001
Elaterinum (U. S. P., 1880),	$\frac{1}{60}$ to $\frac{1}{12}$ grain.	0.001 to 0.005
Elaterium (U. S. P., 1870),	$\frac{1}{10}$ to $\frac{1}{6}$ grain.	0.006 to 0.01
Emetina and salts (emetic),	$\frac{1}{8}$ to $\frac{1}{4}$ grain.	0.008 to 0.015
and salts (diaph.), .	$\frac{1}{120}$ to $\frac{1}{20}$ grain.	0.0005 to 0.003
Emulsio hydrocyan., .	$\frac{1}{2}$ to 1 fl. drm.	2. to 4.
Ergota, ...	15 to 60 grains.	1. to 4.
Ergotinum, . . .	2 to 8 grains.	0.1 to 0.5
Erythrophlœina, . .	$\frac{1}{16}$ to $\frac{1}{4}$ grain.	0.004 to 0.008
Eserina and its salts, .	$\frac{1}{64}$ to $\frac{1}{16}$ grain.	0.001 to 0.008
Ethyl iodidum (inhalation)	5 to 20 minims.	0.31 to 1.3
Europhen	$\frac{1}{4}$ to 2 grains.	0.016 to 0.13
Exalgin, ...	2 to 6 grains.	0.1 to 0.4
Extr. aconiti fol. (Engl.), .	$\frac{1}{3}$ to $\frac{1}{6}$ grain.	0.02 to 0.01
aconiti fol. (U. S. P., 1870),	$\frac{1}{3}$ to $\frac{1}{6}$ grain.	0.02 to 0.01
aconiti fol. fluid., .	1 to 5 minims.	0.06 to 0.35
aconiti rad. (U. S. P., 1880),	$\frac{1}{12}$ to $\frac{1}{4}$ grain.	0.005 to 0.015
aconiti [rad.] fluid., .	$\frac{1}{2}$ to $2\frac{1}{2}$ minims.	0.03 to 0.1
aletridis fl., . .	15 to 30 minims.	1. to 2.
alni rubræ fl., . .	15 to 30 minims.	1. to 2.
aloës aquos, . .	$\frac{1}{2}$ to 3 grains.	0.03 to 0.2
alston. constr. fl., .	1 to 4 fl. drms.	4. to 16.
angelicæ rad. fl., .	30 to 60 minims.	2. to 4.
angusturæ fl., . .	15 to 45 minims.	1. to 3.
anthemidis, . . .	2 to 10 grains.	0.1 to 0.65
anthemidis fl., . .	30 to 60 minims.	2. to 4.
apocyni andros fl., .	8 to 50 minims.	0.5 to 3.
apocyni cannab. fl., .	8 to 30 minims.	0.5 to 2.
araliæ hisp. fl., .	30 to 60 minims.	2. to 4.
araliæ nudic. fl., .	30 to 60 minims.	2. to 4.
araliæ racem. fl., .	30 to 60 minims.	2. to 4.
araliæ spin. fl., . .	30 to 60 minims.	2. to 4.
arecæ fl., . . .	45 to 75 minims.	3. to 5.
arnicæ flor., . .	3 to 8 grains.	0.2 to 0.5
arnicæ fl., . . .	5 to 15 minims.	0.35 to 1.
arnicæ rad., . .	2 to 5 grains.	0.1 to 0.35
arnicæ rad. fl., .	5 to 15 minims.	0.35 to 1.
aromat. fl., . .	30 to 60 minims.	2. to 4.
ari triphylli fl., .	15 to 30 minims.	1. to 2.
asari fl., . . .	15 to 30 minims.	1. to 2.
asclep. incarn. fl., .	15 to 30 minims.	1. to 2.
asclep. syr. fl., .	15 to 30 minims.	1. to 2.
asclep. tuber. fl., .	15 to 30 minims.	1. to 2.
aspidii fl., . .	1 to 4 fl. drms.	4. to 16.
aspidospermæ fl., .	15 to 45 minims.	1. to 3.
aurantii cort. fl., .	$\frac{1}{4}$ to $2\frac{1}{2}$ fl. drms.	1. to 8.
azedarach fl., . .	15 to 75 minims.	1. to 5.
baptisiæ fl., . .	7 to 30 minims.	0.50 to 2.
bellad. alcohol, .	$\frac{1}{6}$ to $\frac{1}{2}$ grain.	0.01 to 0.03
bellad. fol. (Engl.), .	$\frac{1}{6}$ to $\frac{2}{3}$ grain.	0.01 to 0.03
bellad. fol. fl., . .	3 to 6 minims.	0.2 to 0.4
bellad. rad., . .	$\frac{1}{8}$ to $\frac{1}{4}$ grain.	0.008 to 0.015
bellad. rad. fl., .	1 to 3 minims.	0.06 to 0.2
berber. aquifol. fl., .	15 to 30 minims.	1. to 2.
berber. vulg. fl., .	15 to 30 minims.	1. to 2.
boldi fl., . . .	3 to 15 minims.	0.2 to 1.
braycræ fl., . .	2 to 4 fl. drms.	8. to 16.
bryoniæ fl., . .	15 to 60 minims.	1. to 4.
buchu fl., . . .	$\frac{1}{2}$ to $2\frac{1}{2}$ fl. drms.	2. to 8.
cactus grandiflor. fl., .	5 to 10 minims.	0.31 to 0.62
calami fl., . . .	15 to 60 minims.	1. to 4.

REMEDIES.	DOSE.	GRAMMES.
Extr. calend. fl.,	15 to 60 minims.	1. to 4.
calumbæ,	3 to 10 grains.	0.2 to 0.65
calumbæ fl.,	15 to 60 minims.	1. to 4.
canellæ fl.,	15 to 60 minims.	1. to 4.
cannab. Amer. fl.,	3 to 15 minims.	0.2 to 1.
cannab. ind.,	⅛ to ½ grain.	0.01 to 0.03
cannab. ind. fl.,	3 to 6 minims.	0.2 to 0.4
capsici fl.,	1 to 3 minims.	0.06 to 0.2
cardam. comp. fl.,	15 to 45 minims.	1. to 3.
cardui bened. fl.,	15 to 60 minims.	1. to 4.
carnis,	15 to 60 grains.	1. to 4.
cascaræ sagrad. fl.,	10 to 20 minims.	0.65 to 1.3
cascarillæ fl.,	¾ to 2½ fl. drms.	3. to 8.
castaneæ fl.,	¾ to 2½ fl. drms.	3. to 8.
catariæ fl.,	¼ to 1¼ fl. drms.	1. to 4.
catechu liquid.	8 to 30 minims.	0.5 to 2.
caulophylli fl.,	15 to 30 minims.	1. to 2.
chelidonii fl.,	15 to 30 minims.	1. to 2.
chelonis fl.,	30 to 60 minims.	2. to 4.
chimaph. fl.,	¾ to 1¼ fl. drms.	3. to 5.
chionanthi fl.,	¾ to 2½ fl. drms.	3. to 8.
chirettæ fl.,	½ to 1¼ fl. drms.	2. to 4.
cimicifugæ fl.,	8 to 30 minims.	0.5 to 2.
cinchoniæ,	15 to 30 grains.	1. to 2.
cinchoniæ, fl.,	30 to 60 minims.	2. to 4.
cinchoniæ arom. fl.,	30 to 60 minims.	2. to 4.
cinchoniæ comp. fl.,	½ to 1¼ fl. drms.	2. to 5.
cocæ,	1 to 2 drachms.	4. to 8.
cocculi fl.,	1 to 3 minims.	0.06 to 0.2
colch. rad.,	⅓ to 1½ grains.	0.02 to 0.1
colch. rad. fl.,	2 to 4 minims.	0.1 to 0.25
colch. sem. fl.,	1½ to 6 minims.	0.1 to 0.4
collinsoniæ fl.,	30 to 60 minims.	2. to 4.
colocynth,	1½ to 5 grains.	0.1 to 0.35
colocynth comp.,	1½ to 5 grains.	0.1 to 0.35
condurango fl.,	8 to 30 minims.	0.5 to 2.
conii fol. (Engl.),	1 to 4 grains.	0.06 to 0.25
conii fol. alc. (U. S. P., 1870),	½ to 1 grain.	0.03 to 0.06
con. [fr.] alc. (U. S. P., 1880),	⅓ to 1 grain.	0.02 to 0.06
conii fol. fl.,	1 to 2 minims.	0.06 to 0.1
con. [fr.], fl. (U. S. P., 1880),	1½ to 5 minims.	0.1 to 0.35
convallariæ rad. fl.,	15 to 30 minims.	1. to 2.
coptidis fl.,	30 to 60 minims.	2. to 4.
corn. flor. fl.,	30 to 60 minims.	2. to 4.
corydalis fl.,	15 to 30 minims.	1. to 2.
coto fl.,	3 to 15 minims.	0.2 to 1.
cubebæ fl.,	15 to 30 minims.	1. to 2.
cypripedii fl.,	15 to 60 minims.	1. to 4.
damianæ fl.,	½ to 2½ fl. drms.	2. to 8.
delphinii fl.,	1 to 3 minims.	0.06 to 0.2
digitalis,	⅛ to ½ grain.	0.01 to 0.03
digitalis fl.,	1 to 6 minims.	0.06 to 0.4
dioscoreæ fl.,	15 to 30 minims.	1. to 2.
ditæ fl.,	1 to 4 fl. drms.	4. to 16.
dracontii fl.,	30 to 60 grains.	2. to 4.
droseræ fl.,	5 to 10 minims.	0.35 to 0.65
dulcamaræ,	5 to 15 grains.	0.35 to 1.
dulcamaræ fl.,	1 to 2 fl. drms.	4. to 8.
ergotæ,	½ to 8 grains.	0.03 to 0.5
ergotæ fl.,	15 to 60 minims.	1. to 4.
eryodictyi fl.,	15 to 30 minims.	1. to 2.
erythroxyli fl.,	½ to 2 fl. drms.	2. to 8.
eucalypti fl.,	15 to 60 minims.	1. to 4.
euonymi fl.,	15 to 60 minims.	1. to 4.
eupatorii fl.,	30 to 60 minims.	2. to 4.
euphorb. ipec. fl.,	5 to 30 minims.	0.35 to 2.
ferri pom.,	3 to 15 grains.	0.2 to 1.
frangulæ fl.,	½ to 2½ fl. drms.	2. to 8.

REMEDIES.	DOSE.	GRAMMES.
Extr. frankeniæ fl., . . .	8 to 15 minims.	0.5 to 1.
gallæ fl., ...	¾ to 2 fl. drms.	3. to 8.
gelsemii, ...	2 to 8 minims.	0.1 to 0.5
gelsemii fl., . . .	5 to 20 minims.	0.35 to 1.3
gent. fl., ...	30 to 60 minims.	2. to 4.
gent. com. fl., . . .	30 to 60 minims.	2. to 4.
gent. quinque fl., . .	15 to 30 minims.	1. to 2.
geranii fl., ...	15 to 30 minims.	1. to 2.
gei fl., ...	15 to 30 minims.	1. to 2.
gilleniæ fl., . . .	15 to 30 minims.	1. to 2.
gossypii fl., . . .	15 to 45 minims.	1. to 3.
granati rad. cort. fl., .	¾ to 2 fl. drms.	3. to 8.
grind. rob. fl., . . .	30 to 60 minims.	2. to 4.
grind. squarr. fl., . .	30 to 60 minims.	2. to 4.
guaiaci ligni fl., . .	30 to 60 minims.	2. to 4.
guaranæ fl., . . .	15 to 30 minims.	1. to 2.
hæmatoxyli, . . .	8 to 30 grains.	0.5 to 2.
hæmatoxyli fl., . .	30 to 60 minims.	2. to 4.
hamamelid. fl., . . .	30 to 90 minims.	2. to 6.
helleb. nigris, . .	½ to 3 grains.	0.03 to 0.2
helleb. nigris fl., . .	5 to 15 minims	0.35 to 1.
heloniæ fl., . . .	8 to 30 minims.	0.5 to 2.
hepaticæ fl., . . .	30 to 60 minims.	2. to 4.
humuli, ...	3 to 15 grains.	0.2 to 1.
humuli fl., ...	30 to 60 minims.	2. to 4.
hydrangeæ fl., . .	30 to 60 minims.	2. to 4.
hydrastis, ...	3 to 10 grains.	0.2 to 0.65
hydrastis fl., . . .	8 to 30 minims.	0.5 to 2.
hyoscyami (Engl.) . .	1 to 4 grains.	0.06 to 0.25
hyoscyami alc., . .	1 to 2 grains.	0.06 to 0.1
hyoscyami fol. fl., .	3 to 15 minims.	0.2 to 1.
hyoscyami sem. fl., . .	2 to 8 minims.	0.1 to 0.5
ignatiæ, ...	¼ to ½ grain.	0.015 to 0.03
ignatiæ fl., . . .	1 to 6 minims.	0.06 to 0.35
ipecac. fl., . . .	3 to 60 minims.	0.2 to 4.
iridis versicol., .	3 to 6 grains.	0.2 to 0.35
irid. versicol. fl., .	15 to 30 minims.	1. to 2.
jaborandi fl., . . .	10 to 60 minims.	0.65 to 4.
jalapæ (U. S. P., 1870),	5 to 10 grains.	0.35 to 0.65
jalapæ alc., . . .	3 to 6 grains.	0.2 to 0.4
jalapæ fl., . . .	15 to 30 minims.	1. to 2.
juglandis, ...	15 to 30 grains.	1. to 2.
juglandis fl., . . .	¾ to 2 fl. drms.	3. to 8.
junip. fl., ...	30 to 60 minims.	2. to 4.
kamala fl., . . .	30 to 60 minims.	2. to 4.
kino, liquid . . .	15 to 30 minims.	1. to 2.
krameriæ, ...	5 to 15 grains.	0.35 to 1.
krameriæ fl., . . .	30 to 60 minims.	2. to 4.
lactucæ, ...	5 to 15 grains.	0.35 to 1.
lactucæ fl., . . .	15 to 60 minims.	1. to 4.
lactucarii fl., . . .	8 to 30 minims.	0.5 to 2.
lappæ fl., ...	1 to 2 fl. drms.	4. to 8.
laricis fl., . . .	½ to 2 fl. drms.	2. to 8.
leonuri fl., . . .	30 to 60 minims.	2. to 4.
leptandræ, . . .	3 to 10 grains.	0.2 to 0.65
leptandræ fl., . .	30 to 60 minims.	2. to 4.
lobeliæ fl., . . .	1 to 5 minims.	0.06 to 0.35
lupulini fl., . . .	5 to 15 minims.	0.35 to 1.
lycopi fl., ...	5 to 30 minims.	0.35 to 2.
malti, ...	1 to 2½ drachms.	4. to 8.
manzanitæ fl., . . .	½ to 2 fl. drms.	2. to 8.
marrubii fl., . . .	1 to 2 fl. drms.	4. to 8.
matico fl., ...	30 to 60 minims.	2. to 4.
matricariæ, . . .	8 to 30 minims.	0.5 to 2.
menispermi fl., . .	30 to 60 minims.	2. to 4.
methystice fl., . .	15 to 60 minims.	1. to 4.
mezerei.	½ to 1 grain.	0.03 to 0.06
mezerei fl., . . .	3 to 10 minims.	0.2 to 0.65

REMEDIES.	DOSE.	GRAMMES.
Extr. micromeriæ,	15 to 60 minims.	1. to 4.
mitchellæ fl.,	30 to 60 minims.	2. to 4.
myricæ fl.,	30 to 60 minims.	2. to 4.
nectandræ,	1 to 4 fl. drms.	4. to 16.
nuc. vom.,	⅛ to ½ grain.	0.008 to 0.03
nuc. vom. fl.,	1 to 5 minims.	0.06 to 0.35
nuphar fl.,	5 to 15 minims.	0.35 to 1.
nymphææ fl.,	5 to 15 minims.	0.35 to 1.
œnotheræ fl.,	15 to 30 minims.	1. to 2.
opii,	⅙ to ½ grain.	0.01 to 0.03
papaveris,	½ to 2 grains.	0.03 to 0.1
papaveris fl.,	15 to 45 minims.	1. to 3.
pareiræ fl.,	30 to 60 minims.	2. to 4.
petroselina fl.,	1 to 2 fl. drms.	4. to 8.
phellandrii fl.,	1 to 2 fl. drms.	4. to 8.
phoradendri fl.,	½ to 1 fl. drm.	2. to 4.
physostigmæ,	1/16 to ⅙ grain.	0.004 to 0.01
physostigmæ fl.,	1 to 3 minims.	0.06 to 0.2
phytolaccæ baccar fl.,	5 to 30 minims.	0.35 to 2.
phytolaccæ rad.,	1 to 3 grains.	0.06 to 0.2
phytolaccæ rad. fl.,	5 to 30 minims.	0.35 to 2.
pilocarpi fl.,	15 to 60 minims.	1. to 4.
pimentæ fl.,	15 to 45 minims.	1. to 3.
piper. nigr. fl.,	15 to 45 minims.	1. to 3.
piscidiæ fl.,	15 to 60 minims.	1. to 4.
podophylli,	½ to 1½ grains.	0.03 to 0.1
podophylli fl.,	8 to 30 minims.	0.5 to 2.
polygoni fl.,	15 to 30 minims.	1. to 2.
polygonati fl.,	5 to 15 minims.	0.35 to 1.
populi fl.,	30 to 60 minims.	2. to 4.
prinos fl.,	30 to 60 minims.	2. to 4.
prun. virg. fl.,	30 to 60 minims.	2. to 4.
pteleæ,	15 to 30 minims.	1. to 2.
pulsatillæ fl.,	2 to 5 minims.	0.1 to 0.35
quassiæ,	1 to 5 grains.	0.06 to 0.35
quassiæ fl.,	30 to 60 minims.	2. to 4.
quercus fl.,	30 to 60 minims.	2. to 4.
rhamni cath. fl. fl.,	30 to 60 minims.	2. to 4.
rhamni pursh cort. fl.,	30 to 120 minims.	2. to 8.
rhei,	5 to 15 grains.	0.35 to 1.
rhei fl.,	15 to 45 minims.	1. to 3.
rhois arom. fl.,	15 to 60 minims.	1. to 4.
rhois glab. cort. fl.,	30 to 60 minims.	2. to 4.
rhois glab. fruct. fl.,	30 to 60 minims.	2. to 4.
rhois toxicod. fl.,	1 to 6 minims.	0.06 to 0.4
ricini fol. fl.,	½ to 2 fl. drms.	2. to 8.
rosæ fl.,	½ to 2 fl. drms.	2. to 8.
rubi fl.,	15 to 60 minims.	1. to 4.
rumicis fl.,	30 to 60 minims.	2. to 4.
rutæ fl.,	15 to 30 minims.	1. to 2.
sabbatiæ fl.,	30 to 60 minims.	2. to 4.
sabinæ fl.,	5 to 15 minims.	0.35 to 1.
salicis fl.,	½ to 2 fl. drms.	2. to 8.
salviæ fl.,	½ to 2 fl. drms.	2. to 8.
sambuci fl.,	½ to 2 fl. drms.	2. to 8.
sanguin. fl.,	5 to 15 minims.	0.35 to 1.
santali citr. fl.,	1 to 2 fl. drms.	4. to 8.
santonicæ fl.,	15 to 60 minims.	1. to 4.
sarsap. fl.,	½ to 2 fl. drms.	2. to 8.
sarsap. comp. fl.,	½ to 2 fl. drms.	2. to 8.
sassafras fl.,	½ to 2 fl. drms.	2. to 8.
scillæ fl.,	1 to 5 minims.	0.06 to 0.35
scillæ comp. fl.,	1 to 5 minims.	0.06 to 0.35
scoparii fl.,	½ to 1 fl. drm.	2. to 4.
scutellariæ fl.,	½ to 2 fl. drms.	2. to 8.
senecionis fl.,	1 to 2 fl. drms.	4. to 8.
senegæ fl.,	8 to 15 minims.	0.5 to 1.
sennæ fl.,	1 to 4 fl. drms.	4. to 16.

REMEDIES.	DOSE.			GRAMMES.		
Extr. serpent. fl.,	30	to	60 minims.	2.	to	4.
simarubæ,	15	to	30 minims.	1.	to	2.
solidag. fl.,	30	to	60 minims.	2.	to	4.
spigeliæ fl.,	15	to	60 minims.	1.	to	4.
spigeliæ et sennæ fl.,	½	to	2 fl. drms.	2.	to	8.
stillingiæ fl.,	½	to	2 fl. drms.	2.	to	8.
stillingiæ comp. fl.,	½	to	2 fl. drms.	2.	to	8.
stramonii (Engl.),	½	to	1 grain.	0.03	to	0.06
stramonii fol. alc.,	½	to	⅔ grain.	0.02	to	0.03
stramonii sem.,	⅛	to	½ grain.	0.01	to	0.03
stramonii fl.,	1	to	6 minims.	0.06	to	0.35
sumbul fl.,	15	to	60 minims.	1.	to	4.
syzygii jambolini fl.,	5	to	10 minims.	0.3	to	0.7
taraxaci,	5	to	15 grains.	0.35	to	1.
taraxaci fl.,	½	to	2 fl. drms.	2.	to	8.
thujæ fl.,	8	to	15 minims.	0.5	to	1.
toxicodendri fl.,	1	to	5 minims.	0.06	to	0.35
trifol. prat. fl.,	1	to	2 fl. drms.	4.	to	8.
trillii fl.,	½	to	2 fl. drms.	2.	to	8.
trit. rep. fl.,	1	to	4 fl. drms.	4.	to	16.
tussilag. fl.,	30	to	60 minims.	2.	to	4.
urticæ rad. fl.,	5	to	15 minims.	0.35	to	1.
ustilag. maid. fl.,	15	to	60 minims.	1.	to	4.
uvæ ursi fl.,	30	to	60 minims.	2.	to	4.
vaccin. crassifol. fl.,	30	to	60 minims.	2.	to	4.
valerian,	5	to	15 grains.	0.35	to	1.
valer. fl.,	30	to	60 minims.	2.	to	4.
veratr. vir. fl.,	2	to	8 minims.	0.1	to	0.5
verbenæ,	15	to	60 minims.	1.	to	4.
viburni opuli fl.,	1	to	2 fl. drms.	4.	to	8.
viburni [prunifol.] fl.,	1	to	2 fl. drms.	4.	to	8.
wahoo	1	to	5 grains.	0.06	to	0.35
xanthoxyli cort. fl.,	15	to	30 minims.	1.	to	2.
xanthoxyli fruct. fl.,	15	to	30 minims.	1.	to	2.
zingiberis fl.,	8	to	30 minims.	0.5	to	2.
Fel bovis purif.,	3	to	6 grains.	0.2	to	0.4
Ferri arsen.,	¹⁄₂₆	to	½ grain.	0.003	to	0.03
benzoas.,	1	to	5 grains.	0.06	to	0.35
bromid.,	1	to	5 grains.	0.06	to	0.35
carb. sacch.,	4	to	15 grains.	0.25	to	1.
chlorid.,	1	to	3 grains.	0.06	to	0.2
citr.,	5	to	10 grains.	0.35	to	0.65
et ammon. citr.,	5	to	10 grains.	0.35	to	0.65
et ammon. sulph.,	5	to	10 grains.	0.35	to	0.65
et ammon. tartr.,	5	to	15 grains.	0.35	to	1.
et cinchonid. citr.,	5	to	10 grains.	0.35	to	0.65
et pot. tartr.,	15	to	60 grains.	1.	to	4.
et quin. citr.,	5	to	10 grains.	0.35	to	0.65
et strychn. citr.,	1	to	5 grains.	0.06	to	0.35
hypophosphis,	5	to	10 grains.	0.35	to	0.65
iodidum	1	to	5 grains.	0.06	to	0.35
iodidum sacch.,	2	to	3 grains.	0.1	to	0.2
lactas,	1	to	3 grains.	0.06	to	0.2
oxalas,	1	to	3 grains.	0.06	to	0.2
oxid. magnet.,	5	to	10 grains.	0.35	to	0.65
oxid. hydrat.,	½	to	2 ounces.	16.	to	64.
phosphas,	1	to	5 grains.	0.06	to	0.35
pyrophosphas,	1	to	5 grains.	0.06	to	0.35
subcarb.,	5	to	30 grains.	0.35	to	2.
sulphas	1	to	3 grains.	0.06	to	0.2
sulphas exsiccat.,	½	to	1½ grains.	0.03	to	0.1
valer.,	1	to	3 grains.	0.06	to	0.2
Ferrum dialys.,	1	to	15 minims.	0.06	to	1.
redact.,	1	to	5 grains.	0.06	to	0.35
Gallobromol,	5	to	10 grains.	0.32	to	0.65
Gamboge,	1	to	4 grains.	0.06	to	0.25
Gaultheria, oil of,			10 minims.	0.65		
Guaiacol (internally),	¼	to	1 grain.	0.015	to	0.06

228

REMEDIES.	DOSE.	GRAMMES.
Guaiacol (topically),	10 to 60 minims.	0.65 to 4.
benzoas,	1/2 to 10 grains.	0.03 to 0.65
carbonas,	1/2 to 10 grains.	0.03 to 0.65
valerianas,	2 to 20 grains.	0.13 to 1.3
Guarana,	8 to 30 grains.	0.5 to 2.
Helleborein,	1/10 to 1/4 grain.	0.006 to 0.015
Hydrarg. chlor. corros.,	1/64 to 1/10 grain.	0.001 to 0.006
chlorid. mite,	1/6 to 8 grains.	0.01 to 0.5
iodid. flav.,	1/6 to 1 grain.	0.01 to 0.06
iodid. rubr.,	1/50 to 1/10 grain.	0.0013 to 0.006
iodid. vir.,	1/6 to 1 grain.	0.01 to 0.06
subsulphas flav.,	1/4 to 1/2 grain.	0.015 to 0.03
c. creta,	3 to 8 grains.	0.2 to 0.5
Hydrastin,	5 to 10 grains.	0.35 to 0.65
Hydrogen dioxidum (10 vol. sol., locally),		
(internally),	30 to 120 minims.	2. to 8.
Hyoscine,	1/100 to 1/6 grain.	0.0006 to 0.001
Hyoscyamina and salts,	1/125 to 1/32 grain.	0.0005 to 0.002
Hypnone,	1 minim.	0.06
Ichthalbin,	2 to 5 grains.	0.13 to 0.32
Ichthyol,	3 to 4 grains.	0.2 to 0.25
(topically),	10 to 50 per cent.	
Infusum brayerӕ,	2 to 8 fl. ounces.	64. to 256.
digitalis,	2 to 4 fl. drms.	8. to 16.
sennӕ comp.,	1 to 2 fl. ounces.	32. to 64.
Iodoformum,	1 to 3 grains.	0.06 to 0.2
Iodol,	1/6 to 1/2 grain.	0.01 to 0.03
Iodum,	1/10 to 1/4 grain.	0.006 to 0.015
Ipecacuanha { expect., emet.,	1/6 to 1 grain.	0.01 to 0.06
	15 to 30 grains.	1. to 2.
Jalapa,	15 to 30 grains.	1. to 2.
Kairin,	8 grains.	0.5
Kamala,	1 to 2 drachms.	4. to 8.
Kino,	8 to 30 grains.	0.5 to 2.
Lactophenin (antipyretic),	8 to 15 grains.	0.5 to 1.
Lactucarium,	8 to 15 grains.	0.5 to 1.
Lawinin,	50 per cent. sol.	
Liq. ammon. acet.,	2 to 8 fl. drms.	8. to 32.
acidi arseniosi,	2 to 7 minims.	0.1 to 0.50
arsen. et hydr. iod.,	2 to 7 minims.	0.1 to 0.50
ferri chloridi,	2 to 10 minims.	0.1 to 0.65
ferri dialys.,	1 to 15 minims.	0.06 to 1.
ferri nitrat.,	8 to 15 minims.	0.5 to 1.
nitroglycerin. (1 per cent.), trinitrin, spts. glonoin,	1 m. (increasing).	0.06
pepsini,	2 to 4 fl. drms.	8. to 16.
potassӕ,	5 to 30 minims.	0.35 to 2.
potassii arsenit.,	3 to 7 minims.	0.2 to 0.50
potassii citrat.,	2 to 4 fl. drms.	8. to 16.
sodӕ,	5 to 30 minims.	0.35 to 2.
sodii arseniatis,	3 to 7 minims.	0.2 to 0.50
Lithii benzoas,	2 to 5 grains.	0.1 to 0.35
bromid.,	1 to 3 grains.	0.06 to 0.2
carb.,	2 to 6 grains.	0.1 to 0.4
citr.,	2 to 5 grains.	0.1 to 0.35
salicylas,	2 to 8 grains.	0.1 to 0.5
Lupulinum,	5 to 10 grains.	0.35 to 0.65
Magnesia,	15 to 60 grains.	1. to 4.
Magnesii carb.,	15 to 60 grains.	1. to 4.
citr. gran.,	2 to 8 drachms.	8. to 32.
sulphas,	2 to 8 drachms.	8. to 32.
sulphis,	8 to 30 grains.	0.5 to 2.
Malakin (analg., antipyr.),	15 to 20 grains.	1. to 1.3
Manganese binox.,	2 to 4 grains.	0.1 to 0.25
Mangani sulphas,	2 to 10 grains.	0.1 to 0.65
Manna,	1 to 2 ounces.	32. to 64.
Massa copaibӕ,	5 to 30 grains.	0.35 to 2.

REMEDIES.	DOSE.	GRAMMES.
Massa ferri carb.,	5 to 15 grains.	0.35 to 1.
hydrarg.,	1 to 15 grains.	0.06 to 1.
Methylene-blue (with nutmeg),	1 to 5 grains.	0.06 to 0.3
assafœtidæ,	4 to 8 fl. drms.	16. to 32.
chloroformi,	1 to 2 fl. drms.	4. to 8.
cretæ,	1 to 2 fl. ounces.	32. to 64.
ferri comp.,	½ to 2 fl. ounces.	16. to 64.
ferri et amm. acet.,	½ to 1 fl. ounce.	16. to 32.
glycyrrh. comp.,	1 to 4 fl. drms.	4. to 16.
magnes. et assafœt.,	1 to 4 fl. drms.	4. to 16.
potassii citr.,	½ to 2 fl. ounces.	16. to 64.
rhei et sodæ,	½ to 1 fl. ounce.	16. to 32.
Morphina and its salts,	1/16 to ½ grain.	0.004 to 0.03
Morrhuol,	3 to 60 minims.	0.2 to 4.
Moschuol,	1 to 5 grains.	0.06 to 0.35
Moschus,	2 to 15 grains.	0.1 to 1.
Naphtholinum,	2 to 10 grains.	0.1 to 0.65
Naphthol,	2 to 5 grains.	0.1 to 0.35
Narceina,	1/6 to ½ grain.	0.01 to 0.03
Nitroglycerinum,	1/100 to 1/20 grain.	0.0006 to 0.003
Nux vomica,	5 grains.	0.06 to 0.35
Oleoresina aspidii,	15 to 60 grains.	1. to 4.
capsici,	1/6 to ½ grain.	0.01 to 0.03
cubebæ,	5 to 20 minims.	0.35 to 1.3
filicis,	30 to 60 minims.	2. to 4.
lupulini,	2 to 5 grains.	0.1 to 0.35
piperis,	1 to 3 grains.	0.06 to 0.2
zingiberis,	1 to 3 grains.	0.06 to 0.2
Oleum copaibæ,	8 to 15 minims.	0.5 to 1.
cubebæ,	15 to 30 minims.	1. to 2.
eriger.,	5 to 15 minims.	0.35 to 1.
eucalypti,	5 to 10 minims.	0.35 to 0.65
phosphoratum,	1 to 3 minims.	0.06 to 0.2
sabinæ,	1 to 3 minims.	0.06 to 0.2
terebinth.,	5 to 30 minims.	0.35 to 2.
tiglii,	1/6 to 1½ drops.	0.01 to 0.1
Opium (14 per cent. morphine),	1/6 to 1½ grains.	0.01 to 0.1
Ouabaine (in Pertussis),	1/1000 to 1/250 grain.	0.00006 to 0.00025
Pancreatin,	10 to 20 grains.	0.65 to 1.3
Papayotin,	1 to 5 grains.	0.06 to 0.35
Paracotin,	1 to 3 grains.	0.06 to 0.2
Paraldehyde,	20 to 60 grains.	1.3 to 4.
Pareirin hydrochlor.,	1/16 to 1 grain.	0.004 to 0.05
Pelleterine,	5 to 10 grains.	0.35 to 0.65
Pepsinum purum,	15 grs. to ½ ounce.	1. to 16.
saccharatum,	30 grs. to 1 ounce.	2. to 32.
Phenacetin,	5 to 10 grains.	0.35 to 0.65
Phenocolli hydrochloras,	8 to 15 grains.	0.5 to 1.
Phosphorus,	1/128 to 1/50 grain.	0.0005 to 0.0013
Physostigminæ salic.,	1/120 to 1/32 grain.	0.0005 to 0.002
sulphas,	1/128 to 1/64 grain.	0.0005 to 0.001
Picrotoxinum,	1/64 to 1/8 grain.	0.001 to 0.008
Pilocarpina and salts,	1/64 to ½ grain.	0.001 to 0.03
Pil. aloes,	1 to 3 pills.	
et assafœt.,	2 to 5 pills.	
aloes et ferri,	1 to 3 pills.	
aloes et mast.,	1 to 3 pills.	
aloes et myrrhæ,	2 to 5 pills.	
antim. comp.,	1 to 3 pills.	
assafœtidæ,	1 to 6 pills.	
cathart. comp.,	1 to 4 pills.	
ferri comp.,	2 to 5 pills.	
ferri iodidi,	1 to 4 pills.	
galbani comp.,	1 to 5 pills.	
opii,	1 to 2 pills.	
phosphori,	1 to 4 pills.	

REMEDIES.	DOSE.	GRAMMES.
Pil. rhei,	2 to 5 pills.	
rhei comp.,	2 to 5 pills.	
Piperazin,	15 grains (daily).	1.
Piperinum,	1 to 8 grains.	0.06 to 0.5
Plumbi acetas,	½ to 3 grains.	0.03 to 0.2
iodidum,	½ to 3 grains.	0.03 to 0.2
Potassa sulphuret.,	1 to 10 grains.	0.06 to 0.65
Potassii acetas,	15 to 60 grains.	1. to 4.
bicarb.,	8 to 60 grains.	0.5 to 4.
bitartr.,	1 to 2 grains.	0.06 to 0.1
bromid.,	8 to 60 grains.	0.5 to 4.
carb.,	8 to 30 grains.	0.5 to 2.
chloras,	8 to 30 grains.	0.5 to 2.
citras,	15 to 60 grains.	1. to 4.
cyanid,	1/16 to 1/8 grain.	0.004 to 0.008
et sodii tartr.,	½ to 1 ounce.	16. to 32.
hypophosphis,	5 to 15 grains.	.35 to 1.
iodid.,	2 to 15 grains.	0.1 to 1.
nitras,	8 to 15 grains.	0.5 to 1.
sulphas,	1 to 4 drachms.	4. to 16.
sulphidum,	1 to 10 grains.	0.06 to 0.65
sulphis,	15 to 30 grains.	1. to 2.
tartras,	1 to 8 drachms.	4. to 32.
Pulv. antimonialis,	1 to 3 grains.	0.06 to 0.2
aromat.,	8 to 30 grains.	0.5 to 2.
cretæ comp.,	8 to 30 grains.	0.5 to 2.
glycyrrh. comp.,	30 to 60 grains.	2. to 4.
ipecac. comp.,	5 to 15 grains.	0.35 to 1.
jalapæ com.,	30 to 60 grains.	2. to 4.
morphinæ comp.,	8 to 15 grains.	0.5 to 1.
rhei com.,	30 to 60 grains.	2. to 4.
Pyridin,	2 to 5 drops.	0.1 to 0.35
Quinidina and salts,	1 to 30 grains.	0.06 to 2.
Quinina and salts,	1 to 30 grains.	0.06 to 2.
Quininæ arsenias,	1/6 to 1 grain.	0.01 to 0.06
Resina copaibæ,	2 to 10 grains.	0.1 to 0.65
guaiaci,	10 to 30 grains.	0.65 to 2.
jalapæ,	2 to 5 grains.	0.1 to 0.35
podophylli,	1/8 to ½ grain.	0.008 to 0.03
scammonii,	2 to 10 grains.	0.1 to 0.65
Resorcin,	2 to 5 grains.	0.1 to 0.35
Rheum,	2 to 30 grains.	0.1 to 1.
Saccharin,	½ to 4 grains.	0.03 to 0.25
Salacetol (intest. antisept.),	20 to 40 grains.	1.3 to 2.6
Salicinum,	8 to 30 grains.	0.5 to 2.
Salipyrin (antipyretic, anti-neuralgic),	8 to 15 grains.	0.5 to 1.
Salol	10 to 15 grains.	0.65 to 1.
Salophen (antipyretic, anti-rheum.),	15 to 20 grains.	1. to 1.3
Santonica,	8 to 60 grains.	0.5 to 4.
Santoninum,	1 to 5 grains.	0.06 to 0.35
Sapo,	5 to 30 grains.	0.35 to 2.
Scammonium,	3 to 15 grains.	0.2 to 1.
Scoparine,	½ to 1 grain.	0.03 to 0.06
Scopolaminæ hydrochloras,	1/240 to 1/6 grain.	0.00027 to 0.011
Senna,	8 to 60 grains.	0.5 to 4.
Sodii acetas,	15 to 60 grains.	1. to 4.
arsenias,	1/64 to 1/10 grain.	0.001 to 0.006
benzoas,	5 to 15 grains.	0.35 to 1.
bicarb.,	8 to 30 grains.	0.5 to 2.
bisulphis,	8 to 30 grains.	0.5 to 2.
boras,	8 to 30 grains.	0.5 to 2.
bromid.,	8 to 30 grains.	0.5 to 2.
carb.,	8 to 30 grains.	0.5 to 2.
carb. exsicc.,	5 to 15 grains.	0.35 to 1.
chloras,	5 to 30 grains.	0.35 to 2.
hypophosphis,	8 to 15 grains.	0.5 to 1.

REMEDIES.	DOSE.	GRAMMES.
Sodii hyposulphis, . . .	8 to 30 grains.	0.5 to 2.
iodidum, ...	5 to 15 grains.	0.35 to 1.
phosphas, ...	2 to 15 grains.	0.1 to 1.
salicylas, ...	5 to 30 grains.	0.35 to 2.
santoninas, . . .	2 to 10 grains.	0.1 to 0.65
sulphas, ...	1 to 2 grains.	0.06 to 0.1
sulphis, ...	8 to 30 grains.	0.5 to 2.
Somnal, ...	30 to 45 grains.	2. to 3.
Sparteine sulph., . . .	½ to 4 grains.	0.03 to 0.25
Spiritus ætheris compositus,	30 to 60 minims.	2. to 4.
æther. nitrosi, . . .	½ to 2 fl. drms.	2. to 8.
ammoniæ, ...	8 to 30 minims.	0.5 to 2.
ammoniæ arom., . .	15 to 60 minims.	1. to 4.
camphoric, . . .	8 to 30 minims.	0.5 to 2.
chloroformi, . . .	15 to 60 minims.	1. to 4.
lavend. comp., . .	30 to 60 minims.	2. to 4.
menth. pip., . . .	30 to 60 minims.	2. to 4.
Strontium (and salts), . .	5 to 30 grains.	0.32 to 2.
Strophanthin, . . .	1/100 to 1/100 grain.	0.0003 to 0.0006
Strychniæ (and salts), . .	1/64 to 1/12 grain.	0.001 to 0.005
Sulphonal, ...	5 to 20 grains.	0.35 to 1.3
Sulphur, ...	½ to 4 drachms.	2. to 16.
Syr. calcii lactophos., . .	1 to 2 fl. drms.	4. to 8.
calcis, ...	15 to 30 minims.	1. to 2.
ferri bromidi, . . .	15 to 60 minims.	1. to 4.
ferri iodidi, . . .	15 to 40 minims.	1. to 3.
ferri oxidi, . . .	1 fl. drachm.	4.
ferri hyposulph., . .	1 fl. drachm.	4.
ferri quin. et str. phos., .	1 fl. drachm.	4.
hypophosphit., . .	1 fl. drachm.	4.
hypophosph. c. fer., .	1 fl. drachm.	4.
ipecac., ...	½ to 1 fl. drm.	2. to 4.
krameriæ, . . .	½ to 4 fl. drms.	2. to 16.
lactucarii, . . .	1 to 3 fl. drms.	4. to 12.
rhei, ...	1 to 4 fl. drms.	4. to 16.
rhei arom., . . .	1 to 4 fl. drms.	4. to 16.
rosæ, ...	1 to 2 fl. drms.	4. to 8.
sarsap. com., . . .	1 to 4 fl. drms.	4. to 16.
scillæ, ...	½ to 1 fl. drms.	2. to 4.
scillæ comp., . .	15 to 60 minims.	2. to 4.
senegæ, ...	1 to 2 fl. drms.	4. to 8.
sennæ, ...	1 to 4 fl. drms.	4. to 16.
Tannalbin, ...	5 to 15 grains.	0.32 to 1.
Tannigen, ...	5 to 15 grains.	0.32 to 1.
Tannoform, . . .	5 to 15 grains.	0.32 to 1.
Terebene, ...	5 to 10 minims.	0.35 to 0.65
Terpine hydrate, . .	2 to 5 minims.	0.1 to 0.35
Tetra-ethyl-ammonium, .	1 to 2 grains.	0.06 to 0.12
Tetronal, ...	15 to 60 grains.	1. to 4.
Thallin, ...	3 grains.	0.2
Theine (hypo.), . . .	½ grain.	0.03
Theobromin. sodio-salicylas .	5 to 30 grains.	0.32 to 2.
Thymacetin, . . .	8 to 15 grains.	0.5 to 1.
Thymol, ...	½ to 5 grains.	0.03 to 0.35
Tinct. aconiti fol., . . .	8 to 16 minims.	0.5 to 1.
aconiti rad., . . .	1 to 5 minims.	0.06 to 0.30
aconiti rad. (Fleming's),	⅔ to 2½ minims.	0.03 to 0.1
aloes (1880), . . .	½ to 2 fl. drms.	2. to 8.
aloes et myrrh., . .	1 to 2 fl. drms.	4. to 8.
arnicæ flor., . . .	8 to 30 minims.	0.5 to 2.
arnicæ rad., . . .	15 to 30 minims.	1. to 2.
assafœtidæ, . . .	30 to 60 minims.	2. to 4.
belladonnæ, . . .	8 to 15 minims.	0.5 to 1.
bryoniæ, ...	15 to 30 minims.	1. to 2.
cactus grandiflor., . .	15 to 20 minims.	1. to 1.3
calendulæ, . . .	15 to 30 minims.	1. to 2.
calumbæ, ...	1 to 4 fl. drms.	4. to 16.
cannabis ind., . . .	15 to 30 minims.	1. to 2.

REMEDIES.			DOSE.		GRAMMES.	
Tinct. cantharid.,	.	.	8 to	15 minims.	0.5	to 1.
capsici,	.	.	8 to	15 minims.	0.5	to 1.
catechu comp.,	.	.	½ to	2 fl. drms.	2.	to 8.
chirretta,	.	.	15 to	60 minims.	1.	to 4.
cimicifugæ,	.	.	30 to	60 minims.	2.	to 4.
cinchonæ,	.	.	½ to	2 fl. drms.	2.	to 8.
cinchonæ comp.,	.	.	½ to	2 fl. drms.	2.	to 8.
colchici rad.,	.	.	5 to	15 minims.	0.35	to 1.
colchici sem.,	.	.	6 to	15 minims.	0.4	to 1.
conii,	.	.	5 to	30 minims.	0.35	to 2.
croci,	.	.	1 to	2 fl. drms.	4.	to 8.
cubebæ,	.	.	1 to	2 fl. drms.	4.	to 8.
digitalis,	.	.	6 to	15 minims.	0.4	to 1.
ferri acet.,	.	.	15 to	30 minims.	1.	to 2.
ferri chloridi	.	.	15 to	30 minims.	1.	to 2.
ferri chloridi æther,	.		15 to	30 minims.	1.	to 2.
ferri pomati,	.	.	20 to	60 minims.	1.3	to 4.
gallæ,	.	.	½ to	2 fl. drms.	2.	to 8.
gelsemii,	.	.	8 to	15 minims.	0.5	to 1.
guaiaci,	.	.	30 to	60 minims.	2.	to 4.
guaiaci ammon.,	.		30 to	60 minims.	2.	to 4.
hellebori,	.	.	10 to	15 minims.	0.65	to 1.
humuli,	.	.	1 to	2½ fl. drms.	4.	to 9.
hydrastis,	.	.	30 to	90 minims.	2.	to 6.
hyoscyami fol.,	.	.	15 to	30 minims.	1.	to 2.
hyoscyami sem.,	.	.	15 to	30 minims.	1.	to 2.
ignatiæ,	.	.	5 to	15 minims.	0.35	to 1.
iodi,	.	.	5 to	15 minims.	0.35	to 1.
ipecac. et opii,	.	.	5 to	15 minims.	0.35	to 1.
jalapæ,	.	.	½ to	2 fl. drms.	2.	to 8.
kino,	.	.	½ to	2 fl. drms.	2.	to 8.
krameriæ,	.	.	½ to	2 fl. drms.	2.	to 8.
lavend. comp.,	.	.	½ to	2 fl. drms.	2.	to 8.
lobeliæ,	.	.	15 to	45 minims.	1.	to 3.
lupulini,	.	.	½ to	2 fl. drms.	2.	to 8.
matico,	.	.	½ to	2 fl. drms.	2.	to 8.
moschi,	.	.	15 to	60 minims.	1.	to 4.
nux vomicæ,	.	.	8 to	20 minims.	0.5	to 1.3
opii,	.	.	8 to	15 minims.	0.5	to 1.
opii camph.,	.	.	8 to	75 minims.	0.5	to 5.
phytolaccæ,	.	.	8 to	60 minims.	0.5	to 4.
physostigmatis,	.	.	5 to	15 minims.	0.35	to 1.
pyrethri,	.	.	8 to	30 minims.	0.5	to 2.
quassiæ,	.	.	½ to	2 fl. drms.	2.	to 8.
rhei,	.	.	1 to	8 fl. drms.	4.	to 32.
rhei arom.,	.	.	30 to	75 minims.	2.	to 5.
rhei dulc.,	.	.	1 to	4 fl. drms.	4.	to 16.
sanguinariæ,	.	.	15 to	60 minims.	1.	to 4.
scillæ,	.	.	8 to	60 minims.	0.5	to 4.
serpentariæ,	.	.	½ to	2 fl. drms.	2.	to 8.
stramon. fol.,	.	.	8 to	15 minims.	0.5	to 1.
stramon. sem.,	.	.	6 to	15 minims.	0.4	to 1.
strophanthus,	.	.	2 to	15 minims.	0.1	to 1.
sumbul,	.	.	8 to	30 minims.	0.5	to 2.
valer.,	.	.	½ to	2 fl. drms.	2.	to 8.
valer. ammon.,	.	.	½ to	2 fl. drms.	2.	to 8.
veratr. vir.,	.	.	3 to	10 minims.	0.2	to 0.65
zingiberis,	.	.	15 to	60 minims.	1.	to 4.
Tolypyrin (antipyretic, anti- rheum.),	.	.	5 to	20 grains.	0.32	to 1.3
Tolysal (antipyretic, antirheu- matic),	.	.	5 to	20 grains.	0.32	to 1.3
Trimethylamina,	.	.	2 to	15 grains.	0.1	to 1.
Trional (hypnotic),	.	.	15 to	60 grains.	1.	to 4.
Tritur elaterina,	.	.	¼ to	½ grain.	0.008	to 0.03
Uranil nitras,	.	.	5 to	10 grains.	0.3	to 0.65
Urethran.,	.	.	10 to	15 grains.	0.65	to 1.
Veratrina,	.	.	1/60 to	1/10 grain.	0.001	to 0.006

REMEDIES.	DOSE.			GRAMMES.		
Vin. aloes, ...	. 1	to	2 fl. drms.	4.	to	8.
antim. { exp. et alt.,	. 1	to	8 minims.	0.06	to	0.5
antim. { cmet., . .	. 30	to	75 minims.	2.	to	5.
colch. rad., . .	. 8	to	20 minims.	0.5	to	1.3
colch. sem., . .	. 5	to	30 minims.	0.35	to	2.
ergotæ, . . .	. 1	to	3 fl. drms.	4.	to	11.
ferri amar., . .	. 1 fl. drachm.			4.		
ferri citrat., . .	. 1 fl. drachm.			4.		
ipecac. { expect.,	. 5	to	15 minims.	0.35	to	1.
ipecac. { emet., .	. 3	to	6 fl. drms.	11.	to	23.
opii, ...	. 5	to	15 minims.	0.35	to	1.
rhei, . . .	. 1	to	2 fl. drms.	4.	to	8.
Xylolum, . .	. 5	to	15 grains.	0.35	to	1.
Zinci acet., . .	. 1	to	2 grains.	0.06	to	0.1
bromid., . .	. ½	to	2 grains.	0.03	to	0.1
cyanid., . .	. $\frac{1}{16}$	to	⅛ grain.	0.004	to	0.008
iodid., . .	. ½	to	3 grains.	0.03	to	0.2
oxid., . .	. 1	to	10 grains.	0.06	to	0.35
phosphid., . .	. $\frac{1}{16}$	to	½ grain.	0.006	to	0.01
sulphas cmet., .	. 15	to	30 grains.	1.	to	2.
valerianas, . .	. 1	to	6 grains.	0.06	to	0.4

234

INCOMPATIBLES.

Acacia (gum) with alcohol, iron, lead-water, and mineral acids.

Acids (mineral), with alkalies and relatively weak salts of other acids—such as bromides, chlorides, and iodides.

Alkalies, with acids, and with relatively weak salts.

Antipyrin and antifebrin should be given with alcohol or water only.

Arsenic, with tannic acid, salts and oxide of iron, and lime and magnesia.

Bitter infusions and tinctures, with salts of iron and lead.

Bromides, with acids, acid salts, or alkalies,

Calomel, with antipyrin, alkalies, lime-water, salts of iron and lead, and potassium iodid.

Camphor (spirit of), with water.

Carbonates, with acids and acid salts.

Chloral, with cyanids.

Chlorids, with silver-salts, lead-salts, and alkalies.

Chloroform (except in minute quantity) with water.

Corrosive sublimate, with alkalies, lime-water, salts of iron and lead, potassium iodid, albumin, gelatin, and vegetable astringents. (It may, however, be advantageously combined with tincture of ferric chlorid and liq. acidi arseniosi, or with potassium iodid.)

Digitalis, with iron and preparations containing tannic acid.

Iron (salts), with anything containing tannic acid.

Tincture of ferric chlorid, with alkalies, carbonates, mucilages, and preparations containing tannic acid.

Mucilages, with acids, iron salts, and alcohol.

Potassium chlorate and potassium permanganate should not be rubbed up with tannic acid or other organic oxidizable substance.

Potassium (iodid), with all strong acids and acid salts. (See *corrosive sublimate.*)

Spirit of nitrous ether, with antipyrin, sulphate of iron, tincture of guaiacum, and most of the carbonates.

Vegetable preparations holding tannic acid, with salts of iron and lead.

Alkaloids are precipitated or destroyed by tannic acid, alkalies, iodin or iodids, and chlorinous compounds.

235

Approximate Measures.

1 minim varies from			1 to 2 drops.
1 fluidrachm	equals about		1 teaspoonful.
2 fluidrachms	"	"	1 dessertspoonful.
4 fluidrachms	"	"	1 tablespoonful.
2 fluidounces	"	"	1 wineglass.
4 fluidounces	"	"	1 teacup.

The Metric System

has as its unit the Meter (39.37 inches), which is the ten millionth part of the distance from the pole to the equator. From this as a basis all other measures and weights are formed. The sytem is arranged on a decimal scale—that is, all the divisions are connected by the multiple ten, in exactly the same way as the coins in the United States monetary system. The names given to the different divisions and multiples of the unit are formed in each case by a certain prefix, derived from the Latin or Greek, which is placed before the name of the unit. It is the custom in all countries where the metric system is used, in writing prescriptions, to express all quantities by weight, fluids as well as solids being expressed in this way. We have only to do, then, with the *gram* and its decimal divisions, that being the name given to the unit of weight. A *gram* is the weight of *one cubic centimeter* of water at 39° Fahr. The subdivisions of the gram are as follows :—

1 gram	= weight of 1 cc. water at 39° F. written		1.
1 decigram	= 1-10 of a gram	"	.1
1 centigram	= 1-100 "	"	.01
1 milligram	= 1-1000 "	"	.001

In practice the decigram is disregarded, and everything expressed in terms of *grams* and *centigrams :* in the same way as we disregard our dimes and express money values in terms of dollars and cents. In writing prescriptions for solids, then, one has only to know the dose in terms of grams, the mathematical calculation being practically the same as when the apothecaries' weight is employed, only simplified by the use of the decimal system.

Table of Approximations.

Apothecaries'.		Grams (nearly).		Grams (exactly).
Grain i,	=	.06	or	.06479
Ði,	=	1.30	"	1.2958
Ʒi,	=	4.	"	3.8874
℥i,	=	31.	"	31.103

From the preceding Table may be easily deduced the following

RULES FOR EXPRESSING QUANTITY BY WEIGHT OF THE APOTHECARIES' SYSTEM IN METRIC TERMS.

RULE I. *Reduce the quantity to grains and divide by 15 ; the quotient expresses the same quantity [nearly] in grams.*

RULE II. *Reduce the quantity to drachms and multiply by 4 ; the product represents [nearly] the same quantity in grams.*

RULE III. *Reduce each quantity to ounces and multiply by 31 ; the product represents [nearly] the same quantity in grams.*

In changing *fluid measures to grams* the same rules may be employed to get results accurate enough for all practical purposes. But if greater exactness is required, it must be remembered that 1 gram of water measures about 16 minims [exactly 16.231]; consequently [1 fluidounce of water weighs 455.7 grs.]—

1 minim,	=	.06 gram,	exactly	.0616
1 f℥	=	3.70 grams.	"	3.696
1 f℥	=	30.	"	29.576

French System of Length.

1 millimeter	equals	.039368 of an inch
1 centimeter	"	.39368 " "
1 decimeter	"	3.9368 inches.
1 meter	"	39.368 "
1 dekameter	"	393.68 "
1 hektometer	"	3,936.8 "
1 kilometer	"	39,368. "
1 myriameter	"	393,680. "

French System of Weight.

1 centigram	equals	.15434 of a grain.
1 decigram	"	1.5434 grain.
1 gram	"	15.434 grains.
1 dekagram	"	154.34 "
1 hektogram	"	1,543.4 "

French System of Measures.

1 milliliter	equals	16.231 minims or	15.433 grains
1 centiliter	"	2.705 f℥	154.34 "
1 deciliter	"	3.381 f℥	1,543.4 "
1 litre	"	2.113 pints	15,434. "
1 dekaliter	"	2.641 C.	154,340. "
1 hektoliter	"	26.412 C.	1,543,400. "
1 kiloliter	"	264.12 C.	15,434,000. "
1 myrialiter	"	2,641.2 C.	154,340,000. "

Temperature.

1° Fahrenheit = 5·9° Centigrade = 4·9° Reaumur.
To reduce F. to C.: subtract 32° from the F. degrees
given, and divide the remainder by 1.8. *To reduce C. to
F.:* multiply the C. degrees given by 1.8 and then add
32° to the product.

Table of Drops in a Fluid Drachm.

Acid. Hydrocyanic. dilut., 45 ; Acid Sulphuric, Aromat.,
116–148 ; Acid Sulphur., dilut., 49–54 ; Ether, 150 ; Alcohol, 120–143 ; Chloroform, 180–276 ; Liq. Potass. Arsenit., 59–63 ; Acetum Opii, 70–90 ; Ol. Ricini, 55 ; Syrupus
Scillæ, 85 ; Tinct. Aconiti Rad., 118–130 ; Tinct. Ferri
Chloridi, 106–151 ; Tinct. Opii, 106–147. Tinct. Opii.
Camph., 95–110.

Average Weights (avoir.) of the Organs of the Body.

	Male.	Female.
Brain,	49 1-2 ozs.	44 ozs
Cerebrum,	43 ozs., 15 drs.	38 ozs., 12 drs.
Cerebellum,	5 ozs., 4 drs.	4 ozs., 12 1-4 drs.
Pons and Medulla,	15 3-4 drs.	1 oz., 1-4 dr.
Spinal Cord,	1 oz., 4 drs.	1 oz., 4 drs.
Heart,	11 ozs.	9 ozs.
Lung (right),	24 ozs.	17 ozs.
" (left),	21 ozs.	15 ozs.
Thyroid,	1 oz.	2 ozs.
Liver,	53 ozs.	45 ozs.
Pancreas,	3 ozs.	3 ozs.
Spleen,	6 ozs.	5 ozs.
Kidney,	5 1-2 ozs.	5 ozs.
Suprarenal Capsule,	1 dr. to 2 drs.	1 dr. to 2 drs.
Prostate,	6 drs.	
Testis,	1 oz.	
Uterus (virgin),		7 drs. to 12 drs.
Ovary,		1 dr. to 1 1-2 dr.

Apothecaries', or Troy, Weight.

Pound.		Ounces.		Drachms.		Scruples.		Grains.
lb. 1	=	12	=	96	=	288	=	5760
		℥ 1	=	8	=	24	=	480
				ʒ 1	=	3	=	60
						℈ 1	=	20

Apothecaries', or Wine, Measure.

Gallon.		Pints.		Fluidounces.		Fluidrachms.		Minims.
C. 1	=	8	=	128	=	1024	=	61440
		O 1	=	16	=	128	=	7680
				f℥ 1	=	8	=	480
						fʒ 1	=	60

Gargles.

Each to be added to one pint of water.

Acid. carbolici	½ to	3 drachms.
Acid. muriatic	1 to	4 drachms.
Acid. nitric	. .	60 drops.
Acid. tannic	½ to	2 drachms.
Alum	½ to	1 ounce.
Ammon. chlor.	1 to	4 drachms.
Calcis chlorinatæ . . .	1 to	2 drachms.
Catechu (tinct.) . . .	. .	½ ounce.
Cubebæ, fl. ex.	. .	½ ounce.
Ferri chlor. (tinct.) . . .	. .	½ ounce.
Ferri et ammon. sulph. . .	½ to	2 drachms.
Krameriæ, fl. ex. . . .	. .	½ ounce.
Myrrhæ (tinct.)	. .	1 ounce.
Phenol. sodique	½ to	2 ounces.
Potass. chlorat. . . .	½ to	2 ounces.
Potass. permanganat. . . .	1 to	3 scruples.
Quercus alb. fl. ex. . . .	½ to	1 ounce.
Rhois glab. fl. ex. . . .	. .	1 ounce.
Salviæ	½ to	1 ounce.
Sodii borat.	. .	2 ounces.
Sodii hyposulphitis . . .	½ to	2 ounces.
Zinci sulphat.	15 to	60 grains.

Doses of Drugs for Atomization, Inhalation, etc.

Each to be added to one ounce of distilled water.

Acid, tannic	5 to	15 grains.
Acid, sulphurous dil. . .	10 to	20 drops.
Acid, carbolic	10 to	20 drops.
Acid, salicylic	15 to	30 grains.
Acid, citric	. .	1 drachm.
Acetate of lead	1 to	5 grains.
Alum	5 to	25 grains.
Ammon. muriate . . .	5 to	10 grains.
Argenti nitrat.	1 to	10 grains.
Aq. calcis, undiluted.		
Aq. menth. pip., undiluted. .		
Belladonna (Tinct. of) . .	15 to	30 drops.
Cannabis Indica (Tinct. of) .	3 to	15 drops.
Cupri sulph.	1 to	15 grains.
Hammamelis (Tinct. of) . .	. .	20 drops.
Ipecac. (fl. ex.)	. .	20 drops.
Liq. sodii arsenitis . . .	5 to	10 drops.
Morph. sulph.	½ to	1½ grains.
Opii deodorat. (tinct.) . . .	20 to	30 drops.
Potass. chlor.	10 to	20 grains.
Potass. permanganat. . .	5 to	10 grains.
Picis liquid. infus. . . .	. .	½ ounce.
Terebinth. ol.	5 to	10 drops,
Zinci sulph. . . .	3 to	15 grains.

Respiration at Various Ages.

	Per minute
First year . .	. 25
Second year .	. 25
At puberty . .	. 20
Adult age . .	. 18

The Pulse at Various Ages.

At birth	. 130–140
First year	. 115–130
Second year . . .	. 100–115
Third year	. 90–100
Seventh year . . .	. 85–90
Fourteenth year . . .	. 80–85
Adult	. 70–75

Table Giving a Fair Comparison Between Temperature and Pulse.

A temperature of 98° F. corresponds to a pulse of 60.

"	"	99°	"	"	"	70.
"	"	100°	"	"	"	80.
"	"	101°	"	"	"	90.
"	"	102°	"	"	"	100.
"	"	103°	"	"	"	110.
"	"	104°	"	"	"	120.
"	"	105°	"	"	"	130.
"	"	106°	"	"	"	140.

Eruption of the Teeth.

DECIDUOUS.—(20 in number.)   Central Incisors, 7th month ; Lateral Incisors, 7th to 10th month ; Ant. Molars, 13th to 14 month ; Canine, 14th to 20th month ; Post. Molars, 18th to 36th month.

PERMANENT.—(32 in number.)   First Molars at 61-2 years ; Two Middle Incisors, 7 years ; Two Lat. Incisors, 8 years ; First Bicuspids, 9 to 10 years ; Second Bicuspids, 10 to 11 years ; Canine, 11 to 12 years ; Second Molars, 12 to 14 years ; Wisdom, 17 to 21 years.

The teeth of the lower jaw usually precede those of the upper jaw by one or two months.

Eruptive Fevers.

Names.	Incubation.	Day of Rash.	Character of Rash.	Rash Fades.	Duration.
Measles. *Rubeola.*	10 to 14 days.	4th day of fever, after 72 hours' illness.	Small red dots, resembling fleabites, first appearing on temples and forehead, forming blotches with semilunar borders.	On 7th day of fever.	6 to 10 days.
Scarlet Fever. *Scarlatina.*	1 to 6 days, occasionally 21 days.	2d day of fever, after 24 hours' illness.	Bright scarlet, rapidly diffused, first on chest and upper extremities.	On 5th day of fever.	8 to 9 days.
Typhus Fever. *Ship Fever.*	1 to 12 days.	4th to 7th day.	Mulberry colored macula, general and abundant over abdomen, extending to extremities.	— —	14 to 21 days.
Typhoid Fever. *Enteric Fever.*	10 to 14 days, or suddenly.	7th to 14th day.	Rose-colored papules, elevated, few in number, limited to trunk, fresh spots persisting to occur during career.	—	21 to 30 days.
Smallpox. *Variola.*	10 to 14 days.	3d day of fever, after 48 hours' illness.	Small, round, red, hard pimples, forming vesicles (*umbilicated*), then pustules, first appearing on face and wrists.	9th day scabs form, and about 14th day fall off.	14 to 21 days.
Chicken-pox. *Varicella.*	10 to 14 days.	2d day of fever, after 24 hours' illness.	Small rose-colored papules, soon forming vesicles, which do not become pustular.	Slight scab of short duration.	6 to 7 days.
Erysipelas.	3 to 7 days.	2d or 3d day.	Diffused redness, either of a dusky or yellowish hue with swelling.	From 24 to 48 hours.	
Roseola.	6 to 10 days.	After 12 to 36 hours' illness.	Rose-colored spots not elevated, occurring irregularly at different points.		

241

Sylvester's Method.

Remove from the mouth and nostrils all obstructions to the free passage of air to the lungs, free the body from any clothing that binds the neck, chest, or waist; turn it over upon the face for a moment, thrusting a finger into the mouth and sweeping it round, to bring away anything that may have gotten in or accumulated there. Then lay the body flat on the back, with something a few inches high under the shoulders, so as to cause the neck to be stretched out and the chin to be carried from the chest. Draw the tongue well forward out of the mouth and let it be held by an assistant. (If there be no one present, a pencil or small stick may be thrust across the mouth on top of the tongue and back of the last teeth, to keep the mouth open and the tongue out of the throat.) Place yourself on your knees behind the head, seize both arms near the elbows and sweep them round horizontally, away from the body and over the head till they meet above it; give a good, strong pull, and keep it up for a few seconds.

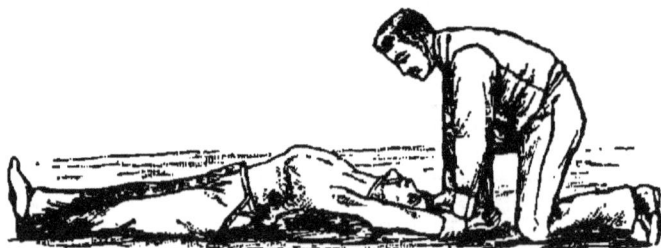

Fig. 1.

After this return the arms to their former position alongside the chest, and make strong pressure against the lower ribs, so as to drive the air out of the chest and effect an act of expiration. Rhythmic traction of the tongue also may be practised.

This plan, regularly carried out, will make about 16 complete acts of respiration in a minute. It should be kept up for a long time, and not abandoned until the heart has ceased to beat. It should be remembered that cessation of the pulse at the wrists amounts to nothing as a sign of death; and life is present when only a most acute ear can detect the sound of the heart. In a mod-

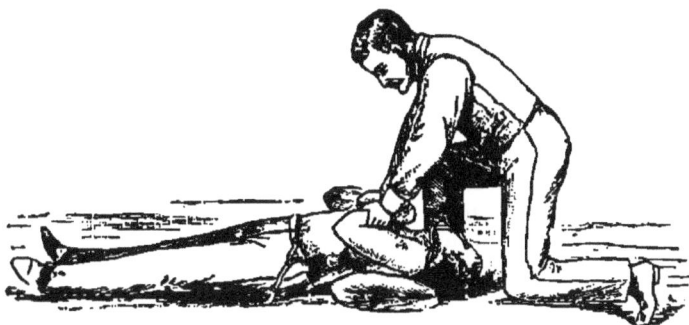

FIG. 2.

erately thin person deep pressure with the finger-ends just below the lower end of the breastbone may sometimes reveal pulsation in the aorta when it cannot be found anywhere else.

These notes were published in the *Medical Times and Register*, and are from the pen of an eminent London surgeon.

Abdomen.

Always avoid purgatives in treating a patient who has swallowed a foreign body. Give opium and constipating food—boiled eggs, cheese, puddings, potatoes, etc.

Never close any wound of the abdominal wall till all hemorrhage has ceased.

Never, under any circumstances, apply pressure to a wound of the abdominal wall to arrest hemorrhage.

Never mind increasing a superficial wound of the abdomen in order to remove a foreign body or to secure a bleeding point.

Never probe any wound in the abdominal wall.

Never forget that all abscesses of the abdominal wall should be opened freely and at once.

Never hesitate or delay to open and drain an abscess in the loin due to rupture or injury to the kidney.

Never procrastinate in strangulated hernia. It is not usually the operation which will prove unsuccessful in herniotomy; the danger lies in your allowing the bowel to become irrecoverable.

Never be deceived by an opiate masking the acute symptoms of hernia, obstruction, peritonitis.

Never tap a suspected renal tumor through the abdominal parietes, *i. e.*, through the peritoneum.

Always relax the abdominal wall after suturing.

Never ligature *en masse* in cutting off omentum. Do it piecemeal.

[The constricted edge of the apron of omentum may unravel, and fatal hemorrhage result.]

In protrusion of the viscera never neglect to pass your finger fairly through the wound to make sure that the reduction has been complete.

And be careful never to push the bowel into an interstice between the muscle or into subperitoneal tissue.

Abscess.

Never try fluctuation *across* a limb, always *along* it.

Never forget that:

1. Abscesses near a large joint often communicate with the joint.

2. Abscesses near a large artery sometimes communicate with the artery.

3. Abdominal wall abscesses sometimes communicate with the gut.

Never forget that *early* openings are imperative in abscesses situated :

1. In neighborhood of joints.
2. In the abdominal wall.
3. In the neck, under the deep fascia.
4. In the palm of the hand.
5. Beneath periosteum.
6. About the rectum, prostate, and urethra.

Remember the frequency with which hæmatoma and traumatic aneurism have been mistaken for abscess, and incised ; and remember, also, that in extravasation below the gluteal fascia there is rarely any sign of bruise or injury to the skin. Never incise such without auscultation or exploratory puncture.

Never plunge ; never squeeze in opening abscesses.

Do not forget that your incision should radiate :

1. In abscesses pointing near the nipple.
2. In abscesses near the anus.
3. In scarifying the chemosis of the cornea.

And that your incisions should be longitudinal :

1. In the hand.
2. In the urethra.
3. In the scalp.

Do not forget that incisions in the neck and face should run parallel with the wrinkles and folds.

Do not be afraid of hurting the lacteal tubes in mammary abscess. More harm is done to the gland by the enlargement of the walls of. the abscess than by a free incision.

Never make a palmar incision, except in the middle of the lower third and in the axial line of the fingers, or at the sides of the palm.

Do not open an abscess anywhere near a large artery without first using a stethoscope, and then only by Hilton's method (*i. e.*, director and dressing forceps).

Never, under any circumstances, use for exploratory puncture that surgical abomination, a grooved needle, for it will allow contamination of all the tissues through which it brings the fluids (Thornton).

In opening a deep abscess in the lumbar region, without the projection of an abscess, do not forget to cut down opposite a transverse process, and not between them, for fear of wounding a lumbar artery.

Aneurism.

Never attempt to cure an aneurism by the formation of a thrombus if the patient has any aseptic condition (such as an abscess, sore, suppurating otitis), for such may induce yellow softening of the clot.

Artery-Bleeding.

Always tie both ends of a divided artery in a wound.

Bladder and Urethra.

Never neglect to pass your hand over the patient's belly in typhoid, or any fever, injury, or fracture of the spine, compression, etc. ; for the bladder may be atonic and injuriously distended without distress.

Never use force in passing a catheter in fractured spine, because of the *insensitiveness* of the urethra.

Never pass a urethral instrument upon a man without having first passed one on yourself.

Never pass an instrument if your patient is suffering from an acute inflammation of the testicle—unless you are relieving retention, or unless testitis occurs in a patient habitually using a catheter.

Do not permit yourself to talk glibly of " impassable" stricture. Such cases are rare. Patience and a little sweet-oil often carry an instrument through.

Never do an internal urethrotomy until you ascertain that your patient is free from undue erections, because of hemorrhage. If the organ is irritable, exhibit bromide of potassium for a few days prior to the operation.

Never put on cantharides blister in nephritis because of absorption (use liq. ammon. fort.).

Do not forget that irritability of the bladder is often due to *renal irritation* and reflex actions.

Never inject more than four ounces at a time into the bladder, and that only with care.

Bones.

Always hesitate to diagnose in an off-hand way " rheumatic" pain in young children. Remember acute periostitis simulates acute rheumatism closely.

Never delay in acute periostitis in cutting freely down to a bone as soon as the nature of the case is detected. Every hour of delay will need a month to repair.

Do not forget the three golden rules in acute periostitis :

1. Prompt incision.
2. Free incision.
3. Free drainage.

Remember secondary abscesses may form in acute periostitis. Be on the *qui vive*.

Do not fret if, on making incisions to the bone, you evacuate but little pus in periostitis. It makes no matter, the relief afforded is often the same.

Remember the golden rules for removing segments from long bones after necrosis :

1. Do not wait for the periosteal sheath (new bony sheath) to have acquired strength enough to preserve the continuity of the limb.

2. Always remove the sequestrum as soon as possible, for it is :

   (a) A permanent source of irritation.

   (b) A danger to the adjacent parts.

3. Do not leave any dead bone behind.

4. Always splint carefully and bandage to maintain the parts in apposition and prevent fracture.

Never forget that there is no periosteal sheath in the necrosis of the popliteal space, and that the exfoliated bone lies close under the popliteal artery.

In removing such avoid four things :

1. Joint.

2. Artery.

3. External popliteal nerve.

4. Rough manipulation.

Scratch with finger nail and scalpel of knife. Do not use the knife.

Breast.

Never forget that a "tumor" in a young woman's breast is not unusually a *chronic* abscess.

Never procrastinate about a tumor of the breast in a female over forty.

Never excise a mammary tumor of doubtful character before cutting it across.

Never remove a true carcinoma of the breast without clearing out the axilla.

Never be too anxious to make your flaps meet and look well in removing a cancer of the breast. Your vanity will often tempt you to leave a flap in which cancer may lie concealed.

Burns.

Do not neglect opium for the shock of burns in children, but use it cautiously ; afterwards do not stint fresh air, food, or warmth.

Never give a hypodermic in burns of children ; you cannot recall it. Give it by the mouth.

Beware of strong application of carbolic oil in burns, and if it be used at all, watch the urine for absorption signs.

Do not dress too often ; but never let the dressings foul.

Never uncover the entire wound at once ; do it piece-meal.

Never omit chloroform or opium in the first dressing of extensive burns.

Always have the tracheotomy instruments at hand in burns or scalds of mouth, because of œdema of glottis.

Chest.

Do not be very solicitous in obtaining crepitus of a fractured rib. Treat it as such.

In manipulating either side of the fractured rib to obtain evidence of undue mobility, do not handle portions of two different ribs.

Never forget that all penetrating wounds of the chest, not involving fracture, should be closed at once.

Do not forget that it is a good practice in severe cases of fractured ribs, and those in which the lung is wounded, to strap the chest and apply ice externally.

[Bandage is said to be contra-indicated if there is much comminution or tearing of the parietes of the chest; or,

1. If dyspnœa increases, on its application.

2. If pain is caused by it.]

Do not strap or bandage if there is much surgical emphysema.

Always regard rib injuries in old people with anxiety.

[There may be, and usually are, pre-existing emphysema and bronchitis, which will hamper the breathing greatly.]

Never tap a chest in paracentesis without making certain, by auscultation and percussion, that you are on the right spot.

Do not neglect to secure your drain tube from slipping into the thorax. Let it be sufficiently, and only sufficiently, long to enter the cavity. Longer is needless.

Always use an exhaustion syringe in tapping the chest.

Never forget in this, as in all other aspirations, to run some carbolic or hydrarg. perchlor. solution through your canula and exhaustion bottle before operating.

Always use an exploring syringe first, if you are in doubt.

Do not forget your landmarks (upper border of lower rib).

Always remember that you aim at the lung rising up and taking the place of the fluid you evacuate. If the lungs are bound down by adhesions and attempts are made to exhaust the fluid with considerable force, rupture and hemorrhage take place.

Do not forget, also, that too forcible a suction applied to the vascular false membranes, which often occupy the pleural cavity, may give rise to hemorrhage into the pleura.

Always stop if pain is complained of.

Dislocation.

Never attempt to reduce a dislocation of humerus in an old person without first examining the state of the arteries to inspire you with caution and gentleness.

Never put a *booted* foot in the axilla to reduce dislocation.

Always reduce by some other method if ribs are broken on the same side.

Remember that injuries to the elbow-joint are often very difficult to diagnose if much swelling co-exists ; but,

Never give a positive opinion of an elbow-joint until you have carefully examined the relations of the olecranon, internal and external condyles, and head of radius.

Remember that in dislocation at the elbow the joint becomes rapidly irreducible.

Never forget that a faulty diagnosis may cause loss of motion in the joint.

Never be ashamed to say you "do not know" until the swelling has subsided, and you are able to be certain of the character of the injury.

Do not forget in dislocation of the carpal bones that the great point is to see that the motions of the fingers are early restored.

Ear.

Never forget that rupture of the membrana tympani, or even fatal consequences, may ensue from roughness.

Never forget that vegetable substances swell in the auditory canal on the application of water.

Remember no foreign body in the ear, except living insects or vegetable substances, can do harm. Syringe gently, unless the foreign body is likely to swell.

Erysipelas.

Support and stimulate in erysipelas ; never deplete or depress.

Do not dress operation or fresh wounds or attend midwifery, if you are dressing a case of erysipelas ; or, in fact, any infectious disease.

Eye.

Never prescribe for an inflamed eye without doing three things, viz :—

1. Without examining for a foreign body imbedded in the cornea, or lodged beneath the lids.

2. Without seeing if cornea or iris is implicated.

3. Without determining the presence or absence of tension of globe.

Never use violence in opening the eye, if there be much

swelling or spasm, because if there be a deep ulcer of the cornea present, perforation may take place.

Never apply lead lotion (Goulard water) should there be the slightest abrasion of the corneal epithelium. [Solid particles of oxide or carbonate of lead become deposited and form permanent opacities.]

Never trust the nurse with verbal instructions for washing out the baby's eyes in infantile ophthalmia. Do it yourself.

Never forget that wounds of the ciliary region are most dangerous, and if they involve the lens, or if they are attended with loss of vitreous, they need excision of the eye.

Never put atropine into an eye :

1. Without testing tension.

2. Without examining for locomotor ataxia (for ataxial cases walk by sight).

3. Without due care as to strength in old people.

[N.B.—Beware of atropine, ergot, colchicum in old people.]

Fracture.

Remember that crepitus may not be obtained in :—

1. Riding of fragments.

2. Impaction of fragments.

3. Entire separation of fragments.

4. Muscle or blood-clot interposed between fragments.

Remember that there is a pseudo crepitus, very like true crepitus, in teno-synovitis, joint effusion, and caries of a joint surface.

Do not forget effusion in or around the dislocated head of a bone sometimes leads to a creaking or crepitus closely resembling that produced by a fracture.

Do not be anxious to get crepitus in such fractures in old people.

Always suspect a bone that is fractured on slight violence, i. e., suspect central sarcoma.

Do not forget that in epiphyseal fracture your prognosis must be guarded, because such injuries in the young are followed sometimes by suspended growth of the bone, producing deformity apparently as the result of degeneration of the cartilage after injury, whereby it loses its power of ossification.

Remember in separation of epiphysis the line of fracture is so broad in the upper extremity of the humerus and the lower extremity of the femur, that there will be no shortening, but the fragments will project.

In all fractures of limbs always examine the pulse below at once.

"In setting" fractures never neglect to fix the joint near the fracture.

Never allow the splint to press on the skin, so as to cause ulceration or œdema, far less gangrene.

Do not, in fracture of the acromion, put a pad in the axilla, or bandage the elbow too slightly to the chest, because the head (the natural splint in such fractures) is thrown outward and the fragments separated.

Never forget to examine every case of fracture of humerus high up, in order to ascertain if the head be dislocated or not.

In adapting a sling to the forearm of a patient with fracture through the middle of the shaft, do not let the sling be so short as to press the elbow upward.

Never delay in fracture involving the elbow-joint to commence passive motion the seventh day—at least not later than the fourteenth day.

Always warn your patient of a probable deformity in a Colles' fracture.

In Colles' fracture do not splint the palm of the hand; leave the fingers free, and work them.

Remember that the extracapsular is certainly more common in old age than the intracapsular fracture.

Do not forget that the so-called absorption and change in the neck of the old femur is not so common as is taught.

Never use violence in injuries to the hip, in order to produce crepitus; much injury may be done in separating an impaction.

Do not keep your *old* patients in bed in order to get union in hip fracture. They are almost sure to suffer from sloughing produced by splints or from bedsores, and will very likely die.

Never forget to bandage the entire limb in fractured femur.

Remember the danger of traction by an extension weight if a fracture be transverse above the condyle [the popliteal artery is brought into contact with the sharp edge of the lower fragment.]

Always shampoo the quadriceps in a fractured patella, provided the state of the soft parts permits it.

Never place fractures in plaster-of-Paris splints, or other splints, which withdraws the seat of fracture from the surgeon's observation, if there be bruising, or until such has subsided, and guard against subsequent swelling by padding.

Never use this treatment without explaining the danger to the patient, and obtaining his consent.

Gangrene.

In gangrene do not mistake the line of discoloration for the line of demarcation. The former may move; the latter never.

Do not neglect the only drug of use—opium.

Do not hurry separation of sloughs in frost-bite gangrene.

General.*

Never use a hypodermic syringe in a secondary syphilitic patient.

Never permit a wet-nurse to be employed without examining into her history and state of health.

Never permit a healthy wet-nurse to suckle a syphilitic child, or child of syphilitic parents.

Never be hasty in suspecting "malingering" in any disease, certainly never in head injuries.

Never neglect to carefully bandage the *entire* limb if you have encircled it at any one point to keep up pressure upon a wound.

Always shampoo gradually and with caution, as early as seems prudent, and at first with prolonged intervals of rest.

Remember three drugs are tolerated well in proportion to their need, viz., opium, mercury, and iodide of potassium.

Always inject ergotine or mercury into muscle, but morphine or brandy under the skin.

Never inject morphine without first testing the urine for albumen or a low S. G.

Never leave a sprain too long at rest. Too long rest is by far the most frequent cause of delayed recovery after injuries of the joints.

Avoid cathartics, deprivation of nourishment, loss of blood by incision in the broken down.

Be careful of abstracting blood from a drunkard or a child.

Be careful of opium in delirium tremens when the pupils are contracted.

Never examine any female under any circumstances without having first obtained her consent, and in the presence of one (or more) reliable witness.

Never examine any female prisoner without consent—without cautioning her that the examination will be taken down in evidence, and without a female companion being present.

Never administer chloroform without a third person being present, nor allow it to be administered in your house, nor until all artificial teeth have been removed.

Do not form hasty opinions, and if you have formed a false opinion, admit your error at once.

* I always recommend dressers to read Surgical Disasters in "Paget's Clinical Lectures."

252

Genital—Penis.

Never sanction a lengthened or adherent prepuce—circumcise.

Never despise any skin in stitching up scrotal wounds—the worst flap will heal.

[Warm a wound of the scrotum before uniting it with sutures.]

Always slit the urethra downwards in amputation of the penis, and stitch the angles outward.

Always keep a catheter in position continuously in injuries to the penis, if the urethra is divided.

Do not tap a hydrocele without examining the position of the testicle with the light.

Do not strap a testicle without shaving the scrotum.

Do not give a decided prognosis of a solid slow-growing tumor of the testicle in which hydrocele co-exists, before you have tapped the hydrocele and examined the gland carefully. It may be non-malignant. If any doubt exists after this, advise a free incision.

Gonorrhœa.

Never neglect to warn your patient about his eyes in treating a *"first"* attack of gonorrhœa.

In giving a *"first"* case of gonorrhœa copaiba, always warn your patient of the possibility of the eruption.

Never neglect in treating gonorrhœal rheumatism to cure the discharge as speedily as possible.

In examining the cause of a knee synovitis of a young man never omit to examine the penis for gonorrhœa or gleet.

In inquiring into a history of syphilis do not hastily judge of the statement of the patient that a rash was syphilitic ; inquire about copaiba.

Never use an injection if there is much pain, scalding, or inflammation, unless it be cocaine.

Never forget many gleets are due to slight contractions of the canal, and may be cured by a steel bougie.

Hand and Foot.

Do not forget that it is wiser in cases of supposed needle in hand or foot, when the patient is not suffering much inconvenience, not to cut down unless the end of the needle is felt.

Never estimate the amount of flat foot when your patient is *sitting*, because the weight is taken off the arch.

Do not forget that the foot may be amputated for supposed strumous disease of the tarsus when, on examination, the affection might have been proved to be limited to one of the tarsal bones, and the patient might have been cured by a less extensive mutilation.

Do not despise or neglect corns, bunions, or ulcers of the leg in the aged, or diabetic. They often start gangrene.

Head.

Do not forget that an injury to the head is never too slight to be despised, and never too severe to be despaired of.

Never be precipitate in opening a hæmatoma of the scalp.

Never close a scalp wound until or unless all dirt is or can be removed.

Never hesitate to suture contused and lacerated wounds, but in doing so do not forget the drainage.

Never pnt stitches in deeply ; there is no reason to wound the tendon.

Beware of cellulitis of the scalp when the dangerous layer of the scalp has been opened. In such cases do not be afraid of incisions, only let them be run from before backwards, be 2 inches in length, and down to the bone. In these cases beware of depletion or deprivation, because they occur in the broken down.

Never neglect to examine the sub-occipital glands as an index to :—

1. Erysipelas of scalp.
2. Pediculosis.
3. Syphilis.

Do not hesitate to trephine if the skull cap is exposed —if there are definite signs of localized paralysis, and if there is no suspicion of general pyæmic infection.

Never forget that a blow on one side of the skull often produces its main effects on the opposite side of the skull.

Do not mistake the depressed centre of an extravasated blood-clot or congenital malformation, or atrophy, for depressed fracture, or the sutures for a linear fracture.

Remember that the more a fracture approaches the punctured form the greater the need for the trephine. Do not forget the rule :—

If the depression is slight,
If the extent is considerable,
If no symptoms are present,
leave it, or *vice versa*, operate.

Remember that the operation for the removal of frag-ments, which have been pressing on the brain, is rarely complete, spiculæ being often left behind.

Remember in trephining the skull that you are to consider the bone under your instrument to be the *thinnest* you have encountered.

Never undervalue the use of calomel and opium in head injuries.

Never treat a case of vomiting without inquiring about hernia and examining abdominal rings.

Do not diagnose a "strangulated" hernia without first feeling, in the male, for each testis.

Never be satisfied with the reduction of a hernia without putting your finger fairly into and through the ring, and ascertaining by comparison of the two sides that no unnatural fulness is left.

Remember that no age is too young for a truss, and that no hernial protrusion should be without one.

In cases of strangulated hernia, if you are in doubt as to the advisability of operating, do not hesitate, but operate.

Do not hesitate to return the gut in herniotomy in all stages of inflammation short of gangrene.

Never procrastinate in cases which will certainly require colotomy.

Joints.

Do not be hasty with a knife in dealing with fluctuating swellings near a joint.

[There are changes in the synovial membrane which produce thickening and suppurating, which can with difficulty be distinguished from an external circumscribed abscess.]

Never forget that synovial tissue of these embracing tendons, may pour out a considerable amount of fluid or even pus.

[The accumulation of fluid in a joint or in the layers of the synovial membrane, or in tendons and bursæ, rarely affect the integument. Therefore, unless there is external redness, never use the scalpel hastily.]

Never probe the joint in clean cut wounds opening a joint, unless a foreign body is known to be lodged therein.

Always persevere with rest and counter-irritation in disease of the shoulder joint as long as there be pain produced by motion, but no longer.

[Too long confinement is apt to produce adhesion of the lower part of the capsule, and to permanently deprive the patient of the power to raise the arm.]

Always trace all sinuses near the shoulder to their source, because the tendons often direct the pus to some point distant from the joint.

Always consider the chance of subacromial bursal disease before you diagnose disease of the shoulder-joint.

Do not hesitate to aspirate a joint for diagnosis, but remember it is criminal to do so without strict aseptic precautions.

Never neglect to put all strumous joints at rest.

[Rest should be maintained for three months after all signs of disease have vanished, and active exercise must even then be very gradually renewed.]

Never neglect early movement in chronic rheumatic arthritis; never allow early movement in strumous arthritis.

Never forget to warn your patient about stiffness in ankylosis of joints after strumous disease.

Never open a joint without rigid asepsis.

Never insist on a lengthy confined position of joints in the treatment of accident or disease of the limb itself.

Never forget whilst breaking adhesion down—

1. The atrophy of rest.
2. The buried bacillus.
3. The fragility of the child's bone.

Hence, in breaking down adhesions do not omit to hold the bones as near the joints as possible. Do not do too much at once. Rupture adhesion by short movements in the way of flexion. Divide contracted tendons some days before breaking down adhesions, and put on ice-bag in every case afterwards.

Beware of employing a Brisement forcé in tubercular joints. [Numerous cases are recorded where this procedure was followed within a few days by general miliary tuberculosis and a speedy death.]

Never attempt to overcome muscular contraction in contraction of joint by forcible extension—tenotomise.

Never let a child wearing a Thomas's splint have a hard bed, for the splint on a hard mattress is thrown out into relief, and causes painful pressure.

Never forget that in serious disease of joint the rapid loss of tissue observed about a joint is never seen in hysterical joint.

Beware of the insidious onset of tubercular arthritis.

Never treat the case of a limping child lightly.

Never omit to examine the hip when pain is complained of in apparently healthy knee.

Never forget that proof of knee disease is no proof of the absence of hip disease of the same side.

Mouth.

Never leave hare-lip pins, in hare-lip operation, longer, *if you use them*, than forty-eight hours.

Always stop to guard your thumbs before you reduce a dislocation of the jaw.

Always use blunt scissors in operating on the frænum linguæ.

Do not forget in ranulæ to search for stone in the duct.

Never think lightly of any ulcer of the tongue or lips of a patient after middle life.

Nose.

Always suspect a foul discharge in a child to result from a foreign body, if the discharge be from one nostril.

Œsophagus.

Always remove all artificial teeth before giving an anæsthetic.

Never forget that when a foreign body, though only of moderate size, has become fixed in the commencement of the œsophagus or the pharynx, and has resisted a fair trial for its extraction or displacement, an incision should be made at once, and it should be removed, although no urgent symptoms are present.

Remember catgut sutures are used for wounds of the œsophagus ; never silk or silver.

Always be certain that your tube enters the œsophagus in using the stomach-pump (especially if the patient be under chloroform or insensible in drink).

Operations.

Never permit a naked light to approach the ether apparatus in anæsthetizing.

Never neglect in all operations which will produce a shock to the urinary system—*e. g.*, varicocele, fistula, piles, radical cure of hernia—to ascertain, before the operation, if the urethral canal be without stricture, for sometimes stricture is found in relieving retention after operation, and you may be unprepared for the obstruction.

Never neglect to examine the lungs in all cases of ischio-rectal disease and fistula in ano.

In inserting plugs or plug appliance for colotomy, gastrostomy, or drainage tubes for abscesses, wounds, especially in thorax, always see that the end of the plug or drain is properly secured.

Never operate without first examining the urine for albumen and sugar.

Never apply an elastic (Esmarch) bandage to render a limb bloodless if tuberculosis or gangrene is present.

Never forget a patient's age in years is not the index to his "vis" or "last." *Vide* "Errors in the Chronometry of Life," "Paget's Old Note Books."

Pelvis.

Never forget to determine the absence of a foreign body in buttock wounds.

Always ligature a bleeding vessel in the buttock at once, even at the risk of a deep dissection.

In fracture of true pelvis do not carry out passive movements very actively, in order to elicit crepitus.

Remember the serious consequences which may ensue from the displacement of a pointed fragment.

In falls on the buttock or rump, in fractured pelvis, or blows in the belly, never omit to empty the bladder, if the patient cannot.

Rectum.

Never forget in fistula in ano to eliminate tertiary syphillitic, strumous, or dysenteric ulceration, stricture and malignant disease of the rectum.

Remember the saying, "No internal opening to a fistula, or a blind fistula is usually a blind surgeon."

Do not forget the probable need for a catheter after an operation on the rectum.

Shock.

In shock and collapse never forget that the essence of successful treatment is to obtain time for your patient to rally. Keep the heart going, but do not trade on its exhausted power ; maintain its action, do not force it.

Sinus.

Never neglect the hint the guardian papillæ give of the irritating focus deeper down.

Never neglect the therapeutics of rest.

Never neglect to slit the forks and the burrows up as well as the sinus.

Spine.

Never forget that in fracture of the spine the tendency to death is due to pneumonia and complications. if the fracture is situated high up, and to urinary inflammation and bedsore, if lower down.

Therefore never forget the atonic bladder or the back. The urethra is insensitive, therefore use your catheter with care and gentleness ; let it be clean and smooth.

Never neglect to see for yourself that the back has been kept clean.

Never puncture a spina bifida in the median line, always at the side, taking in the skin ; *avoid* air, and close puncture securely.

Never suspend by the head alone in adjusting a Sayre's jacket for a Pott's curvature of the spine ; let the toes and armpits help to support the weight.

Never forget that the earlier stages of caries are not accompanied by any decided symptoms. When curvature exists there is no longer any room for doubt, but do not wait for curvature.

Never permit a patient who has sustained an injury to the back to quit the casualty department until he has passed water. [Bloody urine will show at once that the kidney has been injured.]

Syphilis.

Do not adhere to the popular division of "hard" and "soft" sore.

Do not forget a sore may become hard four weeks after coition, because it has been inoculated by a mixed secretion.

Do not forget that no matter what the character of any primary sore may be, the chances are that the sequel will prove that it contained the germ of true syphilis.

Do not believe or rely upon sharply defined rules for the diagnosis of chancre; even with sores which are obviously soft and non-infecting until the incubation period (3–5 weeks) is well passed.

Do not entertain any confidence that induration will not occur; and it would be acting most unwisely to give an absolute opinion on the matter.

Phimosis acquired is so common an accompaniment of the three venereal diseases—acute gonorrhœa, soft sore, hard sore—that you ought never to express a decided opinion until you have got a look at the trouble. Do not hesitate to slit up the prepuce, in order to examine and treat a sloughing sore. If *you* do not do it, the sloughing most probably will.

Always prohibit smoking, and any diet which may lead to diarrhœa while mercury is being given for syphilis.

Never forget occasional idiosyncrasy in patients against taking mercury and iodide.

Remember the one simple rule for successful treatment of syphilis is, keep inunction and fumigation method for exceptional cases, and give small doses of mercury more or less frequently, but never large doses.

Never forget that with a patient confined to bed and on low diet, ptyalism can be produced with half the dose of mercury.

[N.B.—Rapid loss of weight means that mercury is disagreeing with the patient.]

Remember that pot. iod. and mercury, except in the scrofulous and in cachetic patients, are well borne in syphilis if there is need of them.

Never neglect to warn your patient of his gums and his tendency to catch cold, when taking mercury.

For all cases of phagedæna, mercury ought always to be given.

Remember the earlier mercury is exhibited the greater the probability that the symptoms will be wholly prevented or delayed.

Never exercise a syphilitic testis, however bad, even when there is abscess and fungus testis.

Remember in tertiary syphilis whenever a case resists the iodide, and whenever it is important to obtain a rapid result, the mercury should be added to the iodide or the mercury should be given alone.

Never omit to give opium in all gangrene and sloughing wounds which do not prove amenable.

Remember syphilis may imitate all known forms of skin disease, but it can produce no originals. (Hutchinson.)

Never forget that lichen ruber and lichen planus are often dusky and copper tinted, and present all the features which to those of limited experience suggests a confident diagnosis of syphilis.

Remember that in rare instances syphilis imitates variola closely ; there is, however—

1. Persistence.
2. Absence of odor.
3. History to guide you.

Never let a markedly syphilitic mother suckle her child.

Never let a syphilitic child have a wet nurse.

In syphilis do not sanction marriage until two years after the date of infection, and then only if the patient is free from gleet, and has thoroughly and successfully been treated with mercury.

Never assume, as was formerly done, that mercury should be avoided when syphilitic sores ulcerate ; on the contrary, when used with iron, quinine, and opium, it will always prove the means of cure.

Do not forget that the safety of the eye in syphilitic iritis depends, however, mainly upon the promptitude and efficiency with which atropine is employed.

Never forget to examine for retinitis and choroiditis if a syphilitic patient complains of failure of sight or muscæ, and use mercury smartly if you find either.

Never neglect local measures in the lesions of intermediate and tertiary stages of syphilis.

Remember that a node of secondary syphilis usually disappears or is prone to ossify, but a tertiary like other gummata are more liable to suppuration and caries.

Do not open a syphilitic bubo, unless acutely suppurating, or a node of bone ; they usually absorb.

Throat.

In cut throats where the trachea has been opened never neglect to remove all small fragments which hang loose in the trachea, or they will swell and eventually stop respiration.

Never leave a scald of the glottis a minute without tracheotomy tubes and knife placed at hand.

Do not neglect to warn your patient that the food may run away after tracheotomy through the tube for the first few hours.

Never neglect or think lightly of stab wounds of the neck.

In œdema of glottis due to syphilis, erysipelas, wounds of glottis, scalds, always have the tracheotomy instruments by the bedside.

Remember that in stab wounds of the upper part of the neck with arterial bleeding, there is an impossibility in many cases of distinguishing the exact source of the hemorrhage, so numerous are the great vessels in that region. Apply a ligature to common carotid or external carotid if excessive.

Remember that tracheotomy and insertion of tube is especially necessary in wounded epiglottis or arytenoid cartilages.

Always secure your tracheotomy tube by knotting the tape. Little patients are apt to drag at a loop.

Remember diffuse cellulitis of the neck is very fatal.

Avoid sutures in cut throat, when the windpipe is opened.

Never put silk or silver ligatures into a wounded œsophagus ; only use catgut.

Never forget that fractures of the laryngeal cartilages are of serious importance ; the nearer the cords, the acuter the symptoms, the more decisive must be the treatment. If the fragments are displaced and the mucous membrane lacerated or perforated by the fragments (as testified by emphysema and blood spitting) tracheotomy must immediately be performed.

Never neglect in all sudden dyspnœa in a child to pass your finger into the upper part of the larynx to search for a foreign body.

Sanction no delay in removing a foreign body known to be in the larynx. Invert.

Never hesitate in foreign bodies in trachea to invert the patient after the tracheal incision has been made for the extraction of the foreign body. Never use forceps, rather invert the patient, or use a hook, bent probe, or wire snare, inversion, succussion.

But never invert unless you have your tracheotomy instruments ready, for the danger of instant suffocation, through lodging of the foreign body in the glottis, is great

Never forget that lung disease invariably ensues on the retention of a foreign body in the bronchus.

Warnings to Patients and their Friends.

Never forget to warn your patient that a Colles' fracture, even when treated with the greatest care, leaves some deformity.

Never forget to warn a case of fracture of the patella, that the fragments tend to separate.

Always warn your patient that there may be loss of power of deltoid after dislocation of shoulder if much pain is experienced, *i. e.*, the nerves have been pressed upon.

Always warn the patient or his friends of the possibility of suspension of growth, in injury to an epiphyseal cartilage.

Never forget to warn the parents of a hare-lip that one operation is usually inadequate.

Never forget to warn your patient that the loose cutaneous anal tags swell after an operation for piles, or he may suppose you have overlooked them.

Never forget to warn your patient that a Meibomian cyst fills with blood after being scooped out, or he will think that the operation has been performed slovenly.

Always warn the patient's friends that fluid taken by the mouth may run out through a tracheotomy wound for the first few hours, and that such is not due to a wound of the gullet.

FORMULAS AND DOSES FOR HYPODERMIC MEDICATION.

℞ Apomorphinæ, ... gr. j.
   Aq. destillat., ... f℥iiss.
Solve.
One minim = gr. $\frac{1}{150}$. Dose, 5–20 minims. (*Prompt emetic.*)

℞ Atropinæ sulphatis, . . gr. j.
   Aq. destillat., . . . f℥xv.
Solve.
One minim = gr. $\frac{1}{900}$. Dose, 5–20 minims.

℞ Caffeinæ, ... gr. x.
   Alcoholis,
   Aq. destillat., . . . āā f℥iss.
Solve.
One minim = gr. $\frac{1}{18}$. Dose, 4–18 minims.

℞ Camphoræ, ... gr. v.
   Alcoholis, ... f℥j.
Solve.
Dose, 6–30 minims.

℞ Coninæ, ... gr. j.
   Alcoholis,
   Aq. destillat., . . . āā f℥v.
Solve.
One minim = gr. $\frac{1}{600}$. Dose, 5–15 minims.

℞ Chloral hydratis, . . . ℥j.
   Aq. destillat., ... f℥ij.
Solve.
Dose, 4–16 minims.

℞ Daturinæ, ... gr. ss.
   Aq. destillat., ... f℥j.
Solve.
One minim = gr. $\frac{1}{900}$. Dose, 4–10 minims.

℞ Digitalinæ, . gr. ss.
Alcoholis,
Aq. destillat., . āā f℥ij.
Solve.
One minim = gr. $\frac{1}{480}$. Dose, 4–8 minims.

℞ Ergotinæ, . . . gr. xv.
Alcoholis,
Glycerinæ, . . . āā f℥iiss.—M.
One minim = gr. $\frac{1}{20}$. Dose, 5–30 minims.

℞ Extracti ergotæ fluidi, . . q. s.
Filter carefully. Dose, 10 minims.

℞ Hydrargyri chloridi corrosivi,
Ammonii chloridi, . . āā gr. iij.
Misce et solve in—
Aq. destillat., . . f℥iss.
Dein. adde—
Albuminis ovi, . . . f℥iss.
Aq. destillat., . . . f℥v.
Filtra et adjice—
Aq. destillat., . . q. s. ad f℥x.
One minim = gr. $\frac{1}{200}$. Dose, 3–10 minims.

℞ Hydrargyri et sodii iodidi, . gr. iij.
Aq. destillat., . . . f℥iiiss.
Solve.
One minim = gr. $\frac{1}{70}$. Dose, 10 minims every other day.

℞ Morphinæ sulphatis, . . gr. xxiv.
Atropinæ sulphatis. . . gr. j.
Ol. amygdalæ amaræ, . gtt. j.
Aq. destillat., . . . f℥ij.
Solve.
Ten minims contain gr. $\frac{1}{4}$ of morphina and gr. $\frac{1}{96}$ of atropina. (*Diduma's solution.*)

℞ Pilocarpinæ muriatis *vel* nitratis, gr. iij.
Aq. destillat., ... f℥iv.
Solve.
One minim = gr. $\frac{1}{80}$. Dose, 10–20 minims.

℞ Potassii iodidi, ... ℥j.
Aq. destillat., ... f℥iv.
Solve.
Dose, 6–20 minims.

℞ Quininæ sulphatis, . . . gr. xv.
Acid. sulphurici aromatici, . q. s. ad sol.
Aq. destillat., ... q. s. ad f℥iiss.
Fiat solutio.

One minim = gr. $\frac{1}{10}$. Dose, 5–30 minims.

℞ Strychninæ sulphatis, . . gr. j.
Aq. destillat., ... f℥j.
Solve. (Heat in a test-tube, or triturate in a mortar until all the crystals disappear.)

One minim = gr. $\frac{1}{480}$. Dose, 4–15 minims.

℞ Woorariæ, ... gr. j.
Aq. destillat., ... f℥iij.

One minim = gr. $\frac{1}{180}$. Dose, 5–10 minims.

NOTES.—After drawing the required amount of fluid into the syringe, expel the small globules of air by everting the syringe and pressing the piston upwards, until a drop of the liquid appears at the point of the needle.

Draw the skin up and tense at the required place, and press the needle through into the subcutaneous tissues; which done, inject the fluid slowly into them. After the needle has been withdrawn place the finger over the puncture for a short time.

The veins, inflamed spots, and bony prominences are places to be *avoided* in puncturing; the arm, thigh, abdomen, back, and calf of the leg are places *suitable* for puncturing.

In hypodermic medication the dose is about one-half that required by the mouth, and the effects are more rapid, certain, and exact.

This manner of medication should be resorted to when immediate and decided results are required; when medicines otherwise administered fail to do good; when medicines are required which the patient refuses or cannot swallow; when there is an irritable state of the stomach precluding exhibition by the mouth.

Solutions intended for hypodermic use should be neutral, without acid or alkaline reaction, and non-irritating.

The medicines should be rendered perfectly soluble, and the menstruum perfectly free from foreign matters.

Solutions of the alkaloids should be made fresh as required, since they spoil on long keeping.

Filtered rain or spring waters are preferable, as a menstruum, to distilled water which has been kept for some days. BARTHOLOW.

POISONS AND ANTIDOTES.

Acetate of Lead.

Emetics and stomach-pump; magnesium sulphate, dilute sulphuric acid, or the phosphates of soda and magnesia; milk, raw eggs, and water; morphin for pain; iodids to eliminate.

Acid—Acetic, Hydrochloric, Nitric, Oxalic, Sulphuric, Tartaric.

Magnesia, chalk, plaster scraped from a wall, limewater, whiting, soap, milk, oil, demulcents; induce vomiting; avoid stomach-tube; feed by rectum.

Acid, Carbolic.

Powdered chalk, Epsom salts, demulcents, white of egg, milk, dilute sulphuric acid, glycerin, oil; empty stomach; atropin.

Acid, Hydrocyanic.

Empty stomach; potassium permanganate; dilute ammonia-water; atropin; newly precipitated oxid of iron with an alkaline carbonate, chlorin; cold to head and neck.

Aconite.

Emetic of zinc sulphate; stomach-pump; ammonia and brandy; atropin.

Alcohol.

Stomach-pump, emetics, cold to head, ammonium carbonate.

Alkalies—Ammonia, Potash, Soda.

Vinegar, lemon-juice, orange-juice, or citric acid and water, followed by large doses of olive-oil, castor-oil, emetics. If caustic alkalies have been taken, the stomach-pump should not be used.

Antimony, Tartar Emetic.

Tepid water to increase vomiting, vegetable astringents, catechu, tannin, white of egg, magnesia, castor-oil, stimulants.

Arsenic.

Stomach-pump or emetics; hydrated peroxid of iron, or light magnesia with the tincture of the chlorid of iron; chalk and water; follow with milk and demulcents.

Atropin, Belladonna, Hyoscyamus.

Stomach-pump, zinc sulphate, ammonia, and stimulants; tannin; opiates; pilocarpin; physostigmin; artificial heat; artificial respiration; enema of hot, strong coffee.

Baryta, Salts of.

Stomach-pump, emetics, sulphate of soda or magnesia.

Chloroform, Chloral, Amyl Nitrite, Ether.

Fresh air, cold affusions, ammonia to nostrils, artificial respiration, strychnin, counter-irritants, cathartics.

Conium, Hemlock, Nicotini.

Emetics, stomach-pump, tannin, stimulants, respiration.

Copper.

Yellow prussiate of potash or soap; emesis; albumin.

Digitalis.

Stomach pump, emetics, tannin, stimulants : keep in recumbent position ; cathartics.

Hellebore.

Opium, stimulants, ammonia.

Iodine.

Emetics and demulcent drinks, starch or flour mixed in water, opium and external heat.

Irritant Gases—Carbonic Acid, Chlorine, Nitrous Acid, Hydrochloric Acid.

Fresh air, inhalation of ammonia, ether or vapor of hot water; amyl nitrite; nitroglycerin; artificial respiration.

Lead Salts.

Any soluble sulphate, either magnesia or soda, succeeded by emetics, and afterwards opium and milk.

Lobelia.

Stimulants externally and internally, external heat.

Mercury, Corrosive Sublimate.

Albumen, white of egg, flour, milk. Emetics, stomach pump.

Morphia, Opium Preparations.

Emetics, atropin hypodermically, stomach-pump, stimulants externally and internally, brandy and coffee, cold affusion, galvanic shocks, compel patient to move about, inhalations of ammonia, potassium permanganate, oxygen-inhalations, artificial respiration; lingual traction.

Nux Vomica and Strychnin.

Emesis; chloral and bromid, animal charcoal or tannic acid, amyl nitrite. Inhalations of chloroform or ether. Artificial respiration.

Phosphorus.

Copper sulphate as emetic, purgatives; no oil; potassium permanganate.

Silver, Salts of.

Common salt, white of egg, milk, emesis.

Zinc, Salts of.

Sodium carbonate, emetics, warm demulcent drinks.

DIAMETERS OF THE FEMALE PELVIS AND FŒTAL HEAD.

Diameters of the Plane of the Superior Strait and False Pelvis.

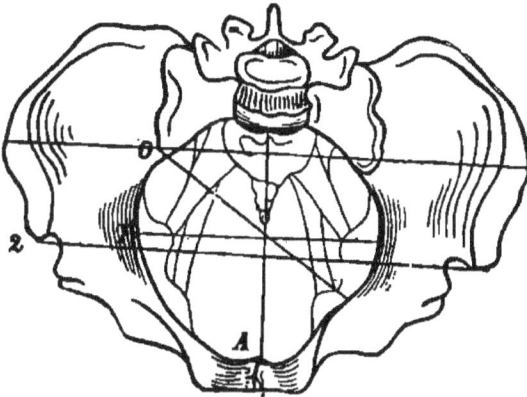

A. ANTERO-POSTERIOR, 11 cm., 4 inches. Extends from the upper part of the posterior surface of the symphysis pubis to the centre of the promontory of the sacrum.

T. TRANSVERSE, 13½ cm., 5¼ inches. Extends from a point midway between the sacro-iliac joint and the ilio-pectineal eminence to a corresponding point on the opposite side.

O. OBLIQUE, 12¾ cm., 5 inches. Extends from the sacro-iliac joint to a point of the brim corresponding with the ilio-pectineal eminence.

CIRCUMFERENCE, 13 inches.

FALSE PELVIS.

1. The TRANSVERSE DIAMETER, from the middle part of the crest of the ilium to the opposite point, measures 29 cm., 11 inches.

2. The distance from the ANTERIOR SUPERIOR SPINOUS PROCESS on one side to a corresponding point on the opposite is 26 cm., 9 inches.

The depth of the FALSE PELVIS, from the top of the crest of the ilium to the level of the PLANE OF THE SUPERIOR STRAIT, is 8.9 cm., 3½ inches.

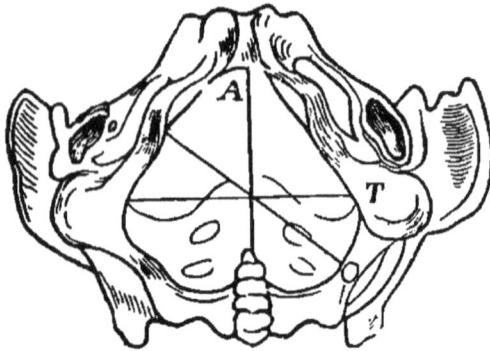

A. ANTERO-POSTERIOR, 9½–11 cm., 4 inches. Extends from the point of the coccyx to the sub-pubic ligament.

T. TRANSVERSE, 11 cm., 4 inches. Extends between the tuberosities of the two ischii.

O. OBLIQUE, 11 cm., 4 inches. Extends from the junction of the rami of the pubis and ischium to the middle of the inferior sacro-sciatic ligament on the opposite side.

CIRCUMFERENCE, 12 inches.

Cavity of Pelvis.

ANTERIOR DEPTH, 3.8 cm., 1½ inches.
LATERAL DEPTH, 8.9 cm., 3½ inches.
POSTERIOR DEPTH, 13 cm., 4½–5 inches.

Diameters of the Fœtal Skull.

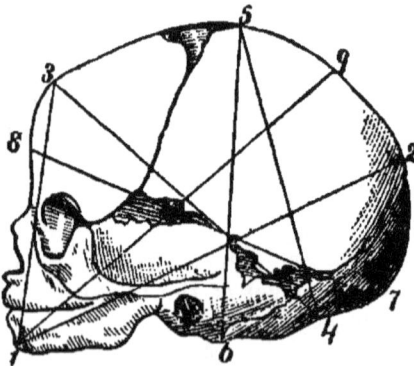

1 to 2. OCCIPITO-MENTAL, 13½ cm., 5 inches. This, the longest diameter of the head, extends from the point of the chin to the posterior fontanelle or occiput.

1 to 3. FRONTO-MENTAL, 7½ cm., 3 inches. Extends from the top of the forehead to the point of the chin.

4 to 5. CERVICO-BREGMATIC, 9½ cm., 3½ inches. Extends from a point midway between the foramen magnum and occipital protuberance to the posterior point of the anterior fontanelle.

5 to 6. TRACHELO-BREGMATIC, 9½ cm., 3½ inches. Extends from the anterior margin of the foramen magnum to the posterior point of the anterior fontanelle.

7 to 8. OCCIPITO-FRONTAL, 11¾ cm., 4 inches. Extends from the occipital protuberance to the os frontis.

1 to 9. SAGITTO-MENTAL, 12½ cm., 4½ inches. Extends from the middle of the sagittal suture to the point of the chin.

3 to 4. CERVICO-FRONTAL, 11¾ cm., 4 inches. Extends from the base of the occiput to the apex of the forehead.

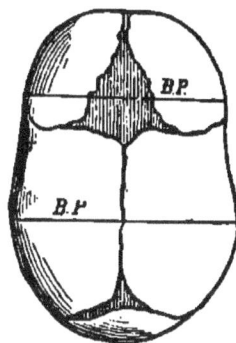

B. P. BI-PARIETAL, 9¼ cm., 3½ inches. Extends between the two parietal protuberances.

B. T. BI-TEMPORAL, 8 cm., 2½ inches. Extends from one side of the os frontis to the other.

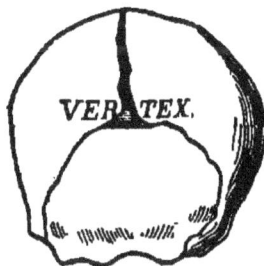

The VERTEX is a circle described around the posterior fontanelle.

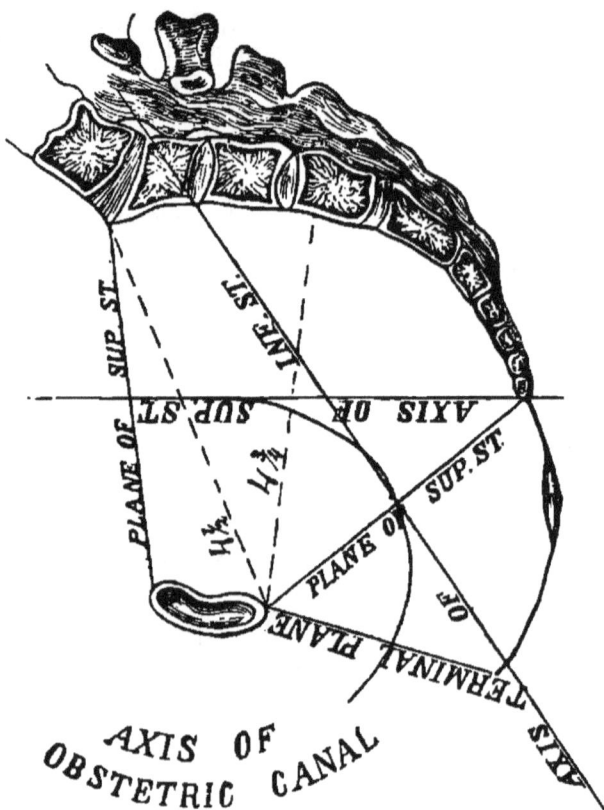

PLANE OF SUP. ST.

AXIS OF SUP. ST.

PLANE OF SUP. ST.

AXIS OF SUP. ST.

4½ 4¾

PLANE OF SUP. ST.

AXIS TERMINAL PLANE

OF

AXIS OF
OBSTETRIC CANAL

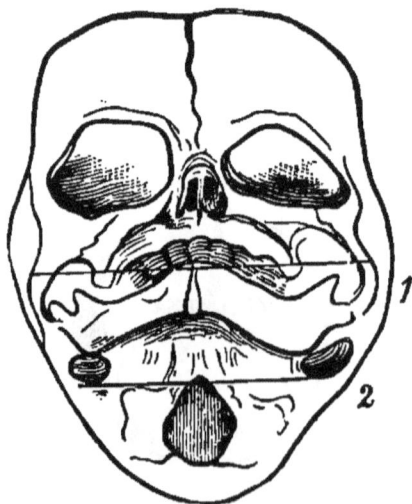

1. Bɪ-ᴍᴀʟᴀʀ, 2½ inches.
2. Bɪ-Mᴀꜱᴛᴏɪᴅ, 2 inches.

DIET TABLE.

BRIGHT'S DISEASE.

Fish.

Raw oysters, raw clams, fresh fish.

Meats.

Beef, mutton, chicken, game, salads.

Bread and Farinaceous Articles.

Good bread, hominy, wheaten grits, rice, toast, oatmeal, gruels.

Vegetables.

Green vegetables generally, spinach, summer cabbage, turnip tops, water-cresses, lettuce, mushrooms, celery.

Desserts.

Rice and milk puddings.

Fruits.

All laxative fruits.

Liquids.

Water abundantly, Poland, Buffalo Lithia, or Vichy water, hot water, milk, skimmed milk, buttermilk.

AVOID

Soups, fried fish, cooked oysters, pork, corned beef, veal, hashes, stews, turkey, heavy bread, batter cakes, potatoes, gravies, lamb, peas, beans.

All made dishes, puddings (except as allowed above), pies, cake, ice-cream, all saccharine dishes and starchy foods, except as allowed. All spices and highly seasoned dishes. Alcoholic drinks, malt liquors, coffee, tobacco.

Scraped beef or mutton.

Mutton and chicken broth, barley, gruel prepared by long boiling, sago, tapioca.

Flour ball: Wheat flour closely packed in a bag, boiled five days, then grated and sifted, and given with boiled milk. Arrowroot and barley flour may be prepared and given in same way.

White of egg and water, expressed juice of meat for infants above the age of six months, whey, brandy.

Pure water abundantly, fresh-boiled milk, plain soda or Vichy water.

In some cases avoid milk entirely; use rice-water. Feed at regular and long intervals as possible (two to six hours), according to age. Give small quantities. Always use stimulants freely.

AVOID

Milk, except that which has been sterilized or boiled, and starchy substances, except as allowed, and unless the starch has been changed into dextrin by the action of dry heat.

CHRONIC RHEUMATISM.

Fish.

All kinds, raw oysters, raw clams.

Meats.

Beef, mutton (once daily only), eggs, chicken, game.

Bread and Farinaceous Articles.

Wheat, corn, or barley bread, rice, brown breads.

Vegetables.

Green vegetables, such as spinach, celery, salads, cresses, peas, summer cabbage, radishes, horse-radish.

Desserts.

Milk puddings, acid fruits.

Drinks and Liquids.

Tea, water, Poland or Vichy water, buttermilk, cocoa shells, claret well diluted, koumiss, milk with lime-water, lemon and lime juice.

An absolute milk diet may be necessary.

AVOID

Fried fish, cooked oysters or clams, pork, veal, turkey, pota-toes. All sweets and starchy substances, except as allowed. All gravies and made dishes. Excess of nitrogenous food. All fried dishes. Beer and all malt liquors, wines.

CONSTIPATION.

Soups.

Clear soups, such as beef, mutton, or chicken broth, oyster and clam soups.

Fish.

All kinds.

Meats.

All fresh meats, poultry, game.

Bread and Farinaceous Articles.

Good bread of all sorts, mush, hominy, oatmeal, wheaten grits, brown bread, corn bread.

Vegetables.

All vegetables if fresh or watery, vegetables with salad oil, boiled spinach, boiled dandelion.

Desserts.

Stewed prunes, stewed figs, tamarinds, baked sour apples, dried fruits, melons, grapes, oranges on rising in the morning, plain puddings, ice-cream.

Drinks and Liquids.

Water abundantly and especially before meals, hot water an hour before meals, buttermilk, koumiss, coffee if half milk, lemonade.

AVOID

All salt or smoked fish or meat, milk, peas, beans, nuts. All milk compounds, pickles, pastry, tea, gin, brandy, cheese.

DIABETES.

Soups.

Animal broth, unthickened only.

Fish.

All kinds, oysters. clams, lobster, shrimps.

Meats.

All kinds, poultry, game, bacon.

Eggs.

Bread and Farinaceous Articles.

Bread and biscuits made with prepared gluten flour.

Vegetables.

Green vegetables, such as summer cabbage, turnip tops, spinach, water cresses, mustard, sauerkraut, lettuce, sorrel, mushrooms, celery, string beans, dandelion, chicory, cold slaw, brussels sprouts, cucumbers, olives, asparagus, truffles, radishes, onions, pickles.

Desserts.

Custards without sugar, eggs, cheese, butter, jellies unsweetened. Nuts, except chestnuts.

Drinks and Liquids.

Water, Poland or Vichy, koumyss, buttermilk, dry wines in moderation, claret, sherry, burgundy, acid fruits, lemons, currants, tea, cream, coffee sweetened with saccharine.

AVOID

Sweet milk, liver, bread, biscuits, toast, farinaceous vegetables, such as potatoes, rice, oatmeal, corn meal, sago, tapioca, arrowroot, etc.; saccharine vegetables, such as turnips, carrots, parsnips, green peas, French beans, beet root, tomatoes, fruits of all kinds; all preserves, syrups, sugars, cocoa, chocolate, cordials, sweet wines; all pastry, puddings, ice cream, honey.

DIARRHŒA.

Meats.

Game, rare meat pulp, sweet breads, fresh meat (sparingly), clam juice.

Bread and Farinaceous Articles, etc.

Bread of all kinds (if stale), dry toast, crackers and butter, macaroni, rice, and rice boiled with milk, flour, long boiled with milk.

Eggs.

Lightly boiled, poached.

Desserts.

Milk and egg pudding (not sweet), hasty pudding of flour and milk.

Drinks and Liquids.

Boiled milk, claret, tea, brandy, water (sparingly), milk punch.

AVOID

Soups. fresh bread, vegetables, fruits, fried dishes, fish, saccharine foods, made dishes, salt meat or fish, veal, lamb, and pork.

DYSPEPSIA.

Soups, etc.

Clear soups, beef, mutton, chicken, or clam broth.

Fish.

Raw oysters, broiled oysters (omitting the hard parts).

Meats.

Beef, mutton, lamb, chicken, game, venison, chopped meat, meat pulp.

Eggs.

Poached, soft boiled, raw.

Bread and Farinaceous Articles.

Bread (one day old), corn bread, rice cakes, stale bread and butter, macaroni, sago, tapioca, cream crackers, dry toast (unbuttered).

Vegetables and Fruits.

Green vegetables, such as spinach, turnip tops, cresses, salads, celery, sorrel, lettuce, string beans, dandelion, chicory, asparagus ; oranges, ripe peaches and pears, apples roasted, and thoroughly cooked dried fruit.

Drinks and Liquids.

Water, Vichy or Poland water, hot water an hour before meals, koumyss, buttermilk, milk and lime-water, milk and seltzer, tea, claret, dry wines, whiskey and water.

AVOID

Rich soups, all fried foods, veal, pork, hashes, stews, turkey, sweet potatoes, all starches and saccharine articles, all gravies, made dishes, sauces, desserts, pies, pastry, puddings, ice cream, sweet wines, malt liquors, cordials, uncooked vegetables.

FEVERS.

Soups, etc.

Beef-tea, clear soup, mutton broth, chicken broth.

Farinaceous Articles, etc.

Indian gruel, Graham flour gruel and oatmeal gruel (if diarrhœa is absent), milk toast, soaked crackers, flax-seed tea, arrowroot, rice and milk.

Drinks.

Water, Vichy, plain soda or Poland water, rice-water, currant jelly-water, lemonade, gum arabic water, orange juice, koumyss, champagne, brandy, whiskey, tea, milk guarded with lime-water.

AVOID

All solids until after crisis. In typhoid no solid food should be given until two weeks after the temperature has become normal, and remains so.

GOUT.

Soups.

Clear soup, clam or oyster broth.

Fish.

Fresh fish, raw oysters, raw clams (little neck).

Meats.

Beef, mutton, chicken, ham, bacon. Meat should be eaten but once daily if possible.

Farinaceous Articles.

Bread, bread from whole wheat, crackers, rye bread, oatmeal, zweibach, cracked wheat, milk toast, rice.

Vegetables.

Potatoes, fresh vegetables.

Desserts.

Milk puddings, fruits of all kinds in moderation if not too acid.

Drinks.

Water plentifully, plain soda or Vichy water, old whiskey well diluted, dry wines, milk, weak tea.

AVOID

Soups, eggs, all made dishes, gravies and spices, pork, veal, turkey, all pies, pastries, and rich puddings, patties, confectionery, sweet wines, burgundy, heavy claret, cordials, malt liquors, tobacco, coffee, asparagus, peas, beans. All acid fruits.

MALNUTRITION.

Soups.

Thick soups, all kinds of broths.

Fish.

Raw oysters, raw clams.

Meats, etc.

Beef, chopped or scraped meat, mutton, chicken, game, butter.

Eggs.

Raw, soft-boiled, poached, and scrambled.

Bread and Farinaceous Articles.

Any amount unless indigestion exists.

Vegetables.

All kinds of ripe and well-cooked vegetables, such as potatoes, spinach, young peas, rice.

Desserts.

Egg and milk puddings, ripe fruits.

Drinks and Liquids.

Pure water, Poland or Vichy water, warm fresh milk, cream, malt preparations, claret, burgundy, port, sherry, tea.

Pork, veal, salt meats (except ham), hashes, stews, thin soups, cooked oysters or clams, turkey, pickles and spices, pies, pastry, and preserves, thick gravies, and all made dishes.

NERVOUS DISEASES.

Soups.

Mutton, beef, chicken, oyster, or clam, clear soup.

Fish.

All kinds, raw oysters, raw clams (little neck).

Meats, etc.

Beef, mutton, chicken, game, chopped meat, butter, salad oil, eggs.

Bread-stuffs.

Wheat bread, rice boiled or as batter cakes, oatmeal, wheaten grits.

Vegetables and Fruits.

Baked white potatoes, spinach, greens, summer cabbage, cresses, lettuce, celery, green peas, asparagus, fresh fruit.

Drinks.

Water freely, plain soda or Poland water, hot water an hour before meals, cocoa, milk, cream, ale and porter, tea or coffee without milk or sugar.

AVOID

Soups generally, stews, hashes, potatoes (white and sweet) starches except as allowed, gravies, macaroni, all made dishes, pies, pastries, and puddings, sweets, distilled liquors, new malt liquors, chocolate, wines, strawberries, raspberries, currants.

OBESITY.

Soups, etc.

Beef, mutton, and chicken broth, free from fat.

Fish.

All kinds.

Meats.

Lean beef, lean mutton, chicken, game.

Eggs.

Vegetables.

Asparagus, cauliflower, onions, celery, cresses, spinach, white cabbage, tomatoes, radishes, lettuce, greens, squash, turnips.

Bread and Farinaceous Articles.

Stale bread and dry toast, gluten biscuits.

Desserts, Fruits, etc.

Grapes, oranges, cherries, berries, acid fruit.

Drinks.

Water, Buffalo lithia or Vichy water, tea or coffee without sugar or milk. Wine occasionally.

Exercise short of fatigue.

AVOID

Fat, thick soups, sauces and spices, hominy, oatmeal, maccaroni, white and sweet potatoes, rice, beets, carrots, starches, parsnips, puddings, pies, cakes, all sweets, milk, water (if urea is in excess), alcoholic drinks, malt liquors. Avoid water in excess.

PHTHISIS.

Soups, etc.

Beef-tea, mutton and chicken broth, clam soup, turtle soup.

Fish.

Fresh fish, raw oysters, raw clams (little neck).

Meats, etc.

Beef rare, scraped meat, bacon, mutton roasted, roasted or broiled poultry, game, soft boiled eggs, beef fat, butter, salad oil, sweet breads.

Bread and Farinaceous Articles.

Wheat bread, Indian bread, rice.

Vegetables and Fruits.

Spinach, asparagus, lettuce, cresses, celery, tomatoes, greens, green peas ; fruits.

Drinks.

Water, Vichy or plain soda water, hot water (a pint an hour before meals), brandy, whiskey, milk, milk punch, wines, malt liquors, cream.

AVOID

Starches and farinaceous foods, as a rule, potatoes, turnips, carrots, all pies and pastries, made dishes, sweets, gravies, puddings.

PREGNANCY.

Soups.

Mutton, chicken, oyster, and clam.

Fish.

Raw oysters, raw clams.

Meats.

Beef, mutton, chicken, game, eggs, butter, fat, sweet breads, ham.

Bread.

Wheat bread, corn bread, oatmeal, wheaten grits, rice.

Vegetables and Fruits.

Baked potatoes, spinach, macaroni, greens, cresses, celery, green peas, lettuce, asparagus, green corn, and oranges, grapes, stewed fruit.

Drinks.

Water (freely), Poland or Vichy water, cocoa, milk, tea and coffee, sour wine.

Desserts.

Plain puddings.

If the stomach should rebel it is well to have the patient breakfast in bed.

AVOID

Pork, veal, stews, hashes, gravies, made dishes, rich desserts.

TABLE FOR CALCULATING THE PERIOD OF UTERO-GESTATION.

Menstruation / Confinement	1	2	3	4	5	6	7	8	9	10	11	12	13	14	15	16	17	18	19	20	21	22	23	24	25	26	27	28	29	30	31	
January / OCTOBER	1/8	2/9	3/10	4/11	5/12	6/13	7/14	8/15	9/16	10/17	11/18	12/19	13/20	14/21	15/22	16/23	17/24	18/25	19/26	20/27	21/28	22/29	23/30	24/31	25/1	26/2	27/3	28/4	29/5	30/6	31/7	NOV.
February / NOVEMBER	1/8	2/9	3/10	4/11	5/12	6/13	7/14	8/15	9/16	10/17	11/18	12/19	13/20	14/21	15/22	16/23	17/24	18/25	19/26	20/27	21/28	22/29	23/30	24/1	25/2	26/3	27/4	28/5				DEC.
March / DECEMBER	1/8	2/9	3/10	4/11	5/12	6/13	7/14	8/15	9/16	10/17	11/18	12/19	13/20	14/21	15/22	16/23	17/24	18/25	19/26	20/27	21/28	22/29	23/30	24/31	25/1	26/2	27/3	28/4	29/5	30/6	31/7	JAN.
April / JANUARY	1/8	2/9	3/10	4/11	5/12	6/13	7/14	8/15	9/16	10/17	11/18	12/19	13/20	14/21	15/22	16/23	17/24	18/25	19/26	20/27	21/28	22/29	23/30	24/31	25/1	26/2	27/3	28/4	29/5	30/6		FEB.
May / FEBRUARY	1/8	2/9	3/10	4/11	5/12	6/13	7/14	8/15	9/16	10/17	11/18	12/19	13/20	14/21	15/22	16/23	17/24	18/25	19/26	20/27	21/28	22/1	23/2	24/3	25/4	26/5	27/6	28/7	29/8	30/9	31/10	MAR.
June / MARCH	1/8	2/9	3/10	4/11	5/12	6/13	7/14	8/15	9/16	10/17	11/18	12/19	13/20	14/21	15/22	16/23	17/24	18/25	19/26	20/27	21/28	22/29	23/30	24/31	25/1	26/2	27/3	28/4	29/5	30/6		APRIL.
July / APRIL	1/8	2/9	3/10	4/11	5/12	6/13	7/14	8/15	9/16	10/17	11/18	12/19	13/20	14/21	15/22	16/23	17/24	18/25	19/26	20/27	21/28	22/29	23/30	24/1	25/2	26/3	27/4	28/5	29/6	30/7	31/8	MAY.
August / MAY	1/8	2/9	3/10	4/11	5/12	6/13	7/14	8/15	9/16	10/17	11/18	12/19	13/20	14/21	15/22	16/23	17/24	18/25	19/26	20/27	21/28	22/29	23/30	24/31	25/1	26/2	27/3	28/4	29/5	30/6	31/7	JUNE.
September / JUNE	1/8	2/9	3/10	4/11	5/12	6/13	7/14	8/15	9/16	10/17	11/18	12/19	13/20	14/21	15/22	16/23	17/24	18/25	19/26	20/27	21/28	22/29	23/30	24/1	25/2	26/3	27/4	28/5	29/6	30/7		JULY.
October / JULY	1/8	2/9	3/10	4/11	5/12	6/13	7/14	8/15	9/16	10/17	11/18	12/19	13/20	14/21	15/22	16/23	17/24	18/25	19/26	20/27	21/28	22/29	23/30	24/31	25/1	26/2	27/3	28/4	29/5	30/6	31/7	AUG.
November / AUGUST	1/8	2/9	3/10	4/11	5/12	6/13	7/14	8/15	9/16	10/17	11/18	12/19	13/20	14/21	15/22	16/23	17/24	18/25	19/26	20/27	21/28	22/29	23/30	24/31	25/1	26/2	27/3	28/4	29/5	30/6		SEPT.
December / SEPTEMBER	1/8	2/9	3/10	4/11	5/12	6/13	7/14	8/15	9/16	10/17	11/18	12/19	13/20	14/21	15/22	16/23	17/24	18/25	19/26	20/27	21/28	22/29	23/30	24/1	25/2	26/3	27/4	28/5	29/6	30/7	31/8	OCT.

283

EXPLANATION.—Find in top line the date of menstruation, the figure below will indicate the date when confinement may be expected, *i.e.*, if date of menstruation is June 1st, confinement may be expected on March 8th, or one day earlier if leap year. (Dr. ELY.)

DRUGS AND MATERIALS USED IN ANTISEPTIC SURGERY.

TOGETHER WITH

GENERAL DIRECTIONS CONCERNING PREPARATIONS FOR
ANTISEPTIC OPERATIONS.

ANTISEPTIC SOLUTIONS.

℞ Acid. carbolic., ... f℥vi¼.
Aquæ, . . . q. s. ad Oj.—M.
Sig.: Solution 1-20 carbolic. LISTER.

℞ Acid. boric., ... ℥iv.
Aq. destillat., ... Oj.—M.
Sig.: Saturated solution, gr. x to f℥j.

℞ Potassii permanganat., . ℥j.
Aquæ, ... f℥j.—M.
Sig.: f℥j to Oj = 1-1000.

℞ Zinci chlorid., ... gr. xl.
Aquæ, . . . q. s. ad f℥j.—M.
Sig.: Apply on a swab to fresh septic wounds.

℞ Hydrarg. chlor. corros.,
Sodii chlor., . . . āā ℥j.
Aquæ, . . . q. s. ad f℥j.—M.
Sig.: f℥j to Oj = 1 to 1000.

℞ Hydrarg. chlor. corros., . . ℥j.
Ammon. chlor., . . . xxxij.
Aquæ, . . . q. s. ad f℥j.—M.
Sig.: f℥j to Oj water = 1 to 1000 solution.

℞ Hydrarg. chlor. corros., . . ℥j.
Acid. tartaric., ... ℥v.
Aquæ, . . . q. s. ad f℥iv.—M.
Sig.: f℥½ to Oj aquæ = 1000.

284

℞ Acidi carbolic., ... f℥j.
Ol. olivæ, ... f℥x.—M.
Sig.: Carbolized oil. Lister.

℞ Iodoform., ... ℥j.
Collodion, ... f℥x.—M.
Sig.: Iodoform collodion. Küster.

℞ Iodoform., ... gr. xxx.
Æther., ... f℥ss.
Aq. destillat., . . q. s. ad f℥j.—M.
Sig.: Iodoform ether. Nussbaum.

℞ Iodoform., ... ℥j.
Æther., ... ℥j.—M.
Sig.: Iodoform ether.

℞ Creolin, . . . f℥j.
Sig.: f℥j to f℥vj to Oj. v. Esmarch.

℞ Hydrogen peroxide, . . . f℥j.
Sig.: Use in hard-rubber atomizer.

SALVES.

℞ Acid. boric., ... ℥iij.
Paraffine, ... ℥x.
Ung. petrolat, ... ℥v.—M.
Sig.: Boric acid salve. Lister.

℞ Acidi salicylic., . . . ℥j.
Paraffine, ... ℥xij.
Cerat. alb., ... ℥xv.
Ol. amyg., ... ℥xij.—M.
Sig.: Salicylic salve. Lister.

℞ Iodoformi, ... ℥j.
Ung. petrolati, ... ℥vj.
Ol. amyg. amar., . . . gtt. ij.—M.
Sig.: Iodoform salve.

℞ Iodoform., ... ℥j to iv.
Ung. petrolat, ... ℥j.—M.
Sig.: Iodoform ointment.

℞ Ol. olivæ, ... f℥j.
Acidi carbolic., . . . gr. xli to xxiv.—M.
Sig.: 1–40 or 1–20 carbolized oil.

R Ung. petrolati, . . . ℥j.
Acidi carbolic., . . . gr. xxiv to xij.—M.
Sig.: 1–20 or 1–40 carbolized vaseline.

LIGATURES.

Take raw catgut; soak in ether for twenty-four hours; keep for twenty-four hours in an alcoholic solution of corrosive sublimate (1–500); wind it on sterile glass rods; and keep in sterile alcohol.

Boil gut in alcohol, and keep in hermetically sealed glass tubes containing alcohol—12 ligatures to the tube.—FOW-LER.

Place the gut for twenty-four hours in ether; at the end of this period place in a solution containing 20 gr. of corrosive sublimate, 100 gr. of tartaric acid, and 6 oz. of alcohol. Keep small gut in this solution for ten minutes, the large gut for twenty minutes. Place for keeping in a mixture containing 1 drop of bichloride of palladium to 8 ounces of alcohol. At time of operation place in a solution one-third of which is 5 per cent. carbolic acid solution, and two-thirds of which are alcohol. —JOHNSTON.

Wind the gut upon glass test-tubes; immerse for twenty-four hours in a 2 per cent. watery solution of formalin; place in flowing water for twelve hours; boil in water for fifteen minutes; cut in pieces; tie in bundles. Place for keeping in the following mixture: 950 parts absolute alcohol, 50 parts glycerin, and 100 parts finely powdered iodoform.—SENN's modification of HOFMEISTER's method.

CHROMICIZED GUT.

Add 200 parts (by weight) of catgut to 200 parts of carbolic acid, 2000 parts of water, and 1 part of chromic acid. Keep the gut in this solution for twenty-four hours, and transfer for keeping to alcohol.—JOHNSTON.

SILK (CZERNY).

The silk should be boiled for one hour in a 1 to 20 carbolic solution, then kept in a 1 to 50 carbolic solution.

Boil in clean water for one hour, then store in an alcoholic solution of sublimate 1–1000.

Rubber tubes, wash clean and keep in a 1 to 20 carbolic solution.

Rubber tubing may be hardened by immersing for five minutes in concentrated sulphuric acid. The tubes are then washed in alcohol and preserved in 1–20 carbolic solution.

Decalcified bones, catgut, horse-hair, silk-worm gut, may all be stored in absolute alcohol containing sublimate 1–1000.

OPERATOR'S HANDS.

Pare nails and clean around and under them with a knife. Clean arms, hands, and nails for one minute with a brush, very warm water, and potash soap (pearline) ; then wash for one minute in stronger alcohol, and then for one minute in 1–1000 or 1–500 bichloride solution or 1–30 carbolic solution. The hands are then allowed to remain wet.

OPERATIVE REGION.

The patient should have a warm bath before the operation, and the operation region must be shaved and covered with cloths dipped in 1–1000 bichloride or 1–30 carbolic, and covered with paraffine paper ; this dressing must remain for several hours previous to the operation. Immediately before the operation the parts are washed and brushed with potash soap, then rubbed with alcohol, ether, or turpentine, and irrigated with 1–500 bichloride or 1–30 carbolic solution. The environs should be covered with towels wet with 1–500 bichloride or 1–30 carbolic, and changed during the operation as often as soiled. The region to be operated upon should also be covered with similar towels until the surgeon commences his incision, and during the entire operation scrupulous care must be exercised to keep every portion of the wound covered except that part which the surgeon must have exposed for the continuance of his work.

INSTRUMENTS.

Brush with 1–20 carbolic solution ; sterilize by roasting, boiling, or by storing for one hour in 1–20 carbolic solution. During operation keep in a 1–40 carbolic solution. To prevent rusting boil in one per cent. sod. carb. solution.

A very effectual method is to place them in metal boxes and heat in an ordinary oven (200° F.) for one-half to one hour ; they may then be used dry.

SPONGES.

If *new*, cleanse in soda solution and immerse for twenty-four hours in water to which is added—

℞ Potassii permanganat., . . gr. 15½.

This turns them brown ; then wash in a bowl of water, to which add—

℞ Acid. hydrochlor., . . . f℥v.
Sodii hyposulphit., . . . f℥iss.—M.

This bleaches them. They are then washed with hot water and potash soap and kept in 1-1000 bichloride or 1-20 carbolic solution.   KELLER.

Infected sponges. Keep in lukewarm water for twenty-four hours, or, better still, in running water for the same time; then wash with potash soap and warm water, and keep in 1-1000 bichloride or 1-20 carbolic. It is better, however, to use sterile gauze for sponging.

THE WOUND.

Unless it is infected, the wound need not be flushed or irrigated with irritating antiseptic solutions. If the mechanical effect of irrigation is necessary, sterilized water containing three-quarter per cent. of common salt may be employed.

If the wound is probably infected, irrigate with 1-500 bichloride solution, subsequently flushing out with a weaker lotion varying in strength from 1-2000 to 1-5000.

In operations about the mouth, bladder, intestines, etc., boric acid solution or the sterilized salt solution may be used.

STERILE GAUZE.

Boil in water containing washing-soda ; rinse out the soda; boil for fifteen minutes in water, or place in a steam sterilizer for the same time.—DaCOSTA.

IODOFORM-GAUZE.

Make a mixture containing equal parts (by weight) of iodoform, glycerin. and alcohol. Add corrosive sublimate in the proportion of 1 part to 1000 of the mixture. Let the mixture stand for three days. Take moist bichloride gauze, saturate with the mixture, let it drip for a time, and keep it in sterilized and covered glass jars.—JOHNSTON.

Boil cheese-cloth in water made alkaline by the addition of washing-soda, wring out in hot water, again boil in water without the addition of the soda, run it through a bichloride solution of 1–200, and pack away moist in jars that have been previously washed in the same solution. This gauze should be wrung out in a solution of bichloride 1–1000 immediately before being applied to the surface of the body.

℞ Gauze, ... 15,500 gr.
   Hydrarg. chlor. corros., . . 77 gr.
   Sodii chloridi, ... 7750 gr.
   Glycerinæ, ... 1550 gr.
   Aquæ, ... 68 f℥.—M.
                                        MAAS.

LISTER'S DOUBLE CYANIDE GAUZE.

Wash *all utensils* used in preparing this gauze in—

℞ Sol. of bichlor., 1–500,
   Sol. carbol. acid, 1–20,   āā   equal parts.—M.

Then add gr. c. of double cyanide of mercury and zinc (Lister) to four pints of a 1 to 4000 solution of bichloride of mercury.

(Keep this well stirred, since it does not form a solution ; the double cyanide is only in suspension in the bichloride solution.)

Run plain gauze through it and pack away moist.

The double cyanide salt is prepared as follows :—

℞ Cyanide of potassium, . . gr. 130.
   Cyanide of mercury, . . gr. 252.
   Mix and dissolve in water, . . f℥xss.

Add this solution to—

℞ Zinc sulphate, ... gr. 287.
   Water, ... f℥iv.—M.

Collect the resulting precipitate and wash with water f℥viii divided into two portions. Diffuse the precipitate by means of mortar and pestle in distilled water f℥viii containing hæmatoxylin gr. 1½, and a drop of a solution made by adding stronger ammonia f℥j to distilled water f℥xv ; let this mixture stand for several hours. The dyed salt is then drained and dried at a moderate heat.

SOLUTION FOR CARBOLIZED GAUZE.

℞ Resin, ... ℥iv.
   Alcohol, ... f℥xx.
   Castor oil, ... f℥ᵌ.
   Carbolic acid, . . . f℥ii⅔.—M.

Run gauze though this solution and hang up to dry.